The Biology of Disease

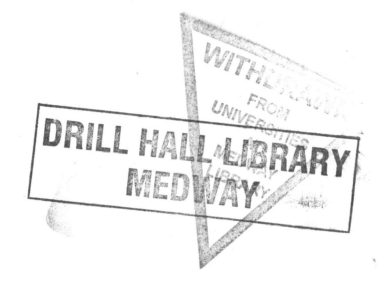

ASSOCIATE EDITOR TEAM

Professor J Crocker (Department of Histopathology, Birmingham Heartlands Hospital, Birmingham UK)
Professor RF Ambinder (Johns Hopkins School of Medicine, Baltimore USA)
Professor EL Jones (Department of Pathology, University of Birmingham, Birmingham UK)
Professor LS Young (CRC Institute for Cancer Studies, University of Birmingham, Birmingham UK)

Dedication: This is in memory of Professor Jaroslav Dušek who tragically died during the preparation of this book. His contribution to the teaching and practice of the medical sciences in the Czech Republic was great and he is sadly missed by his colleagues and friends.

The Biology of Disease

EDITED BY

Jonathan Phillips
School of Health Sciences
University of Wolverhampton
Wolverhampton UK

Paul Murray
Department of Pathology
Division of Cancer Studies
The Medical School
University of Birmingham
Birmingham UK

Paul Kirk
School of Health Sciences
University of Wolverhampton
Wolverhampton UK

SECOND EDITION

Blackwell
Science

© 1995, 2001
Blackwell Science Ltd
Editorial Offices:
9600 Garsington Road, Oxford OX4 2DQ
350 Main Street, Malden
   MA 02148 5020, USA
54 University Street, Carlton
   Victoria 3053, Australia

Other Editorial Offices:
Blackwell Science KK
MG Kodenmacho Building
7–10 Kodenmacho Nihombashi
Chuo-ku, Tokyo 104, Japan

Iowa State University Press
A Blackwell Science Company
2121 S. State Avenue
Ames, Iowa 50014-8300, USA

First published 1995
Second edition 2001
7   2009

Set by Graphicraft Limited, Hong Kong
Printed and bound in Malaysia
by KHL Printing Co Sdn Bhd

The Blackwell Science logo is a
trade mark of Blackwell Science Ltd,
registered at the United Kingdom
Trade Marks Registry

A catalogue record for this title is
available from the British Library

ISBN 978-0-6320-5404-6

Library of Congress
Cataloging-in-Publication Data

The biology of disease / edited by
Jonathan Phillips, Paul Murray,
Paul Kirk.—2nd ed.
       p. ;   cm.
   Includes bibliographical references
and index.
   ISBN 978-0-6320-5404-6
   1. Pathology.   2. Diseases.
I. Phillips, Jonathan, Ph.D.
II. Murray, Paul, Ph.D.   III. Kirk,
Paul DPhil
   [DNLM: 1. Disease. QZ 140 B6145
2001]
RB111.B48   2001
616.07—dc21

                00-041405

DISTRIBUTORS

Marston Book Services Ltd
PO Box 269
Abingdon, Oxon OX14 4YN
(*Orders*:   Tel: 01235 465500
               Fax: 01235 465555)

USA
Blackwell Science, Inc.
Commerce Place
350 Main Street
Malden, MA 02148-5020
(*Orders*:   Tel: 800 759 6102
                    781 388 8250
             Fax: 781 388 8255)

Canada
Login Brothers Book Company
324 Saulteaux Crescent
Winnipeg, Manitoba R3J 3T2
(*Orders*:   Tel: 204 837 2987)

Australia
Blackwell Science Pty Ltd
54 University Street
Carlton, Victoria 3053
(*Orders*:   Tel: 3 9347 0300
             Fax: 3 9347 5001)

For further information on
Blackwell Publishing, visit our website:
www.blackwellpublishing.com

Contents

List of Contributors

Numbers in [   ] denote authors of chapter or case study.

R.F. Ambinder
MD PhD
James B. Murphy Professor of Oncology,
389 Bunting Blaustein Cancer Research Building,
Johns Hopkins School of Medicine,
Baltimore MD 21231,
USA [CS12]

J.G. Ayres
BSc MD FRCP
Professor of Respiratory Medicine
(University of Birmingham)
Birmingham Heartlands Hospital,
Birmingham, B9 5SS [3]

D. Bareford
MD FRCP FRCPath
Consultant Haematologist,
Department of Haematology,
City Hospital NHS Trust,
Dudley Road,
Birmingham, B18 7QH [CS21]

K. Baumforth
BSc PhD
Research Fellow,
School of Health Sciences,
University of Wolverhampton,
62–68 Lichfield Street,
Wolverhampton, WV1 1DJ [4,22,23]

J. Biddulph
BSc PhD
Research Fellow,
School of Health Sciences,
University of Wolverhampton,
62–68 Lichfield Street,
Wolverhampton, WV1 1DJ [3]

S.J. Bowman
PhD, FRCP
Senior Lecturer,
Department of Rheumatology,
University of Birmingham,
Birmingham, B15 2TT [CS13]

A. Broomfield
BA MA
Clinical Molecular Geneticist,
DNA Laboratory,
Birmingham Women's Health Care Trust,
Birmingham, B15 2TG [27]

D. Burnett
PhD FRCPath
Micropathology Ltd,
The University of Warwick Science Park,
Barclays Venture Centre,
William Lyons Road,
Coventry, CV4 7EZ [5]

C.K. Campbell
BSc MSc PhD
Deputy Head,
Mycology Reference Unit,
Public Health Laboratory,
Myrtle Road,
Kingsdown,
Bristol, BS2 8EL [7]

R. Carter
BSc PhD
Division of Biological Sciences,
Institute of Cell, Animal and Population Biology,
University of Edinburgh, Ashworth Laboratories,
West Mains Road,
Edinburgh, EH9 3JT [CS5]

I.P.L. Coleman
BSc PhD CBiol MIBiol
Principal Lecturer,
School of Health Sciences,
University of Wolverhampton,
62–68 Lichfield Street,
Wolverhampton, WV1 1DJ [18]

P.G. Corrie
PhD FRCP
Oncology Centre,
Addenbrooke's Hospital,
Cambridge, CB2 2QQ [24,CS28]

R. Cramb
MB ChB MSc FRCPath
Consultant Chemical Pathologist,
Department of Clinical Biochemistry,
Queen Elizabeth Medical Centre,
Edgbaston,
Birmingham, B15 2TH [17,CS15]

C.B. Crocker
MRCGP
General Practitioner,
The Surgery,
30 Westfield Road,
Birmingham, B27 7TL [CS32]

J. Crocker
MD, FRCPath MRCP
Professor of Histopathology,
Department of Histopathology,
Birmingham Heartlands Hospital,
Bordesley Green East,
Birmingham, B9 5ST [CS20]

C. Davenport
PhD
Medical Writer,
Parexel International Limited,
River Court,
50 Oxford Road,
Denham,
Uxbridge, UB9 4DL [11]

J.E. Digby
BSc PhD
Research Fellow,
School of Health Sciences,
University of Wolverhampton,
62–68 Lichfield Street,
Wolverhampton, WV1 1DJ [15]

J. Dušek
(Deceased)
Formerly Institute of Pathology,
Palacký University,
Olomouc,
Czech Republic [CS16]

S.J. Dunmore
BSc PhD
Senior Lecturer,
School of Health Sciences,
University of Wolverhampton,
62–68 Lichfield Street,
Wolverhampton, WV1 1DJ [15]

D. Edgar
BSc FRCP MRCPath
Consultant Immunologist,
Department of Immunology,
The Royal NHS Trust Hospital,
Grosvenor Road,
Belfast, BT12 6BN [10,CS9]

M.S. Enayat
PhD CBiol MIBiol
Principal Clinical Scientist,
Haematology Department,
Birmingham Children's Hospital NHS Trust,
Steelhouse Lane,
Birmingham, B4 6NH [CS17]

H.T. Hassan
MD PhD
Professor of Oncology,
School of Health Sciences,
University of Wolverhampton,
62–68 Lichfield Street,
Wolverhampton, WV1 1DJ [13,CS10,CS30]

F.G.H. Hill
FRCPath FRCP
Consultant Haematologist,
Haematology Department,
Birmingham Children's Hospital NHS Trust,
Steelhouse Lane,
Birmingham, B4 6NH [CS17]

J.M. Jewsbury
PhD
29 Melloncroft Drive,
Caldy,
Wirral,
Merseyside, CH48 2JA [7]

E.M. Johnson
BSc, PhD
Clinical Scientist,
Mycology Reference Unit,
Public Health Laboratory,
Myrtle Road, Kingsdown,
Bristol, BS2 8EL [7]

E.L. Jones
MD FRCPath
Leith Professor of Oncology,
Department of Pathology,
The Medical School,
University of Birmingham,
Birmingham, B15 2TT [CS31]

N.D. Karunaweera
MB BS PhD
Department of Parasitology,
Faculty of Medicine,
University of Colombo, 8
Sri Lanka [CS5]

D. Killington
PhD
Senior Lecturer
Molecular Virology Group,
School of Biochemistry and Molecular Biology,
University of Leeds,
Leeds, LS9 9JT [9]

J.R. King
BSc MB ChB LRSC MRCPsych
Consultant Psychiatrist,
Worcestershire Community Healthcare,
Hill Crest,
Quinneys Lane,
Redditch,
Worcestershire, B96 7WG [CS1]

P.R. Kirk
MSc DPhil
Associate Dean,
School of Health Sciences,
University of Wolverhampton,
62–68 Lichfield Street,
Wolverhampton, WV1 1DJ [5,6,13]

Z. Kolar
MD, PhD
Professor,
Centre for Molecular Biology and Medicine,
Palacký University,
Olomouc,
Czech Republic [CS33]

S.E. Lawson
MRCP MRCPath
Research Fellow,
Haematology Department,
Birmingham Children's Hospital NHS Trust,
Steelhouse Lane,
Birmingham, B4 6NH [CS17]

H. Lederman
MD PhD
Associate Professor of Paediatrics,
Johns Hopkins University,
School of Medicine,
Johns Hopkins Hospital,
Baltimore, MD 21287–3923,
USA [12]

E.L. Maltby
PhD
Consultant Cytogeneticist,
North Trent Cytogenetics Service,
Sheffield Children's Hospital,
Sheffield S10 2TH [CS25,CS26]

A. Martin
BSc PhD
Senior Lecturer,
School of Health Sciences,
University of Wolverhampton,
62–68 Lichfield Street,
Wolverhampton, WV1 1DJ [24]

D. Maxton
MD FRCP
Consultant Physician and Gastroenterologist,
Department of Gastroenterology,
Royal Shrewsbury Hospital,
Shrewsbury, SY3 8XQ [CS18,CS19]

F. Macdonald
PhD MRCPath
Principal Molecular Geneticist,
DNA Laboratories,
West Midlands Regional Genetics Service,
Birmingham Women's Hospital,
Birmingham, B15 2TG [19,CS22]

P.G. Murray
MSc PhD
Senior Lecturer,
Department of Pathology,
Division of Cancer Studies,
University of Birmingham,
Edgbaston,
Birmingham, B15 2TT [1,3,21,22,23,CS4,CS8,CS29,CS32]

D.H. Myers
BM FRCP FRCPsych
Consultant Psychiatrist,
Shropshire Mental Health Trust,
Bicton Heath,
Shrewsbury, SY3 8DM [CS2]

P.N. Nelson
BSc PhD PGCE
Senior Lecturer,
School of Health Sciences,
University of Wolverhampton,
62–68 Lichfield Street,
Wolverhampton, WV1 1DJ [CS13]

K. Nye
MB ChB FRCPath
Consultant Microbiologist,
Public Health Laboratory,
Birmingham Heartlands Hospital,
Bordesley Green East,
Birmingham, B9 5SS [8,CS6,CS7]

J. Palefsky
MD
Professor,
Department of Laboratory Medicine,
University of California,
San Francisco, USA [CS4]

S.A. Perera
MSc PhD
Senior Lecturer in Biomedical Sciences,
School of Health Sciences,
University of Wolverhampton,
62–68 Lichfield Street,
Wolverhampton, WV1 1DJ [7]

J.D. Phillips
BSc PhD CBiol FIBMS
Principal Lecturer and
Co-ordinator Postgraduate Taught Awards,
School of Health Sciences,
University of Wolverhampton,
62–68 Lichfield Street,
Wolverhampton, WV1 1DJ [1,2,14,16,CS20,CS29,CS32]

C.A. Rea
BSc PhD
Senior Lecturer,
School of Health Sciences,
University of Wolverhampton,
62–68 Lichfield Street,
Wolverhampton, WV1 1DJ [17]

P.B. Rylance
BSc MB FRCP
Consultant Physician,
The Renal Unit,
New Cross Hospital,
Wednesfield Road,
Wolverhampton, WV10 0QP [CS11,CS15]

B.M. Singh
MD FRCP
Consultant in Diabetes and Endocrinology,
Wolverhampton Diabetes Centre,
New Cross Hospital,
Wolverhampton, WV10 8QP [CS15]

K.W.M. Scott
MD FRCPath
Consultant Histopathologist,
Department of Histopathology,
New Cross Hospital,
Wednesfield Road,
Wolverhampton, WV10 0QP [CS34]

M.J. Tarlow
MB MSc FRCP
Formerly Senior Lecturer in Paediatrics and Child Health,
Birmingham Heartlands Hospital,
Birmingham, B9 5ST [CS3]

I. Todd
PhD
Senior Lecturer in Immunology,
Division of Immunology,
Medical School,
University of Nottingham,
Queen's Medical Centre,
Nottingham, NG7 2UH [11]

P.A. Walker
BSc PhD DipEd FLS
Associate Dean,
School of Health Sciences,
University of Wolverhampton,
62–68 Lichfield Street,
Wolverhampton, WV1 1DJ [3]

J.J. Waters
PhD MRCPath
Principal Cytogeneticist,
Regional Cytogenetics Service,
Birmingham Women's Hospital,
Birmingham, B15 2TG [20,CS24]

L.S. Young
PhD DSc FRCPath HonMRCP
Professor of Cancer Biology,
CRC Institute for Cancer Studies,
Cancer Research Campaign Laboratories,
University of Birmingham,
Birmingham, B15 2TA [23,24]

Preface to the Second Edition

We were delighted to be given the opportunity to prepare a second edition of *The Biology of Disease*. Its appearance is timely in that, in the five years or so since the first edition, significant advances have been made in the basic sciences of cell biology and immunology, and in our understanding of the molecular mechanisms of disease. These developments are reflected in the relevant chapters. A new edition also offers the opportunity to review the aims of the book, though these still remain to produce a succinct volume with sufficient detail to enable a good understanding of the principles of disease biology.

In planning the second edition, we were keen to build upon the successful aspects of the first, particularly the use of case studies to amplify the points made in the chapters and to show how an understanding of the biology of disease translates into clinical practice. We have expanded the number of case studies to include a greater range of conditions and have reorganized some chapters to reflect this more clinically oriented approach. This is in line with developments in the medical curricula where students are exposed to clinical teaching at an early stage, and there is increased emphasis on clinically oriented problem solving. We anticipate that the revised book will also appeal to students on a range of other courses in the Health Sciences, including biomedical science, physiotherapy and other paramedical subjects, complementary therapies and nursing.

Finally, we would like to express our thanks to the Associate Editor team, to our colleagues in our respective Institutions, to the production team at Blackwell Science and not least to our families. All of these have supported us throughout, demonstrating good humour and patience at difficult times, and made significant contributions to the achievement of our goals.

Jonathan Phillips
Paul Murray
Paul Kirk
June 2000

Preface to the First Edition

The Biology of Disease aims to present the basic principles of disease processes in a form readily accessible to students trying to assimilate large volumes of information from a variety of sources. In conceiving this book, we recognized a need for a succinct volume that would give a broad yet sufficiently detailed account of the biology of disease. Acknowledging the expertise which lies in our medical and scientific colleagues (some working in education, some in research and others in clinical practice), we have drawn upon the experience and enthusiasm of a wide range of authoritative contributors. We feel that the book has benefited from this diversity of expertise, which has enabled us to cover many of the important topics in medicine today. Equally importantly, we were keen to adopt an accessible style of presentation and a common writing style, and we are grateful to all our contributors for their help in enabling us to achieve this aim.

From the outset, we felt it important to integrate the biological principles of disease processes with their clinical manifestations—the signs and symptoms which enable a diagnosis to be made. We have achieved this by ensuring that the principal chapters are clinically relevant and, where possible, that they bridge any gap between the biological and clinical features of disease. In addition, we have included clinical case studies in all the major sections of the book, each of which emphasizes the link between our current understanding of the basic science of the relevant condition and its clinical presentation. There is inevitable overlap and integration of topics in different sections of the book , so we have indicated cross-references where appropriate.

We anticipate that this book will be of use to a wide range of readers, particularly medical students approaching their clinical studies, students of clinical and biomedical sciences, and students of other paramedical subjects. Sections of the book cover major areas of clinical science including epidemiology, immunology, infection, disorders of the blood, genetic diseases, oncology and mental health. Each section is complete in itself, enabling the book to be used selectively for the study of individual topics. We have tried to provide a succinct, yet comprehensive, overview of each topic and we hope that readers will be stimulated to seek out further, more detailed information. For this reason each chapter concludes with key points and suggestions for further reading.

We are most grateful to all our contributors whose cooperation and expertise has been invaluable in achieving the aims of the book. We also thank our Associate Editor, John Crocker, for his help and guidance in the early stages of the editing process. Finally, we wish to acknowledge the support of our colleagues in the School of Health Sciences, of the editorial team at Blackwell Science and not least, that of our respective families, all of whom have helped us to nurture this venture to fruition.

Jonathan Phillips
Paul Murray

The Nature of Disease

Definition of health and disease

Health and disease are difficult concepts to define. Health is often defined as the absence of disease and an individual may be in good health if there are no impediments to his functioning or survival. The World Health Organization (WHO) defines health as '. . . a state of complete physical, mental and social well-being and not merely the absence of disease or infirmity'. This latter definition is much broader and it is likely that most of us would not be considered 'healthy' on the basis of these criteria.

Nevertheless, the WHO definition is useful since it acknowledges the importance of psychological and social well-being in the maintenance of health. Perhaps a more realistic definition considers that health is a condition or quality of the human organism which expresses adequate functioning under given genetic and environmental conditions. This definition implies that an individual may be considered healthy even if compromised in some way. An example here would be someone with Down syndrome who might well be considered healthy under the latter definition but not under the former.

Implicit in many of these definitions of health is the concept that efficient performance of bodily functions takes place in the face of a wide range of changing environmental conditions. Health in this context may be regarded as an expression of adaptability and disease a failure thereof. Disease can also be defined as a pattern of responses to some form of insult or injury resulting in disturbed function and/or structural alteration.

Concepts of normality

Individuals who are free from disease are often described as being 'normal'. It is important to recognize that normality does not always indicate health, but is merely an indication of the frequency of a given condition in a defined population. Some diseases occur with such frequency in the population that they might be considered to be 'normal', e.g. dental caries.

If we examine the distribution of an indicator of health, for example blood haemoglobin levels (Fig. 1.1), we can see that they usually follow a *normal distribution* in the population. Applying limits to the distribution curve produces two cut-off points. Below and above these points haemoglobin levels may be considered abnormal. However, the borderline between the normal and abnormal is not so clear cut. For instance, a value within the normal

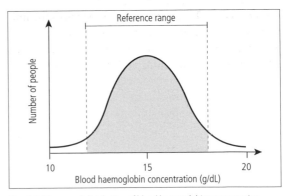

Fig. 1.1 The normal distribution of blood haemoglobin concentration.

range may be considered pathological in a particular individual or under certain circumstances. Likewise, a small percentage of individuals falling within the abnormal zones will remain healthy and suffer no consequences as a result of their slightly 'abnormal' haemoglobin concentration. Furthermore, in adult females, the total blood haemoglobin concentration tends to be lower than in males, due in part to their monthly menstrual blood loss. Taking another example, that of blood cholesterol concentration, the normal distribution in Western countries may not reflect ideal levels for the maintenance of health. For this reason the term *reference range* instead of *normal range* is preferred when defining the desired level of an analyte.

The rigid application of reference ranges can give rise to some confusion, depending on how they are interpreted. For example it is commonplace to show reference ranges for the *differential* white cell count (i.e. the different populations of white blood cell which make up the total leucocyte count) as either a percentage of the total or as the actual (or *absolute*) number in a given volume. When expressed as percentage figures these assume that the total white cell count is normal. Use of absolute numbers is less ambiguous since, if the total white cell count is raised or reduced, the percentage figures may suggest that particular cell populations are normal or abnormal when the reverse is the case. For example, a normal lymphocyte count is in the range $1.5–4.0 \times 10^9/L$ or 20–45% when the total white cell count is normal ($4–11 \times 10^9/L$). If the total white cell count is raised to $15 \times 10^9/L$, a differential count showing lymphocytes as 15% of the total could be interpreted as indicating lymphopenia (reduction in lymphocyte count). In reality the absolute lymphocyte count is normal (15% of $15 \times 10^9/L$ is $2.25 \times 10^9/L$), and the abnormally high cell population here would be neutrophils, accounting for the majority of the raised white cells in circulation. When considering data presented later in the case studies, readers should bear these principles in mind.

Onset of disease

It can be difficult to be precise about the transition from health to disease because pathological changes

with potential to cause disease are present in many apparently healthy people. For example, early *atheromatous* (fatty) deposits (see Chapter 17) are present in the arteries of a substantial proportion of symptom-free middle-aged adults in Western societies, increasing their risk of cardiovascular disease. Most patients with coronary heart disease would date the onset of their illness from the first clinical manifestation (e.g. chest pain), rather than from the blood lipid changes or *hypertension* (increased blood pressure) which may have begun years before and which predisposed them to heart disease.

Causes of disease

A great many agents and stimuli are implicated in the causation (*aetiology*) of human disease. In the majority of cases it is not possible to discover a single causative agent which always causes disease when present. For example, exposure to the microorganism *Mycobacterium tuberculosis* does not invariably result in tuberculosis. A variety of other factors are also important for establishment of infection, including the status of the host immune system and the size of the infective dose. However, tuberculosis cannot occur in the absence of the organism. Exposure to *M. tuberculosis* is therefore the *necessary* causal factor and the other factors may be defined as *subsidiary* causal factors.

Tuberculosis represents an example of a disease for which the causal factors involved are well established. For other diseases, identification of the causal factors has proved more difficult and the search for these factors continues to represent a significant challenge to medical science. Often the initial search for a causal factor begins by the examination of the patterns of disease within human populations. This is epidemiology and is the subject of Chapter 3. Epidemiological studies usually include analysis of mortality (death) and morbidity (illness) rates.

Types of aetiological factors

There is a widespread perception that a disease is an entity that is able to attack humans from the outside rather than a failure of adaptive responses from within. In fact the types of aetiological factors implicated in disease may be broadly divided into *endogenous* factors (those which create a disturbance or imbalance from within) and *exogenous* factors (factors which threaten existence from the outside). Chromosome abnormalities giving rise to genetic disorders may be regarded as endogenous factors, whereas microorganisms are good examples of exogenous aetiological agents. However, there is overlap between these two groups. For example, some chromosome abnormalities have been shown to be the result of parental exposure to mutagens in the environment, e.g. ionizing radiation. Some genetic disorders then, may ultimately be attributed to exposure to exogenous factors.

Classification of disease

Diseases are classified either on the basis of the outward signs produced by disease (*manifestations*) or on the existence of a common aetiological agent. Most diseases are classified on manifestational criteria irrespective of the causative agents involved. Thus, a number of causal factors are implicated in the development of various types of carcinoma of the lung, including cigarette smoke, asbestos, coal smoke and other atmospheric pollutants, but patients with the manifestations of lung cancer are grouped together irrespective of the involvement of one or more of these agents. Conversely, disease caused by *M. tuberculosis* may produce different clinical manifestations in different individuals, yet all are classified as forms of tuberculosis.

Classification of disease on the basis of shared aetiology may follow identification of a new and important aetiological agent, particularly if this offers promise of major therapeutic or preventive advantage. However, this is not always so. The identification of cigarette smoke as the most important cause of lung cancer, for example, did not promote a revision of the classification of lung cancer or of other diseases known to be associated with smoking (e.g. emphysema, bronchitis, atherosclerosis).

The classification of disease into discrete entities enables patients to be assigned to specific groups. The patients may then be treated in a similar fashion to other patients assigned previously to the same group, thus, at least in theory, improving the clinical outcome based on past experience. However, an alternative view is that the development of disease, and its progression and response to treatment should be regarded as unique to the individual.

Identifying disease

We have seen how diseases are classified but have not yet considered how a particular set of features is first designated as a disease state. Doctors use *signs* (what the doctor sees or feels when carrying out a physical examination), *symptoms* (what the patient complains of) and a range of laboratory and clinical tests to determine whether a patient has a given disease. The taking of a thorough clinical history will determine whether there has been exposure to any potential aetiological agents. The existence of certain predisposing conditions may make the development of a disease more likely. Examples of these risk factors include certain genetic disorders, lifestyle, psychological and personality profile, age and environmental factors such as climate and pollution. Furthermore, the presence of one disease (e.g. diabetes mellitus) may predispose a patient to the development of further disease (in this case atherosclerosis).

One of the early steps in identifying a disease is to establish a range of diagnostic possibilities from which the eventual diagnosis will be selected. The final diagnosis may sometimes be established shortly after clinical presentation, in other cases perhaps only after extensive use of laboratory and clinical tests, or occasionally may never be identified during the lifetime of the patient. It must be remembered that disease is a dynamic process and the indicators of disease may vary as the disease progresses. Furthermore, in some patients, particularly those who are elderly, different diseases may coexist, thus confusing the diagnostic processes.

The impact of disease on an individual patient or population group may be measured as morbidity (i.e. its detrimental effects such as pain or disability) or in terms of life expectancy or mortality rate. *Prognosis* is the likely future for the patient in terms of length and quality of life. Prognosis depends on many factors, including the stage the disease has reached and the likely impact of therapy. Once a disease has been identified, treatment aimed at relief of symptoms or, where feasible, cure is usually initiated. Patients may be cured of the disease, or may enter *remission* (a symptom-free period) from which they may either *relapse* (when symptoms of the disease return) or be cured. Some diseases are not amenable to cure, but can be controlled by the administration of drugs, hormones or by surgery. Some patients with advanced disease may receive palliative treatment only with the aim of relieving their symptoms for the remainder of their life.

Mechanisms of disease

Understanding the way in which disease begins and develops is the major focus of research within the biomedical sciences. The assumption is made that an understanding of the biology of disease will contribute to an improvement in health care, both in terms of the prevention of disease and its treatment. In many cases this has proved to be satisfyingly correct. For example, the recognition that type 1 diabetes mellitus results from damage to insulin-secreting cells in the pancreas led to the development of insulin replacement therapy. However, an understanding of the biology of many important diseases (e.g. cancer) is only beginning to emerge and for the most part this has not yet contributed greatly to a decline in mortality rates.

The aim of this book is to instil an appreciation of the biological basis of disease. It does not attempt to be a comprehensive textbook of pathology, but seeks to draw attention to some of the important biological features resulting in disturbed homoeostasis. Subsequent chapters address the fundamental biological aspects of important groups of human disease, while the case studies consider the clinical aspects of selected disease states relating these, where possible, to their underlying biology.

Psychological and Social Aspects of Disease

It is now widely accepted that biological mechanisms have a role in the onset of the major psychoses and other mental illnesses and that in some disorders they may be the most important factors. The use of the term 'biological psychiatry' acknowledges this influence, and recognizes that one of the major challenges facing medical science is the further elucidation of the biology of mental illness. In recent years much progress has been made in identifying genetic, physiological and pathological factors, in addition to the mental and emotional, which contribute to psychological and psychiatric well-being. However, the biological approach does not deny the role of adverse life events and the effects of other psychological and social factors in ill health.

Types of mental illness

Some disorders of mental function have a well-defined basis in physical illness (psychiatric organic states), whereas in others there is no discernible pathology ('functional' psychiatric disorders). Functional mental disorders have traditionally been classified mainly as either neuroses or psychoses, though the distinction between the two groups is not always obvious.

From the viewpoint of biological psychiatry, the classification of mental illness on the basis of symptoms is of less importance than the search for its biological mediators. This chapter reviews some of what is known of the biology of affective disorder, schizophrenia and dementia, and briefly considers some physical factors contributing to psychiatric organic states.

Affective disorders

Affective illnesses are disorders of mood characterized by recurrent periods of depression with or without episodes of mania. The term 'bipolar' affective disorder is reserved for those patients who have experienced at least one manic episode and 'non-bipolar' and 'unipolar' affective disorder for those who have experienced depressive but no manic episodes.

Depressed patients feel gloomy, helpless and hopeless. They usually also experience sleep disturbance: problems in falling asleep, waking early and difficulty in resuming sleep again once they are awake. In contrast, mania is characterized by uninhibited restless activity, excitement, apparent happiness or euphoria, and generation of a succession of ideas, often behaving impulsively or irrationally.

In bipolar disorder, the transition from depression to mania and vice versa can occur in regular cycles lasting from less than 1 day in some patients to months or years in others. However, bipolar disorder is relatively rare, affecting approximately 1 in 1000 of the population in Western societies. Unipolar depression is much more common, with up to 5% of the population experiencing depression at some time in their lives. Family, twin and adoption studies have supported the influence of genetic factors in affective disorders. Research has indicated at least two subgroups of bipolar affective disorder, one X-linked and another transmitted on chromosome 11, though these studies are not conclusive and genes on other chromosomes may be involved.

Biological changes in affective disorder

The search for biological indicators of depression has revealed two procedures which are claimed to help to distinguish endogenous depression (which cannot solely be explained by life events) from reactive depression (e.g. following bereavement). In the dexamethasone-suppression test, the administration of dexamethasone suppresses adrenal release of cortisol in both normal subjects and in those with reactive depression. In endogenous depression there is no suppression of cortisol release by the drug. The second indicator is the speed of entry to rapid eye movement (REM) sleep: those with endogenous depression enter this phase of sleep much more rapidly than normal subjects or those with reactive depression. These functional differences, though not completely reliable or consistent, support the view that biological factors contribute to endogenous depression.

It has been shown that depression is associated with several other biological abnormalities, which range from hormonal deficiencies to a relative inactivity of the left hemisphere of the brain. In addition, research has indicated the possibility that viruses or other infectious agents may be linked to a small proportion of cases of depression. However, most research has focused on well-recognized alterations in neurotransmitters in mental illness, though it is recognized that such changes may be secondary to other factors.

Neurotransmitters in depression

The discovery that mood can be influenced by pharmacological agents which alter neurotransmission adds weight to the theory that the affective disorders have a biological basis. Depressed patients tend to have abnormal transmission at noradrenalin, dopamine or serotonin (also known as 5-hydroxytryptamine) synapses, though the precise causes of these abnormalities have not yet been fully explained. However, the common antidepressants ('tricyclic' drugs and monoamine oxidase inhibitors) are known to prolong the synaptic effect of catecholamines and serotonin, though their clinical effect often takes some time to become evident. A particular class of drug (the selective serotonin reuptake inhibitors) act by inhibiting the synaptic reuptake of serotonin, thus prolonging its effect.

Lithium in bipolar affective illness

Lithium salts are used prophylactically in the long-term management of bipolar affective disorder and research into the mode of action of lithium has provided much impetus to the search for biological factors in this illness. Lithium is of particular interest because, at therapeutic doses, it exerts a range of diverse physiological and biochemical effects. However, its precise mode of action in controlling mood swings in manic depressive illness has yet to be elucidated, though it is likely that lithium modulates intracellular signalling mechanisms. One hypothesis proposes that lithium exerts its effect through intracellular cyclic adenosine monophosphate (cAMP) and phosphatidyl inositol metabolism to induce adrenergic and cholinergic balance. However, of the very many theories to explain the pharmacological action of lithium, none has yet withstood the test of time.

Schizophrenia

Schizophrenia affects around 1% of the population in most developed countries. There are no reliable physiological or biochemical tests for the disorder, diagnosis of which relies on psychiatric evaluation. The symptoms of schizophrenia are described as 'positive' (e.g. delusions and auditory hallucinations) or 'negative' (e.g. withdrawal, blunted emotions and lack of motivation). In certain patients either positive or negative symptoms predominate, but it is unclear whether these are manifestations of different syndromes or whether they represent different points in the spectrum of a single disorder.

There is some evidence that structural abnormalities of the brain are more closely associated with negative symptoms, yet the positive symptoms appear to respond more satisfactorily to antipsychotic drugs.

Biological features

The aetiology of schizophrenia remains obscure, though research has indicated the following four features in the majority of cases—a genetic influence, seasonal differences, central nervous system (CNS) abnormalities, and involvement of dopamine receptors.

A genetic component
It has long been recognized that schizophrenia runs in families. However, this does not necessarily imply a genetic basis to the disorder, since social, cultural and environmental factors are all shared within families. Support for the hypothesis that genes contribute to the aetiology of schizophrenia comes from adoption and twin studies, with concordance of 40–50% demonstrated between monozygotic twins. It is likely that several genes are involved, and that they are partially, but not necessarily fully, responsible for most cases of schizophrenia.

Season of birth
It has been shown that patients with schizophrenia are more likely to have been born in the winter months. The increase is slight (5–10%), but statistically significant. The significance of this finding is not clear, but could indicate the involvement of either an infectious agent acquired early in life or seasonal factors affecting ambient temperature, diet, pregnancy or complications in childbirth.

CNS abnormalities
A variety of clinical investigations and imaging techniques have been used to investigate putative CNS abnormalities in schizophrenia, including *computed tomography* (CT), *magnetic resonance imaging* (MRI), *single photon emission computed tomography* (SPECT) and *positron emission tomography* (PET). These have revealed a number of interesting findings, including evidence of cerebral atrophy, left temporal lobe dysfunction, evidence of neuronal loss and disorganization and changes in blood flow and energy metabolism in the brains of affected subjects.

The significance of the diverse and inconsistent CNS abnormalities observed in schizophrenia is a matter of current speculation, and their existence indicates the extent to which the biology of this disease is as yet poorly understood.

Involvement of dopamine receptors
Neuroleptic drugs (drugs with an antipsychotic action), block dopamine synapses in the brain and relieve the positive symptoms of schizophrenia (auditory hallucinations and delusions). However, the pharmacological reduction in dopaminergic neurotransmission occurs much more rapidly than the alleviation of symptoms, so antipsychotic drugs are assumed to exert some of their effects indirectly.

Possible abnormality in glutamate neurotransmission
Abnormalities which will eventually lead to the development of schizophrenia have been suggested to arise early in the development of the brain, perhaps during the second trimester of pregnancy. It is thought that the migration of neurons to their designated sites in the developing brain could be disrupted, leading to abnormal development of the cortex and faulty connections with the limbic system. If such damage occurs, it could be due to genetic or environmental factors, perhaps also involving abnormalities in glutamate neurotransmission. Glutamate is a neurotransmitter released by axons extending from the cortex into the limbic system and it is known that glutamate receptors are involved in the differentiation and migration of young neurons in the developing brain.

Other research has indicated that, in *post mortem* brains from schizophrenic patients there is a reduction in glutamate receptors, particularly in the left temporal lobe. The activity of dopamine synapses is thought to inhibit the release of glutamate, so pharmacological reduction in dopaminergic neurotransmission may gradually increase glutamate activity. If this is demonstrated to be the case, it could explain the delayed clinical response to antipsychotic medication in schizophrenia.

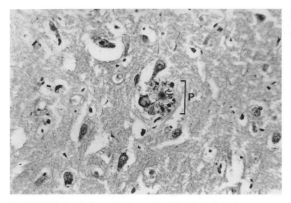

Fig. 2.1 Alzheimer's disease is characterized histologically by the presence of neurofibrillary tangles and of plaques (P) containing amyloid protein.

The dementias

Alzheimer's disease, the most common cause of presenile and senile dementia, is associated with degenerative changes in cortical association areas, particularly those of the hippocampus and the temporal, frontal and parietal lobes. The degenerative changes include plaque and tangle formation (Fig. 2.1), with loss of somatostatin- and glutamate-containing cell bodies in the cerebral cortex. The distribution of lesions suggest that the degenerative process spreads along glutamate-containing association neurons within the cortex. The discovery that plaques contain a high concentration of aluminium, and epidemiological data linking exposure to high levels of aluminium in drinking water to the formation of tangles, suggest that aluminium may have a role in the aetiology of Alzheimer's disease. In addition, there is a strong genetic element in many cases of Alzheimer's disease, possibly involving a gene on chromosome 21.

There is epidemiological evidence to suggest that infectious agents are responsible for certain forms of dementia. In particular, *variant Creutzfeld–Jakob disease* has been linked to *bovine spongiform encephalopathy* (BSE) in cattle and *scrapie* in sheep, both of which have been demonstrated to be due to the infectious agents known as prions (see Chapter 7). The human immunodeficiency virus (HIV) can also infect the brain, where it is associated with the occurrence of distinctive multinucleate giant cells. The condition may progress to cause psychotic symptoms or intellectual deterioration.

Other causes of dementia include cerebral artery atherosclerosis (resulting in cerebral ischaemia), demyelination (as in multiple sclerosis) and neoplasia.

Mental illness and organic disease

Despite the undoubted advances in understanding of disease processes in mental illness it is essential to appreciate that physical illness can also produce psychiatric symptoms. For example, confusional states have a number of possible causes including inflammation, infection, *uraemia* (retention in the blood of waste products including urea) or drug intoxication. Less dramatically, the tiredness and lethargy of anaemia can present as depression, and many patients with thyroid disorders exhibit psychiatric symptoms ranging from depression in hypothyroidism to anxiety in hyperthyroidism.

Psychological and social factors in disease

There is a psychological component to many physical illnesses, particularly those associated with prolonged incapacity or social isolation such as rheumatoid arthritis. Conversely, and somewhat controversially, it has been claimed that specific psychological states of mind may predispose to certain disease states: type A behaviour (excessive ambition, hostility and time urgency) and its proposed link with coronary heart disease is one example. More controversial is the claim that certain psychological traits and behavioural characteristics are associated with a higher prevalence of malignant disease. It is postulated that feelings of depression, hopelessness and other psychological stressors adversely affect the immune system, which in turn influences susceptibility to cancer.

Finally, despite the emphasis in this chapter on the biology of mental illness, it is important not to overlook the influence of social factors on mental health. Poverty, unemployment and poor housing all impact on self image, particularly in societies where expectations are high. It has been estimated that a significant proportion of primary medical consultations are for symptoms associated with anxiety and depression, some of which can be attributed to biological factors and others to social and

---

Key points

1 The precise biological mechanisms underlying the functional psychiatric disorders have yet to be fully elucidated.

2 There is some evidence that endogenous and exogenous forms of depression can be differentiated by biological markers.

3 Abnormalities of catecholamines and serotonin synaptic neurotransmission are a feature of depression.

4 The mode of action of lithium in controlling bipolar affective disorder is not yet understood, but may involve intracellular signalling mechanisms.

5 Schizophrenia is characterized by genetic factors, CNS changes and abnormalities in dopaminergic neurotransmission.

6 Degenerative changes in Alzheimer's disease, the cause of which is unknown, include plaque and tangle formation in the CNS. Certain other forms of dementia are due to infection, demyelination or ischaemia.

7 Physical illness can cause psychiatric symptoms. Conversely, many physical symptoms may have an emotional basis and certain disease syndromes are recognized to have a strong psychological component.

8 In clinical practice, an understanding of the effect of lifestyle and social factors, including poverty, deprivation and social exclusion on the incidence and progression of disease is, in many cases, as important as a consideration of the biological influences.

---

environmental influences or adverse life events. Furthermore, social deprivation has a significant effect on the incidence, morbidity and mortality rates of a wide spectrum of disease, so much so that action to address inequalities in health is currently high on the political agenda.

Summary

The purpose of this chapter has been to introduce some aspects of biological psychiatry and to alert readers to the notion that disease cannot be separated from its broader social context.

Comprehensive coverage of the biology of mental illness is not possible in the space available but the interested reader can pursue the topic by means of the further reading list. Finally, case studies 1 and 2 give a flavour of the challenge of psychiatry in clinical practice, and the need to consider alternative 'physical' diagnoses where patients present with symptoms attributed to 'mental' illness.

Further reading

Harrison P., Geddes J. & Sharpe M. (1998) *Lecture Notes on Psychiatry*. Blackwell Science Ltd., Oxford.

Kalat J.W. (1992) *Biological Psychology* (4th edn). Wadsworth Publishing, Belmont.

Lewis S.W. & Higgins J.N. (1996) *Brain Imaging in Psychiatry*. Blackwell Science Ltd., Oxford.

Lishman W.A. (1997) *Organic Psychiatry*. Blackwell Science Ltd., Oxford.

Owen F. & Itzhaki R. (1994) *Molecular and Cell Biology of Neuropsychiatric Diseases*. Chapman & Hall, London.

Rose N. (1994) *Essential Psychiatry*. Blackwell Scientific Publications, Oxford.

CHAPTER 3

Principles of Epidemiology

Epidemiology is the study of the distribution of health and disease in populations. Epidemiologists use descriptive and analytical methods to determine the existence and extent of correlations between the distribution of disease and well-being, and agents which may affect this, such as degree of exposure to environmental influences or the biological and sociological characteristics of individuals in populations. If the studies are precise enough it may be possible to suggest causal links.

Epidemiology is fundamental in determining the aetiology of disease or ways of enhancing health. Its methods allow the assessment of disease burdens and trends providing administrators and legislators with a rational basis for planning the management and development of health services from local to global levels. The subject is essential in the evaluation of regimens of treatment by clinical trials, and in efficient delivery of health care.

This chapter introduces some of the basic concepts of epidemiology and outlines the more elementary methods it employs. These are further illustrated using as examples colorectal cancer and asthma.

Epidemiological measures of illness and death

For the scientific study of disease and health in populations and comparisons between populations anecdotal evidence and the simple counting up of numbers of cases are inadequate. Even to reach the stage of natural history requires the use of rates. To know that there are 100 cases of disease in population A and 1000 in population B enables no sensible conclusion as to whether A or B has a more serious problem. In fact if the population of A is 1000 and that of B is 1000 000 the problem is worse in A than B since the rate for A = 100/1000 and for B = 1000/ 1000 000, or 0.1 compared to 0.001. For easy comparison of rates, and to avoid awkward decimal fractions, rates are usually multiplied by a factor. In this example 1000 would be reasonable so that the rates become (100/1000) × 1000 and (1000/1000 000) × 1000 or 100 per thousand for A and 1 per thousand for B. The rates show the real difference between the two populations. Any other factor could have been used, the choice is arbitrary and for convenience.

Morbidity rates

These are measures of the illness in the population and are usually expressed as either *incidence rates* or *prevalence rates*. The *incidence* of a disease is the number of new cases occurring over a specified time period. The *incidence rate* per 10 000 would therefore be:

$$\frac{\text{no. of } new \text{ cases of a disease in a given time period}}{\text{total population } at \ risk \text{ over the same time period}} \times 10\ 000$$

Incidence is a measure of the risk of contracting a disease since it concerns new cases.

Not all members of a population may be at risk and should not be included in the denominator. For instance, in calculating incidence rates for ovarian cancer, it would be misleading to include males in the total population, since only females can be at risk of contracting this disease. The population at risk may be decided on a variety of features besides sex. The most important are age, social class, ethnic group, occupation and geographical location.

Prevalence is the number of cases existing in a population over a given time period.

$$\frac{\text{Prevalence rate}}{\text{per 10 000}} = \frac{\text{No. cases existing during given period}}{\text{Total population } at \ risk \text{ during that time}} \times 10\ 000$$

Prevalence may be expressed in two ways, *point prevalence* or *period prevalence*. As the term suggests point prevalence is the number of cases of disease at a point in time. Period prevalence is the number of cases over an extended length of time. Figure 3.1 shows the difference between these.

Relation between incidence and prevalence

Each new case of a disease joins an already existing number of cases and thus adds to the prevalence pool. The prevalence pool will remain at a given size if the number of new cases added is matched by old cases leaving the pool by recovering, being cured or dying. A low incidence will lead to a high prevalence if a disease has low rates of recovery, cure or death. Crudely, the *prevalence = incidence × duration of disease*. The situation is analogous to a dripping tap keeping water level in a sink at a certain level depending on how fast water is draining from the sink.

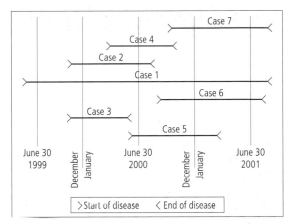

Fig. 3.1 Duration of cases of a disease over a 2-year period illustrating the meaning of prevalence and incidence. Cases of disease recorded from 30 June 1999 to 30 June 2001 from a total population at risk of 100. Period prevalence from 1 January 2000 to 31 December 2000 is 7 (cases 1–7). Point prevalence on 30 June 2000 is 4 (cases 1, 2, 4 and 5). The incidence for the year 2000 is 4 (4, 5, 6 and 7). The incidence rate for the year 2000 is 4/100.

Mortality rate

Death rates may be useful indicators of the frequency of disease. If a disease has a very high case-fatality, or lasts only a short time from onset to death, the mortality rate is a good measure of the incidence of the disease. The most generalized form of mortality rate is that calculated from all causes of death over a given period (usually a year). This is represented as:

$$\frac{\text{total no. of deaths in the population over a defined period}}{\text{no. in the population at mid period}}$$

The use of such crude rates can be misleading, because they collapse a mass of demographic data into a single statistic. Table 3.1a gives the crude death rates for two developed and two developing countries in 1994. Contrary to expectation the developed countries have higher death rates than the undeveloped ones.

The explanation is that the demographic structures of the two pairs are very different. Table 3.1b shows that both Germany and the UK have more than three times the proportion of people aged 65 years old or more than Brunei or Costa Rica. The

Table 3.1 (a) Crude death rates for two developed and two developing countries. From WHO (1994). (b) Populations of two developed and two developing countries stratified by age for 1994. From WHO (1994) *World Health Statistics Annual for 1994*. WHO, Geneva. (c) Age-specific death rates for the UK 1996. From Office for National Statistics.

(a)

Developed countries death rate per 1000		Undeveloped countries death rate per 1000	
UK	11.4	Brunei	3.1
Germany	11.6	Costa Rica	3.7

(b)

Age group	Population (%)			
	Germany	UK	Brunei	Costa Rica
0–14	16.2	19.0	34.3	33.5
15–64	68.7	65.0	62.1	62.1
65+	15.1	15.5	3.6	4.4

(c)

Age group	Death rate per 1000
Under 1	6.1
1–4	0.3
5–14	0.1
15–24	0.5
25–34	0.7
35–44	1.4
45–54	3.4
55–64	9.8
65–74	27.7
75–84	68.1
85+	164.4

chance of dying over any one year is much greater on average the older a person becomes, once past early childhood (Table 3.1c). Because the proportion of old people is higher in the two Western countries their death rates are inflated and do not reflect the better living conditions and state of health obtaining in those countries. It would not be unreasonable to compare Germany and the UK in terms of their crude death rates, because their demographic structures are similar, but it is meaningless to compare either with Costa Rica or Brunei in this way. For such a comparison age-specific death rates would need to be calculated so that the rates in each age cohort could be directly compared.

The use of specific mortality (or morbidity) rates is often too clumsy in practice. A more convenient way of obtaining a fair comparison between countries is to *standardize* the crude rates using appropriate demographic factors which have a major bearing on health. The two chief factors used for adjustment of rates are age and sex.

Standardization of rates

Standardizing removes the bias described above, while retaining a single figure statistic for comparing each population. Standardization may be calculated indirectly or directly. The *standardized mortality ratio* is an indirect method calculated by using the expression:

$$\frac{\text{observed deaths in a population over a given time period}}{\text{expected deaths in a standard population over the same period}} \times 100$$

Table 3.2 gives an example of such a calculation.

Standardized incidence ratios may also be calculated by replacing mortality figures with incidence in the expression.

Rates can be directly standardized for age or other features. In comparing two populations the age (or other feature) specific rates found within them are applied to a third reference (standard) population. The recalculated rates are those which would have been found in each had they had the same demographic structure as the reference population. The consequence is that the rates so adjusted for the two populations can then be directly (and fairly) compared with each other.

The reference population chosen is arbitrary, since we are first comparing 1 to 3 and then 2 to 3 to finally compare 1 with 2 the benchmark is of little significance. In practice, however, workers normally use published reference populations such as the world standard population, or the European standard population (demographically a relatively ageing population) found in World Health Organ-

Table 3.2 Calculation of standardized mortality ratio for lung cancer (ICD 162) in men in England and Wales (1995 compared to 1993) in the age range 55–85+. The SMR indicates an improvement in death rates for lung cancer in this age range over the 2-year period. From Office of National Statistics.

Age group	Death rate from lung cancer England and Wales 1993 per million (SP)	Population for England and Wales 1995 (thousand) (PI)	Expected deaths (SP × PI)	Observed deaths
55–59	1.02	1321.6	1348.0	1288
60–64	1.98	1204.0	2383.9	2161
65–69	3.51	1107.2	3886.3	3533
70–74	4.86	970.3	4715.7	4519
75–79	6.15	622.2	3826.5	3602
80–84	7.11	409.6	2912.3	2099
85+	6.58	240.1	1579.9	1447
Total			20 652.6	18 649

SMR = observed/expected × 100 = (18 649/20 652.6) × 100 = 90.3%.

PI, population investigated; SP, standard population.

ization (WHO) yearbooks. This is considered further on p. 23.

Epidemiological studies

Epidemiologists, like other scientists, employ study methods ranging from descriptive through observational to experimental (or intervention) studies.

Descriptive studies

To elucidate possible patterns of association between agents which may affect health positively or negatively, it is necessary to collect and collate data which relates such agents to different sectors of a population, e.g. age group, social class, periods of time when they are affected and the geographical areas over which the agent is distributed.

Often such studies rely on data which are routinely collected by government statistical services, authorities within the NHS, case records and so on. Such data may show how rates of disease change among people in different occupations, parts of a city or region over periods of time. This can lead to the discovery of important trends in disease and health and the identification and quantification of new and existing factors detrimental or advantageous to the health of a population. Figures 3.2–3.4 show examples of such data. The data may then be used to generate hypotheses on causation which

may be tested by observational or experimental studies.

As can be seen in Fig. 3.2 the trends for the two forms of cancer are different: melanoma has increased in incidence and is more common in women. Lung cancer incidence rate has fallen in men but is rising in women. Death rates for melanoma have remained steady indicating improved survival; for lung cancer death rates parallel the incidence rates, i.e. there is no improvement in survival. The lung cancer figures indicate that more men are stopping smoking while more women are taking it up.

The histograms in Fig. 3.3 show the association of coronary heart disease mortality with social class in males in England and Wales. Premature deaths are more common in the lowest social grouping. In this group mortality has hardly changed over 23 years of records; mortality in the highest social group has shown a considerable decrease.

The distribution of standardized mortality ratios (SMRs) shown in Fig. 3.4 indicates possible conditions adverse to health in the north and west, and parts of London.

Descriptive studies are economical, but can be no better than the raw data on which they are based. Records are not always adequately kept and there may be inaccuracy or lack of consistency in the diagnosis of disease between practitioners and between different countries. Morbidity figures record only

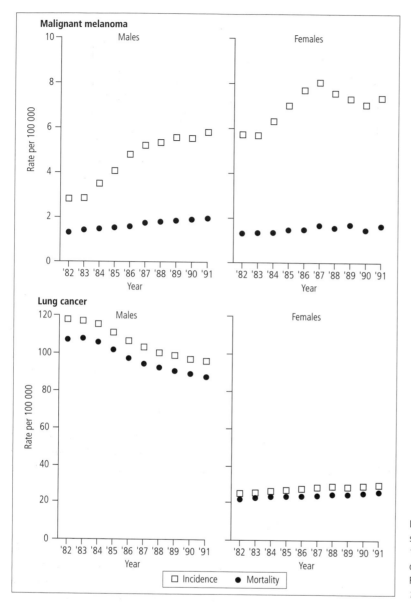

Fig. 3.2 Three-year rolling directly standardized incidence and mortality rates per 100 000 (European population) for two forms of cancer over 12 years in the West Midlands. From W. Midlands RHA *Public Health Report 1995*.

those people presenting for medical advice; other cases for various reasons may not seek medical help and will not be recorded. Even records of mortality depend on the accuracy of the certification of cause of death. Changes in the definition of disease may occur. WHO's international classification of diseases (ICD) is revised every 10 years, so that, for example, a particular cancer may move from one classification group to another in line with medical advances.

Observational studies

Cross-sectional studies

Sometimes available descriptive data may not be

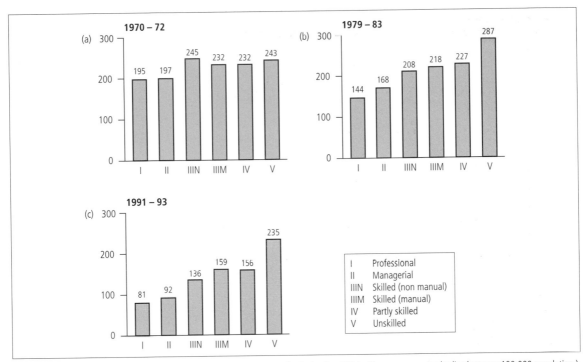

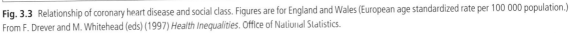

Fig. 3.3 Relationship of coronary heart disease and social class. Figures are for England and Wales (European age standardized rate per 100 000 population.) From F. Drever and M. Whitehead (eds) (1997) *Health Inequalities*. Office of National Statistics.

adequate to meet the purposes of an epidemiological study, and *cross-sectional studies* of a population may be devised. These survey a sample of a population at a given point in time with respect to its health condition in relation to an agent suspected of being associated negatively or positively with the health of the population.

Such studies are economical to perform but are unable to establish cause directly since they determine the state of health and risk factor at the same time. They give a measure of the prevalence of a condition, and are able, if repeated, to show trends in behaviour, such as the amount of smoking or dietary habits, affecting health. Progress towards the attainment of health targets is usefully monitored in this way, and can provide helpful information to improve health promotion.

Cross-sectional surveys give a snapshot or series of snap shots of the health of a population and associated risk factors. To ascertain causal effects,

longer term *longitudinal studies* are needed. If the survey is a snapshot these are akin to a full-length film. They fall into two types: *case–control* and *cohort studies*.

Case–control studies

These target those members of a population sample (*cases*) who already have the health condition to be investigated. These people are compared to a sample of the population who are currently unaffected by the condition (*controls*). The exposure of the cases and controls to the suspected agent is then determined either from records or by questionnaire and interview techniques.

Case–control studies are relatively inexpensive and completed quickly. They are useful in indicating the aetiology of rare diseases since only small numbers are needed as the cases already exist. Their main disadvantages are that since records and

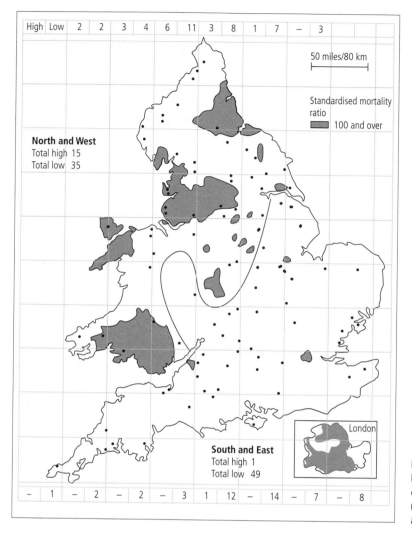

| High | Low | 2 | 2 | 3 | 4 | 6 | 11 | 3 | 8 | 1 | 7 | – | 3 | | |

North and West
Total high 15
Total low 35

50 miles/80 km

Standardised mortality ratio
▇ 100 and over

South and East
Total high 1
Total low 49

London

| – | 1 | – | 2 | – | 2 | – | 3 | 1 | 12 | – | 14 | – | 7 | – | 8 |

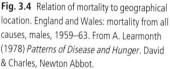

Fig. 3.4 Relation of mortality to geographical location. England and Wales: mortality from all causes, males, 1959–63. From A. Learmonth (1978) *Patterns of Disease and Hunger*. David & Charles, Newton Abbot.

registers were not set up with a particular study in mind they may be deficient in necessary detail or in the way data have been kept. Records may also be destroyed or misplaced. If interviews and questionnaires are used, people may have forgotten key details, they may not always be altogether truthful, particularly if embarrassing or intimate personal details are needed, or conversely may make up details in an attempt, as they see it, to help the investigator. Case–control studies are restrictive in that they can only study one condition at a time (compare with cohort studies, p. 17). A further problem is that risk cannot be directly calculated, since the

cases are an unknown sample of the whole population and incidence cannot therefore be determined.

To work out whether those with the health condition show greater exposure to the suspected aetiological agent numbers of cases and controls and their exposure are tabulated in a 2×2 table (Table 3.3).

The proportion of all the cases in Table 3.3 who have been exposed to the agent is $a/(a + b)$ and for the controls $c/(c + d)$. These ratios might be considered as representing the absolute risk for the cases and the controls. This would follow if the whole population at risk was known and incidence could be calculated. In case–control studies which

Table 3.3 Form of data presentation in a case–control study.

	Exposed	Not exposed	Total
Cases	a	b	a + b
Controls	c	d	c + d
Total	a + c	b + d	

The letters represent the numbers recorded for each group.

are retrospective, the groups a + b and c + d are not the total population exposed and not exposed, the cases and controls are at best a random sample of the total population.

Since absolute risk cannot be calculated, the ratio of risk between the cases and control (i.e. *relative risk*) cannot be directly calculated either. An estimate of relative risk can be made if the cases are a fair sample of all cases, the controls are an unbiased sample of the whole population and the disease is rare. This estimate is called the *odds ratio*, and represents the ratio between odds that a person with the condition has been exposed to the risk factor and the odds that a person without the condition has been exposed. Using the letters found in the 2 × 2 table this can be written as:

$$(a/(a + b)) \div (c/(c + d))$$

If the disease is rare, then a will be very small compared to b, i.e. a + b ≈ b. Similarly, c will be small compared to d and the expression can be rewritten $(a/b) \div (c/d)$ or ad/bc. Figure 3.5 illustrates this diagrammatically.

An odds ratio of 1 would indicate that the odds of having the condition are equal for those exposed or those not exposed, a ratio of 3 would indicate that the odds are three times greater for those exposed, and a figure less than 1 that the odds are less for those exposed, in other words the exposure is beneficial. An example of the use of such statistics, contributing to the case–control study of sporadic Creutzfeldt–Jakob disease in the UK is given in Table 3.4.

The odds ratio expressed in Table 3.4 indicates more than twice the risk for those with a family history of dementia. The result is difficult to interpret: recall bias may have influenced the outcome if

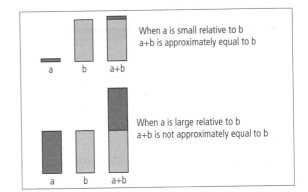

Fig. 3.5 Basis for deriving odds ratio equation.

Table 3.4 Exposure history of 216 cases of sporadic Creutzfeldt–Jakob disease and their controls.

	Family history of dementia	No family history of dementia	
Cases	35	181	
Controls	16	200	N = 216

Odds ratio = (35 × 200) ÷ (16 × 181) = 2.4

relatives of cases (those with dementia) were more likely to remember other relatives with this condition than those of the control population.

Cohort studies

These begin with a defined population at risk, e.g. workers in a particular factory. This cohort of initially disease-free persons is then followed into the future and the effects of exposure to the putative agent recorded for the whole length of the study. Since the whole population is known, incidence rates can be worked out for those suffering exposure and those not suffering exposure. The great advantage of cohort studies is that relative risk and attributable risk can be calculated (see below), to provide the best assessment of the importance of a risk factor as a possible cause of a condition. They can also be used to study several diseases at the same time, or to determine rare causes of a condition.

Such studies are not suitable for investigating rare diseases because a very large population would have to be defined in the first place to ensure that

Table 3.5 Form of data presentation in a cohort study.

	Exposed	Not exposed	Total
Condition present	p	q	p + q
Condition not present	r	s	r + s
Total	p + r	q + s	

sufficient cases cropped up over the study period. They also have the disadvantage of requiring much longer time periods than case–control studies to ensure that sufficient cases are recorded. For these reasons cohort studies have considerable logistical difficulties, and are more expensive in cash terms and in the labour involved than case–control studies. There are further problems related to time length. People may leave the study by migration, refusal to comply, or by death. If these numbers become too high, it becomes impossible to draw meaningful conclusions. Cohort studies are less practicable than case–control studies for conditions with long incubation periods. There are other forms of study design, beyond the scope of this chapter, which combine the advantages of case–control and cohort studies.

Table 3.5 illustrates how the results of a cohort study can be recorded.

Risk may be directly calculated. The *absolute risk* of contracting the condition for persons exposed is $p/(p + r)$

relative risk $= (p/(p + r)) \div (q/(q + s))$

A value of 1 from this calculation would indicate no association between the exposure and the health condition. Figures exceeding 1 indicate an association between the two, the higher the figure the greater the association. A figure less than 1 indicates a beneficial effect if the condition investigated is a form of disease. Briefly, relative risk is a measure of the strength of the association between exposure and the health condition. It may be of little significance, e.g. a risk of 1 in a million is twice the risk relative to a risk of 1 in 2 million but it is still effectively negligible.

To determine how much of the health condition can be put down to a particular agent requires a third measure of risk, the *attributable risk*. This is important in medical practice, particularly public health, because it indicates how much the incidence of the condition may be reduced if the risk factor were eliminated.

Attributable risk = (incidence of disease for those exposed) – (incidence for those not exposed)

Using the symbols in Table 3.5:

attributable risk $= (p/(p + r)) - (q/(q + s))$

For public health purposes a further useful measure is the *attributable fraction in those exposed*. This can be calculated from the formula:

$$\text{attributable fraction} = \frac{\text{(incidence in exposed)} - \text{(incidence in not exposed)}}{\text{incidence in exposed}}$$

Using the symbols in Table 3.5 this becomes:

$$\frac{(p/(p + r)) - (q/(q + s))}{p/(p + r)}$$

Attributable fraction indicates the excess disease arising among those exposed which can be attributed to that exposure. As such it indicates how much disease could be eliminated by getting rid of the agent concerned.

Experimental studies

In observational studies the epidemiologist is able to test hypotheses only passively, being dependent on what data arise or have arisen from circumstance. In science, the strongest tests for hypotheses are those provided when the investigator is able to intervene actively by controlling variables. Randomized clinical trials are examples of such an experimental approach. All proposed new drug treatments are tested in this way and the method can be used to investigate other kinds of medical intervention and health service provision.

In such trials people are allocated randomly to control or intervention groups. A trial for determining the efficacy of a candidate drug for testicular cancer might be formulated as in Fig. 3.6.

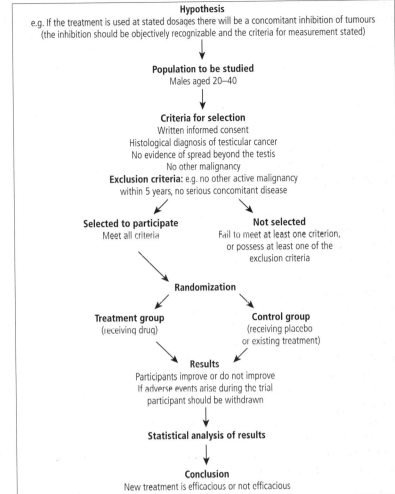

Hypothesis
e.g. If the treatment is used at stated dosages there will be a concomitant inhibition of tumours
(the inhibition should be objectively recognizable and the criteria for measurement stated)

Population to be studied
Males aged 20–40

Criteria for selection
Written informed consent
Histological diagnosis of testicular cancer
No evidence of spread beyond the testis
No other malignancy
Exclusion criteria: e.g. no other active malignancy
within 5 years, no serious concomitant disease

Selected to participate
Meet all criteria

Not selected
Fail to meet at least one criterion,
or possess at least one of the
exclusion criteria

Randomization

Treatment group
(receiving drug)

Control group
(receiving placebo
or existing treatment)

Results
Participants improve or do not improve
If adverse events arise during the trial
participant should be withdrawn

Statistical analysis of results

Conclusion
New treatment is efficacious or not efficacious

Fig. 3.6 Outline of a trial for determining the efficacy of a candidate drug for testicular cancer. Note: there must not be any difference obvious to the participants in the treatment of the two groups, e.g. tablets given to both groups should look the same in size, shape and colour so they are unaware of the group to which they have been allocated (single blinding). The clinical team should not know to which group participants have been allocated, nor be able to distinguish between the tablets (double blinding).

In order to avoid *placebo effects*, it is essential that those in the trial do not know to which group (control or intervention) they have been assigned. To prevent subjective bias by the experimenters it is also preferable that they are unaware of the allocation to groups. This process is called *blinding*.

Bias may arise in further ways. *Selection bias* occurs when those selected to participate are not representative of the population at risk. For example, if a study depends on volunteers from the population bias would occur, if those volunteering represented those who were more concerned about their health than the generality of the population. Such people would be likely to be more careful in their dietary and drinking behaviour and more likely to take exercise and so not necessarily be representative of the whole population.

Bias will occur if people dropping out of a study are not similar to those who remain in it, or if those dropping out of one group of a pair of groups under comparison differ systematically from those dropping out of the other group.

Information bias can arise in retrieving information from subjects or from records (an example was given in Table 3.4). Interactions between interviewers and subjects may affect response rates. Cases might be questioned more carefully by an interviewer than controls, being prompted to ransack their memories about past exposures more than those without the disease. Non-response to questionnaires can give rise to bias if the non-responders differ systematically from the responders.

Confounding

An agent may be correlated strongly with a health condition, but may not be its actual cause, being merely independently correlated with the cause. Such agents are called *confounding variables*. The commonest confounder is age.

A study might show a strong correlation between moderate daily intake of red wine (say 250 mL) and a significant reduction in the risk of cardiac disease. This could be a causal relationship. If, however, wine consumption is itself strongly correlated with a fish-based diet rich in ecasopentaenoic acid, then there will be a necessary correlation of the diet and the reduction of heart disease. This could also be a causal factor. If there were independent evidence of the beneficial effect of this diet, and since red wine consumption is clearly not itself the cause of the fish-based diet, then consumption of wine is a confounder of the true situation (fish-based diet reduces heart disease).

Minimization of confounding effects

Matching
In the example given above the confounding effect of wine consumption could be removed by a study matching wine consumers with non-consumers for diet, age and sex. If too many matching variables are used then the numbers that can be recruited to a study may be reduced below acceptable sample sizes for adequate statistical analysis. If matching is based on a variable which is actually associated with the health condition real differences between groups will be eliminated.

Restriction
If a factor being investigated as a possible aetiological agent and its incidence is greater in say men than women, then sex and the factor will be con-

founded. This can be avoided by restricting the study to one sex.

Stratification
To resolve the confounding between the effects of moderate intake of red wine and the effect of the fish-based diet on rates of heart disease, the data could be stratified as shown in Table 3.6.

Correlation or cause?

Even if an epidemiological study has shown a strong association between an agent and an health condition, it is not necessarily true that the agent is a *cause* of the condition. Statistical analysis may show that the correlation is significant, but this is not *proof* of actual cause.

Association may arise by chance, bias or confounding. If in using evidence allowing rejection of a null hypothesis, probability levels are set too high the hypothesis may be falsely rejected (*type I error*). If the level is set too low the null hypothesis may be falsely retained (*type II error*).

In simple terms A causes B if and only if:
- A always precedes B in time.
- Changing A *always* changes B.
- The correlation of A and B is not due to both being independently correlated with a further agent C.

In practice, it is impossible to be certain that there is no further underlying agent such as C, and it is impossible to perform the infinite number of observations of the relation between A and B which are needed to give absolute proof of cause.

Even such guides as Koch's postulates for infectious disease may not give the cause of disease, since disease is often multifactorial in genesis. It is not possible to suffer from tuberculosis unless the bacillus is present (*necessary cause*), but the presence of the bacillus is not a *sufficient cause* for clinical manifestation of disease. This may depend on other characteristics in the infected person, e.g. genetic susceptibility, a compromised immune system, overcrowded living conditions or malnutrition.

Although only imperfect knowledge can be available in the real world, decisions still have to be made on regimens of treatment, or the delivery of health care or development of health promotion. Bradford

Table 3.6 Stratification of heart disease against red wine consumption and diet. (a) Expected type of distribution of rates if moderate wine consumption is the agent. (b) Expected type of distribution of rates if fish consumption is the agent.

(a)

Amount of fish consumed per day	Heart disease rate/wine consumed per day			
	No wine consumed	250 mL	500 mL	1000 mL
No fish	High	Low	Moderate	High
100 g	High	Low	Moderate	High
200 g	High	Low	Moderate	High
300 g	High	Low	Moderate	High
400 g	High	Low	Moderate	High

(b)

Amount of fish consumed per day	Heart disease rate/wine consumed per day			
	No wine consumed	250 mL	500 mL	1000 mL
No fish	High	High	High	High
100 g	Moderate	Moderate	Moderate	Moderate
200 g	Moderate	Moderate	Moderate	Moderate
300 g	Low	Low	Low	Low
400 g	Very low	Very low	Very low	Very low

Hill in 1965 devised nine criteria for making practical decisions on causality. These are guidelines and not absolute criteria.

Temporality

Cause must always precede effect in time. This is logically necessary, but not certainly provable.

Strength

What is the relative risk or odds ratio? The greater it is, the greater is the likelihood of causal association.

Consistency

If different studies, in different populations using different study designs corroborate the conclusion then cause becomes more likely. Inconsistency, however, does not eliminate cause, since some effects may manifest only on rare occasions.

Specificity

When a particular agent is associated with a particular health condition it may be held to be causal. However, the multifactorial aetiology of disease renders the finding of such specific agents unlikely since the causes may logically also have more than one effect. Smoking, for example, is associated not only with lung cancer, but also other lung diseases, cardiovascular disease and other pathologies. Many authors would now dismiss this as a useful criterion.

Dose–response relationship

Increasing exposure to the suspected agent will lead to an increase in disease if the agent is harmful or an increase in health if it is beneficial. Since confounding may produce the same response, cause is again not certainly proved.

Plausibility

Does the postulated cause fit in with generally accepted scientific knowledge? This assumes that current scientific knowledge contains enough information to preclude the supposed cause. This can be misleading, since it assumes that current scientific knowledge is a full description of the possibilities which could exist.

Coherence

The association should not conflict with what is known of the natural history and biology of the condition. In effect this is an opposite case to plausibility (above), and should be treated with the same caution.

Experiment

Experimentally changing exposures to the agent consistently changes the level of disease or health. Such correlation cannot logically provide proof of cause, but lack of it may cast doubt on a causal association.

Analogy

A very weak criterion. Simply because use of a particular drug can lead to cancer does not necessarily imply that use of a similar one will do the same.

Apart from temporality which is a logically necessary criterion, these criteria are hedged about with exceptions and cannot provide irrefutable evidence of cause.

Summary

Measuring rates of disease and health in popula-

Key points

1 Epidemiology is the study of the distribution of health and disease in populations.

2 The distribution is measured by calculation of rates. Examples are given for the calculation of incidence, prevalence and mortality rates and how these rates may be indirectly or directly standardized.

3 Descriptive studies elucidate patterns of association between agents affecting health and sectors of populations or among populations.

4 Observational and experimental studies allow quantification of risk and may suggest causal relationships between exposure to possible aetiological agents and health status.

5 Strong associations are not invariably causes and may only be correlations due to errors such as bias or not eliminating confounding factors in the study design. Criteria which may *in corroboration* indicate cause are listed.

---

tions allows comparisons between them to be made and trends to be detected. Data collected is helpful in rational decision making on the distribution of health and medical services, as well as suggesting further ideas for investigation in the aetiology of disease and the promotion of health.

Descriptive, observational and experimental studies can be used to test hypotheses derived from such data accumulation. The degree of risk associated with suspected aetiological agents can then be quantified. Statistically significant correlations between risk and health condition may indicate a causal relation, but even after allowance is made for possible bias and confounding effects a degree of uncertainty may remain in attributing actual cause to a particular agent.

Further reading

Beaglehole R., Bonita R. & Kjellström T. (1993) *Basic Epidemiology*. WHO, Geneva.

Bradford-Hill A. (1965) The environment and disease: association or causation? *Proceedings of the Royal Society of Medicine* **58**: 295–300.

Hansson L. *et al.* (1999) Effect of angiotensin-converting enzyme inhibitors compared with conventional therapy on cardiovascular morbidity and mortality in hypertension. *Lancet* **353**: 611–616.

Jefferson T. & Demichelli V. (1999) Experimental and non experimental study designs. HB vaccines: a case study. *Journal of Epidemiology and Community Health* **53**: 51–54.

National CJD Surveillance Unit and Department of Epidemiology and Population Studies (1999) *Creutzfeldt–Jakob Disease surveillance in the UK. Seventh Annual Report 1998*. London School of Hygiene and Tropical Medicine, London.

WORKED EXAMPLE 1: THE EPIDEMIOLOGY OF COLORECTAL CANCER

Approximately 15 000 people die from colorectal cancer each year in England and Wales. Histological examination classifies 90% of these as adenocarcinomas. The precise histological classification of a cancer at a common site is important because a difference in histology may imply a difference in the *aetiological* (causal) factors (see also case study 34).

Diet is believed to influence the risk for colorectal cancer. A high fibre and low fat diet has been recommended to reduce the risk from these cancers. However, without the knowledge of the precise dietary factors that play a critical role, it seems unlikely at present that the incidence will be reduced to any great extent by *primary prevention* through dietary modification.

It is generally accepted that the majority of [colorectal] adenocarcinomas develop within pre-existing adenomas. This line of progression is commonly known as the 'adenoma–carcinoma' sequence. This implies a method for *secondary prevention* of this disease by the removal of the precursor lesions.

The *screening* of asymptomatic adults is considered the best means at present to decrease mortality from colorectal cancer. A reduction in mortality from this disease may be achieved through secondary prevention, and possibly, through the detection of cancers at an earlier stage, which may be associated with improved prognosis.

Classification of the disease: ICD system

The *'ICD, Injuries and Causes of Death'* published by WHO assigns a classification code (ICD code) to each disease. At the three-digit level of the ninth revision of the ICD (*ICD-9*), the term 'colorectal cancer' is often used to describe cancers of ICD-9 153 (cancers of the 'colon') and ICD-9 154 (cancers of the 'rectum'). The ninth revision has now been superseded by the tenth revision (ICD-10), and this has been in general use from around 1997. However, many statistics will still rely on data that is coded to the ninth revision.

The magnitude of the problem

The Office for National Statistics (ONS) produces statistics using the ICD system, including yearly figures on the incidence of cancer by site (i.e. by ICD code) and mortality by underlying cause of death (i.e. by ICD code) in England and Wales. The statistics on cancer incidence have been published approximately 3–7 years from the year of interest — hence incidence figures for 1990 were published in 1997. However, the statistics on mortality have been published 1–2 years from the year of interest

Table 3.7 The three most frequent sites of cancer in England and Wales in 1990. From ONS (1997a).

ICD-9 code and site		Number of cancer registrations
Males		
162	Lung	25 020
153–154	Colorectal	13 972
185	Prostate	13 320
140–208	All sites of cancers*	103 566
Females		
174	Breast	29 145
153–154	Colorectal	13 850
162	Lung	11 545
140–208	All sites of cancers*	105 865

* Excluding ICD-9 173, non-melanoma skin cancer; 16 686 cases in males and 15 459 cases in females

Table 3.8 The three most frequent causes of cancer deaths in England and Wales in 1995. From ONS (1997b).

ICD-9 code and site		Number of cancer deaths
Males		
162	Lung	20 498
185	Prostate	8 866
153–154	Colorectal	7 991
140–208	All sites of cancers*	72 443
Females		
174	Breast	12 543
162	Lung	11 129
153–154	Colorectal	7 758
140–208	All sites of cancers*	66 276

* Excluding ICD-9 173, non-melanoma skin cancer; 264 deaths in males and 175 deaths in females.

so mortality figures for 1995 were also published in 1997.

Using data from the England and Wales ONS, colorectal cancer is the *second* most common site of cancer in each sex (Table 3.7) and the *third* leading cause of death from cancer in each sex (Table 3.8). The three most frequent sites of cancer account for 51% of cancers registered (from Table 3.7), and 50% of deaths from cancers (from Table 3.8).

In Table 3.7, cases of non-melanoma skin cancer (ICD-9 173) have been excluded because it is believed that the number of cases are inaccurate due to serious under-registration (ONS, 1997a). Deaths from these cancers have also been excluded from Table 3.8 for consistency with Table 3.7.

Standardization of epidemiological data

When considering the incidence of disease in a given population it is important to consider demographic factors. For example, when the incidence of a disease increases with age, the population incidence can be greater in a country with a higher proportion of elderly people, and lower in a country with a higher proportion of younger people.

Direct standardization of the incidence rates

Age standardization is used to eliminate differences between population disease rates that are due to differences in the age distribution of the populations. A number of *standard populations* exist and include the African, world and European standard population. All are hypothetical populations. The African standard population has the smallest proportion of old people and the European the highest proportion.

The method of calculation of the incidence rate of colorectal cancer in males in England and Wales age standardized to world population is shown in Table 3.9. It can be seen from this how a change in the age distribution can have a large effect on the calculated population disease rates; the rate for all ages has changed from 56.2 per 100 000 to 34.1 per 100 000.

Incidence rates of cancers of the colon, rectum and colorectum in each sex in England and Wales for 1990, age standardized to the world population are given in Table 3.10. From this it can be seen that the incidence of cancer of the colon is similar in males and females, with a rate ratio close to unity (1.2). However, the incidence rate of cancer of the rectum in males is almost double that of females, the male to female rate ratio being 1.8.

A difference in the male to female rate ratio for cancer of the colon compared with cancer of the rectum might imply a difference in the aetiological

Table 3.9 Calculation of age standardized incidence rates.

Age i	Incidence rate per 100 000 males in E & W per year* (R_i)	No. of persons in standard (world) population† (W_i)	Expected cases in standard population $E_i = (R_i \times W_i)/100\,000$
0–4	0.0	12 000	0.00
5–9	0.1	10 000	0.01
10–14	0.3	9 000	0.03
15–19	0.1	9 000	0.01
20–24	0.6	8 000	0.05
25–29	0.8	8 000	0.06
30–34	2.1	6 000	0.13
35–39	5.1	6 000	0.31
40–44	11.9	6 000	0.71
45–49	22.9	6 000	1.37
50–54	48.6	5 000	2.43
55–59	82.9	4 000	3.32
60–64	130.4	4 000	5.22
65–69	202.0	3 000	6.06
70–74	276.9	2 000	5.54
75–79	386.2	1 000	3.86
80–84	439.9	500	2.20
85+	557.5	500	2.79
All ages	56.2	100 000	34.10

* E & W, England and Wales. Source of incidence rates: ONS (1997a).
† Source of world population: Muir *et al*. (1987).
Standardized rate = 34.10 per 100 000 males.

Table 3.10 Incidence rates of cancers in England and Wales, 1990, age standardized to the world population (rate per 100 000).

	Colon	Rectum	Colorectum
Males	19.44	14.68	34.10
Females	15.58	8.01	23.60
M to F ratio	1.2	1.8	1.4

factor(s) for each cancer and different exposures to the aetiological factor(s) between males and females.

Geographical comparisons

The incidence of colorectal cancer varies between countries and within countries. The observation that high incidence rates occur in Westernized societies suggests that environmental factors influence the risk of colorectal cancer. Importantly, the finding that within a geographical region, ethnic and racial subgroups that maintain isolated and distinct life-styles exhibit risks that often differ from the surrounding population, implies that the causal factor is not in the shared physical environment but a lifestyle factor. Epidemiologists have surmised that diet is the most important lifestyle factor.

Time trends

Divergent temporal (over time) trends in the incidence of colon and rectal cancer suggests that the aetiological factors may differ between cancers at each site. For example, the incidence of colon cancer has been shown to increase whilst, concurrently, rectal cancer has been decreasing in the same country.

Screening for the disease

Population screening for colorectal cancer by using a biennial (every other year) screen with a faecal occult blood (FOB) test is being evaluated by a *randomized controlled trial* in the UK (Hardcastle *et al.*, 1996).

A randomized controlled trial is an example of a *longitudinal* or *cohort* study because cohorts (groups of people) are *followed over time*. In a randomized controlled trial of screening, the screen test is offered to individuals who are randomized and allocated to the *intervention* (screening) group. Those who are allocated to the control group will not be offered, by the trial, the screen test. After a period of follow-up (time from entry into the screening trial), ratios (intervention group to control group) of the incidence of and mortality from the disease being screened for are produced.

In this screening trial (Hardcastle *et al.*, 1996), 60% of the intervention group accepted at least one screen test. After a median of 7.8 years of follow-up ('median' because all of the individuals were not entered into the trial at the same time), the rate ratio of the incidence of colorectal cancer was 1.04 and of the mortality from colorectal cancer 0.85. This means that the incidence rate in the intervention group was 4% higher than the control group, and the mortality rate was 15% lower than the control group.

A higher incidence rate in the intervention group for a period of follow-up is always expected. This is, in part, because cancers detected through screening, without intervention, would have surfaced clinically at a time after that period of follow-up and not during that period. *Over-diagnosis* of cancers will also increase the incidence in the intervention group. This occurs when cancers that would never have been found are detected. A lower incidence rate in the intervention group compared with the control group after a period of follow-up may occur if cancers are being prevented, e.g. by the removal of those adenomas that without intervention would have progressed to a cancer and surfaced clinically during that period of follow-up.

Further reading

Breslow N.E. & Day N.E. (1980) *Statistical Methods in Cancer Research* Volume I: *The Analysis of Case–control Studies* (IARC Scientific Publications no. 32). International Agency for Research on Cancer, Lyon.

Breslow N.E. & Day N.E. (1987) *Statistical Methods in Cancer Research*. Volume II: *The Design and Analysis of Cohort Studies* (IARC Scientific Publications no. 82). International Agency for Research on Cancer, Lyon.

Coggon D., Rose G. & Barker D.J.P. (1997) *Epidemiology for the Uninitiated*, 4th edn. BMJ Publishing Group.

References

Hardcastle J.D., Chamberlain J.O., Robinson M.H.E. *et al.* (1996) Randomised controlled trial of faecal occult blood screening for colorectal cancer. *Lancet* **348**: 1472–1477.

Muir C., Waterhouse J., Mack T., Powell J., Whelan S. (eds) (1987) *Cancer incidence in Five Continents*. Volume V (IARC Scientific Publications no. 88). International Agency for Research on Cancer, Lyon, p. 792.

Office for National Statistics (1997a) *Cancer Statistics Registrations. Registrations of Cancer Diagnosed in 1990, England and Wales. Series MB1 no. 23.* The Stationery Office, London.

Office for National Statistics (1997b) *Mortality Statistics Cause. Review of the Registrar General on Deaths by Cause, Sex and Age, in England and Wales, 1995. Series DH2 no. 22.* The Stationery Office, London.

WORKED EXAMPLE 2: EPIDEMIC ASTHMA DAYS IN BARCELONA

Throughout the 1980s, on a number of isolated days in Barcelona, unprecedented high numbers of hospital admissions for acute asthma occurred (Fig. 3.7). These were dramatic events and each day became known as an 'epidemic day'. The cause for the epidemic days was not at all clear at first, although there were a number of interesting clinical features about the attacks that gave some clues. Adults, for instance, were far more likely to be affected than children and some attacks were very rapid in onset, recovery being equally rapid. A high proportion of attacks were so severe that mechanical ventilation on an intensive care unit was required and a higher than expected number of deaths occurred.

Investigations

Investigators considered the possibility of an air-borne cause for these epidemic days and were suspicious that emissions from the industrial area to the west of the city might be the cause. The first step in the investigation was a descriptive study mapping the geographical distribution of the patients at the time the attacks occurred (Fig. 3.8). The cases of asthma did not cluster around the industrial area as had been predicted, but around the docks. In

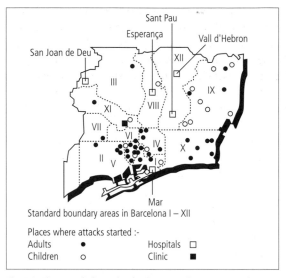

Fig. 3.8 Places at which attacks of asthma started. From Anto *et al.* (1989).

Table 3.11 Unloading of soya bean on epidemic and non-epidemic days. Figures are given as numbers of days.

	Soya		
	Unloading	Not loading	Total
Epidemic days	13	0	13
Non-epidemic days	262	468	730
Totals	275	468	743

the next stage the investigators considered what goods were being unloaded on epidemic and non-epidemic days. Initial analysis pointed to two types of goods—soya bean products and wheat—being unloaded significantly more frequently on epidemic days than on non-epidemic days. Statistical analysis using a 2 × 2 table (Table 3.11) showed that an epidemic day *never* occurred when soya products were *not* being handled, although there were days when soya *was* being unloaded when epidemics *did not* occur.

The relative risk is thus calculated as unquantifiably high (Table 3.11), indicating a very strong association between soya unloading and the pres-

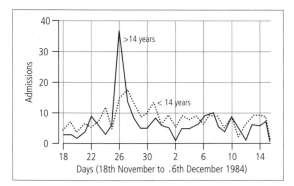

Fig. 3.7 Daily number of adult and children asthma emergency room admissions from November 18 to December 18, 1984. From Anto *et al.* (1989).

ence of an epidemic of acute asthma. In 1965 Bradford Hill identified nine criteria for an association to be regarded as causal (see pp. 21–22). These epidemics were *temporally* related to soya being unloaded, the mechanism was *biologically plausible* and an *analogous* situation already existed, as castor bean dust was known to be a potent aeroallergen.

Having determined a strong epidemiological association the next step was to determine evidence of allergic sensitization to soya in those admitted with acute asthma on epidemic days. A case–control study was undertaken of patients who were admitted with acute asthma on epidemic days (cases) and they were compared to patients admitted with acute asthma but not on an epidemic day (controls). Results from both skin-prick testing and specific immunoglobulin E (IgE) levels (employing the allergenic protein in the husk of the bean as the antigen), showed that cases were 30 times more likely to be sensitized to soya protein than controls.

Diagnosis and intervention

On the basis of the epidemiological evidence and the clinical evidence of allergy, the cause of the epidemic days was thought to be soya bean asthma. At the time of the outbreak soya was being unloaded into two dockside silos, one with and one without a filter cap which prevented loss of soya dust into the atmosphere. When dust released from the uncapped silo was effectively eliminated by the addition of a filter cap (in epidemiological terms an *intervention* to remove an *exposure*) no further epidemic days occurred (Table 3.12), providing ultimate *experimental* proof of a cause and effect relationship.

Table 3.12 Effect of intervention on soya bean epidemic asthma (only days on which soya bean was unloaded are included).

	Total days	Days with high no. of asthma admissions	Epidemic days	Admissions to intensive care/day
Before cap installation	167	29	18	0.26 ± 0.9
After cap installation	133	6	0	0.01 ± 0.12
P value	< 0.001	< 0.001	< 0.001	

Discussion

These unusual epidemic days demonstrate the causal role of airborne allergens from a specific industrial source in causing asthma, in contrast to the more familiar domestic or general sources of allergen (e.g. cat dander in the home, grass pollen during the summer). The cause was identified by the practice of good epidemiology followed by appropriate immunological confirmation. The outcome of the identification of soya as the cause of these epidemic days has been dramatic and epidemic days have been eliminated. Other recognized examples of industrial emissions causing asthma in the surrounding population are few, although a similar effect had been seen previously resulting from emissions from castor bean processing factories in South Africa and North America.

Reference

Anto J.M., Sunyer J., Rodriguez-Roisin R., Suarez-Cervera M. & Vazquez L. (1989) Community outbreaks of asthma associated with inhalation of soyabean dust. *New England Journal of Medicine* **320**: 1097–1102.

CHAPTER 4

The Molecular Basis of Cell Reproduction, Senescence and Death

Cellular reproduction, senescence and death are important physiological responses that are frequently thrown into disorder in a variety of disease states. This chapter describes the processes of cellular reproduction, senescence and death. Cell death is considered with particular reference to apoptosis, increasingly recognized as a fundamental mechanism of physiological cell death. Where appropriate the relevance of these processes to specific disease states will be outlined. However, their contribution to disease pathogenesis is considered in more detail in later chapters.

Cellular reproduction—the cell cycle

The process of cellular reproduction is frequently expressed in terms of the *cell cycle*—a sequence of events that ultimately leads to cell division and the creation of two daughter cells from a single parental cell. The cell cycle is divided into four phases (Fig. 4.1) as follows.
• The *S* (*synthetic*) phase during which the genetic material is replicated.
• The *M* (*mitotic*) phase during which the cell constituents are segregated to each daughter cell.
• The *G1* (*first gap*) phase which precedes the S phase. This represents the period during which the cell is committed to cell cycle progression.
• The *G2* (*second gap*) phase which separates S phase from M phase. This phase is important because it allows cells to repair errors that may have

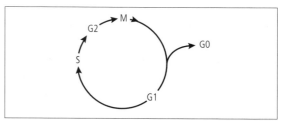

Fig. 4.1 The cell cycle is the process by which cell reproduction occurs. There are distinct phases within the cell cycle. These include the S (synthetic) phase during which the genetic material is replicated and the M (mitotic) phase during which the cell constituents are segregated to each daughter cell. These are separated by two gap phases: G1 (first gap) which precedes the S phase, and G2 (second gap) which separates S phase from M phase. G0 is used to denote cells which have left the cell cycle.

occurred during DNA replication before the cell divides.

A fifth phase, known as *G0*, is used to denote cells, which have left the cell cycle.

Stimulus for cell reproduction

Extracellular growth factors usually provide the external signal for a cell to divide. Thus, when growth factors are present in the extracellular environment, only cells expressing the corresponding receptors for the growth factor will respond and divide. This ensures that growth factor signals are only delivered to those cells required to divide. In addition, when the growth factor is no longer present, these cells will stop dividing. The mechanism

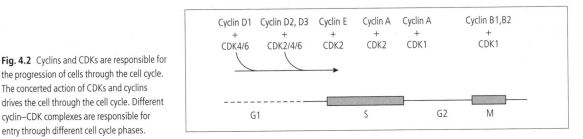

Fig. 4.2 Cyclins and CDKs are responsible for the progression of cells through the cell cycle. The concerted action of CDKs and cyclins drives the cell through the cell cycle. Different cyclin–CDK complexes are responsible for entry through different cell cycle phases.

by which the binding of growth factor to its receptor on a cell ultimately leads to cell divison is complex and is considered in more detail in Chapter 22. However, the general process is described briefly below.

Binding of growth factor to its receptor usually leads to the activation of the receptor. If this is a protein kinase then activation of the receptor may mean that it is now able to phosphorylate other proteins (or itself), in turn activating them and thereby transferring the growth signal. This second set of proteins, which are usually located within the cytoplasm, are often referred to as 'second messengers'. In turn, these activated second messengers activate other proteins and the sequence of activation continues until eventually a group of proteins in the nucleus, known as transcription factors, are activated. The group of transcription factors stimulated by these pathways are able to switch on the expression of the genes required to execute the cell cycle (see below).

Molecular control of the cell cycle

The cell cycle is controlled by three main groups of regulatory proteins: the *cyclin-dependent kinases* (CDKs) of which there are currently nine known members (CDK1 to CDK9); the *cyclins* which comprise at least 15 members (cyclin A to cyclin T); and the *cyclin-dependent kinase inhibitors* (CDKIs).

CDKs phosphorylate other proteins and thereby allow cells to progress through the cell cycle. As their name suggests these kinases are dependent on the cyclins for their activity. Thus, a CDK can only be activated once its partner cyclin is present in sufficient concentration. The CDK is therefore inactivated once levels of its partner cyclin fall below a threshold concentration. Some CDKs are activated

by more than one cyclin, so that CDK activity during the cell cycle may be maintained through the interaction of the CDK with different cyclins. The activation of CDK–cyclin complexes is further controlled by their phosphorylation by a CDK7–cyclin H complex. This latter complex is often referred to as CDK-activating kinase (CAK).

During early G1 phase and as a result of the growth factor stimulation described above, expression of the cyclin D genes is stimulated. There are three cyclin D-type proteins (cyclin D1 to cyclin D3). Cyclin D1 is able to complex with both CDK4 and CDK6, whereas cyclin D2 and cyclin D3 are able to form a complex with CDK2, CDK4 and CDK6 (Fig. 4.2). The activated CDKs are then able to phosphorylate members of the retinoblastoma family of proteins, including pRb protein itself.

In the early part of the G1 phase the pRb protein is present in a hypophosphorylated form and is able to bind to and inactivate members of the E2F family of transcription factors. The E2F transcription factors are responsible for stimulating DNA replication. Therefore, DNA synthesis will only take place once pRb has been fully phosphorylated and E2F released. Activity of the CDKs 2/4/6–cyclin D complexes during early G1 begins the phosphorylation of pRb.

At the onset of the S phase the concentrations of the cyclin D proteins decrease, whereas the concentration of cyclin E peaks, having already begun to rise during early G1. Cyclin E now binds to CDK2, effectively taking over the previous role of the cyclin D proteins in the activation of CDK2. The CDK2–cyclin E complex then completes the phosphorylation of pRb and DNA synthesis can now proceed. Thus, it is believed that cyclin E is responsible for the initiation of the S phase of the cell cycle.

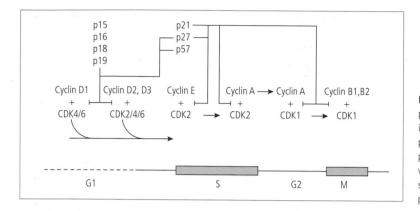

Fig. 4.3 CDK inhibitors inhibit cell cycle progress. There are two main groups of CDK inhibitor: the p21 protein family (comprising p21, p27 and p57) and the INK4 family (p15, p16, p18 and p19). The CDK inhibitors act at various 'checkpoints' within the cell cycle to suppress CDK–cyclin activation and inhibit progress through the cell cycle.

During the S phase, cyclin E is rapidly degraded and the activation of CDK2 is taken over by cyclin A. The cyclin A–CDK2 complex is necessary for the continuation of DNA replication during S phase. However, towards the end of the S phase, cyclin A preferentially activates CDK1. This marks the end of the S phase and the beginning of G2. Following G2, CDK1 activation by the cyclins B1 and B2 initiates and maintains mitosis. However, CDK1 activation at this stage is subject to several control steps, involving phosphorylation and dephosphorylation events. These control measures ensure that mitosis does not begin until DNA synthesis has occurred.

CDK inhibitors

The activation of CDKs by their partner cyclins must be tightly regulated in order to prevent perpetual cell reproduction. This is achieved by the CDKIs which prevent progress through the cell cycle by blocking the activity of the CDKs. CDKIs usually act at specific stages of the cycle, known as 'checkpoints'. The two major checkpoints controlled by the CDKIs are at the transition from G1 to S phase and at the start of mitosis (G2 to M) (Fig. 4.3). There are two major families of CDKIs, the p21 family and the INK4 family.

p21 family

The p21 family consist of p21 itself, p27 and p57. Some of these proteins are known by other names and often these alternative designations are given as a superscript. Thus, p21 is also known as wild-type p53-activated fragment 1 (WAF1) or CDK2-interacting protein 1 (CIP1) and is often written p21[WAF1/CIP1]. Likewise, p27 and p57 are referred to as kinase-inhibiting proteins 1 (KIP1) and 2 (KIP2), respectively. They are often written as p27[KIP1] and p57[KIP2]. The p21 family are able to inhibit a wide range of CDKs.

Following cellular trauma or DNA damage, p21 expression is induced by the p53 protein resulting in cell cycle arrest until the DNA damage can be repaired. Alternatively, if the damage is beyond repair, p53 can induce cell death by increasing expression of proapoptosis proteins such as Bax (see later). The p53-mediated induction of cell cycle arrest is considered in more detail in Chapter 22.

INK4 family

In contrast to the p21-type proteins, members of the INK4 (inhibitor of CDK4) family are more specific in their actions, preferentially inhibiting CDK4 and CDK6 during the G1 phase of the cell cycle. The INK4 family comprises p15[INK4A], p16[INK4B], p18[INK4C] and p19[INK4D]. A related protein encoded from the same gene region as p19[INK4D] and referred to as p19[ARF] plays a role in p53-mediated cell cycle arrest (see below).

Cell senescence

Key experiments have demonstrated that fibroblasts will stop dividing after a finite number of cell doublings. The point at which cells no longer divide is known as *senescence*. It has been shown that most

Table 4.1 Differences between necrosis and apoptosis.

	Necrosis	Apoptosis
Appearances	Large swathes of cells die	Individual cells die
	Cells (and nuclei) swollen	Nuclei and whole cells shrunken, rounded and darkly stained
	Plasma membranes disrupted	Chromatin condensed in demilunes and caps
Causes	Usually pathological	Can be physiological, developmental or pathological
Inflammatory effect	Wide range of cells attracted	Only phagocytic macrophages attracted

normal cells undergo senescence and that structures known as *telomeres* are key to this process.

Telomeres and telomerase

Telomeres are repeated sequences of DNA located at the ends of chromosomes. Without telomeres the chromosome ends would be recognized as DNA breaks and would be repaired. Thus, telomeres prevent chromosome fusion that would ultimately lead to massive genome instability.

Each time the cell divides the telomeres shorten. This is because of something called the *end-replication problem*. Essentially, when DNA is replicated an RNA primer is used. This is a short sequence of RNA, which binds to the telomeres and initiates DNA replication. However, the telomere sequence that binds the RNA primer is not itself replicated. Thus, the telomeres progressively shorten. When the telomeres reach a critical length the cell stops dividing and goes into senescence.

However, some normal cell types are designed not to enter a senescent stage. These include stem cells. These cells possess an enzyme known as *telomerase*. This enzyme is able to maintain telomere length. Some cancer cells express telomerase and it is believed to be one of the reasons why these cells can proliferate indefinitely.

Cell death

Two morphologically different forms of cell death are recognized, *apoptosis* and *necrosis*. Generally, apoptosis refers to *programmed* or *physiological* cell death, whereas necrosis is usually the response to

noxious injury. However, while the terms apoptosis and programmed cell death are often used synonymously, cell death can be programmed without undergoing the morphological characteristics of apoptosis. In addition, there is evidence that programmed cell death can lead to necrosis in some situations.

Necrosis

Necrosis is usually the result of severe injury to cells and can occur in response to a wide range of stimuli. Necrosis is characterized morphologically by mitochondrial swelling, the formation of cell surface 'blebs' and ribosomal disaggregation. These initial changes may be reversible. However, if the noxious stimulus persists and these changes become more pronounced to include extreme 'blebbing' at the cell surface, together with much greater dilation of the mitochondria (high amplitude swelling) then they will inevitably lead to cell death. Eventually, there is membrane disruption, dissolution of organelles, including the nucleus, and lysosomal degeneration followed by activation of an inflammatory response. The induction of inflammation is a characteristic feature of necrosis (Table 4.1). End-stage necrosis involving many cells within a tissue leads to the loss of tissue architecture (Fig. 4.4).

Apoptosis

In the early 1970s it was proposed that cells died 'normally' by a form of cell 'suicide', although it took another 20 years and studies involving the nematode worm *Caenorhabditis elegans* for the fundamental

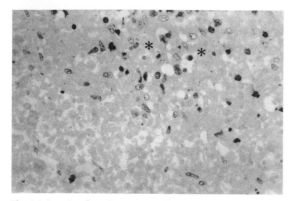

Fig. 4.4 A section of a malignant tumour showing necrosis, with destruction of tissue architecture and a mixed inflammatory infiltrate (asterisks).

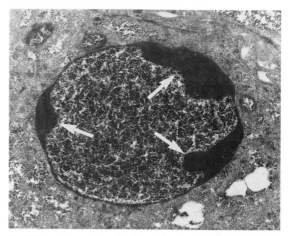

Fig. 4.5 An electron micrograph of an apoptotic nucleus showing crescentic areas (arrowed) of condensed chromatin beneath the nuclear membrane. Courtesy of Professor George Antonokopolous, Department of Pathology, University of Athens.

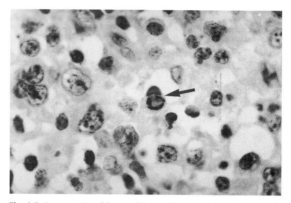

Fig. 4.6 An apoptotic cell (arrowed) in a malignant lymphoma (a cancer of the lymphoid cells) exhibiting partitioning of the nucleus with dense, heavily stained chromatin.

importance of apoptosis or programmed cell death to be recognized. Apoptosis occurs throughout life and plays a key role in homoeostasis. Apoptosis is also crucially important during development. For example, apoptosis is responsible for the loss of tadpole tails and for the removal of the interdigital webs in humans.

In contrast to necrosis, apoptosis does not normally induce an inflammatory response thereby avoiding further tissue damage. The morphological changes that accompany apoptosis are quite different from those seen in necrosis. Firstly, there is loss of cell–cell adhesion and the cells become smaller and rounded, sometimes with lobulations although some organelles remain intact. Cell shrinkage results from loss of water and sodium ions. Within the nucleus the chromatin condenses to form 'half-moon' shaped structures (Fig. 4.5) and the nucleoli appear disorganized. The nucleus itself may break up into multiple fragments (Fig. 4.6). DNA fragmentation (into 180–200 bp pieces) caused by nuclear damage leads to the characteristic formation of apoptotic ladders when the fragments are resolved upon agarose gels and visualized under ultraviolet (UV) light.

Finally, the apoptotic cells are rapidly recognized and phagocytosed by macrophages without leakage of their contents. Apoptotic bodies may be seen within the cytoplasm of the consuming cells for up to 9 h following phagocytosis (Fig. 4.7). The rapid clearance and digestion of dead cells even after large numbers of cells have died may explain why apoptosis was overlooked for so long.

Caspases

Studies involving *C. elegans* identified three genes, two of which were required for apoptosis, *ced-3* and *ced-4*, and a third, *ced-9*, which prevented apoptosis. *Ced-3* encodes a protein which is similar to the human interleukin 1β converting enzyme (ICE), a proteolytic enzyme that cleaves the inactive precursor of IL-1β to an active cytokine. Many proteolytic enzymes were subsequently shown to be

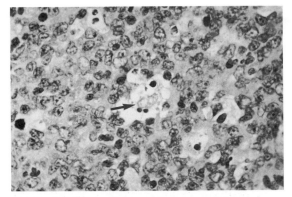

Fig. 4.7 A macrophage (arrowed) containing apoptotic debris, seen as dense, round bodies (so-called 'tingible bodies'). This cell is in a secondary lymphoid follicle of a lymph node. The macrophage has phagocytosed a B lymphocyte deleted by apoptosis as part of the process of affinity maturation.

involved in apoptosis. Collectively, these proteolytic enzymes are known as *caspases* since they all possess cysteine in their active sites and cleave target proteins at specific aspartate residues. Later ICE was redesignated caspase 1.

Caspases are produced as precursor enzymes, known as *proenzymes*, *zymogens* or *procaspases* (Fig. 4.8) and share amino acid and structural homology. They aggregate to form heterodimers and tetramers with more than one active site. All the caspases can be activated autocatalytically (i.e. self-activated) or by other enzymes (usually other caspases).

Caspases cause cell death by a number of mechanisms.

- They inactivate proteins, e.g. bcl-2, which protect cells from apoptosis.
- They directly disassemble cell structures, e.g. nuclear lamina.
- They reorganize and cleave the cytoskeleton.
- They prevent DNA replication and repair by cleaving many proteins important in cell maintenance and repair, such as poly adenosine diphosphate ribose polymerase (PARP) and DNA-dependent protein kinase (DNA-PK). At the same time they activate a DNA fragmentation factor (DFF) which digests DNA.
- They induce signals which mark the cell for phagocytosis.
- They cut off contact with neighbouring cells.
- They disintegrate the cell into apoptotic bodies.

Owing to their ability to induce such changes, caspase activation must be strictly controlled. This is achieved in a variety of ways which include: limiting the availability of substrate, formation of the caspases as inactive procaspases, the presence/absence of caspase inhibitors/cofactors, positive and negative feedback mechanisms, compartmentalization of caspases and their cofactors, and highly stringent substrate specificity.

Caspase activation may be subdivided into two classes: *effector caspase activation* and *initiator caspase activation*. A proapoptotic signal activates an initiator caspase that in turn activates an effector caspase ultimately causing cell death (Fig. 4.9). Different initiator caspases respond to different apoptotic signals, e.g. caspase 8 responds to the activation of

Fig. 4.8 Caspase activation. The enzyme is synthesized as a large inactive procaspase. Oligomerization of the procaspase (with or without the aid of adapter proteins) results in cleavage at two aspartate residues. The prodomains are discarded and the two large and two small subunits form the active caspase. The activating cleavages are usually catalysed by caspase molecules themselves.

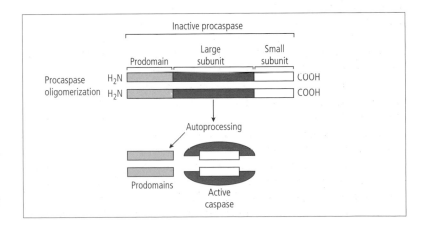

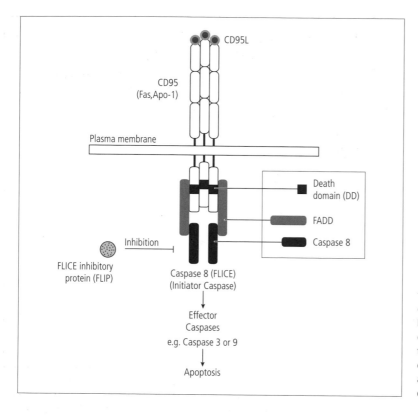

Fig. 4.9 CD95 death receptor signalling. Binding of the trimeric CD95L causes trimerization of CD95 receptor molecules and clustering of their cytoplasmic DDs. FADD binds and recruits/activates caspase 8 (initiator caspase). Caspase 8, also known as FLICE, then activates downstream effector caspases, e.g. caspases 3 or 9, and the cell undergoes apoptotic death. FLIPs negatively regulate caspase activation.

death receptors (see later) and caspase 9 to the presence of cytotoxic agents. Initiator caspase activation relies on the binding of specific cofactors to the procaspase. For example, caspase 8 activation requires Fas-associated death domain (FADD) (see later) whilst caspase 9 activation requires apoptosis protease activating factor (APAF-1), cytochrome C, and adenosine triphosphate (ATP) (see later).

Role of mitochondria in apoptosis

Mitochondria participate in apoptosis by releasing proapoptotic proteins including cytochrome C and apoptosis-inducing factor (AIF). Cytochrome C together with APAF-1 and ATP activate caspase 9 (Fig. 4.10). This in turn leads to the activation of caspase 3 and subsequent cell death. AIF may induce cell death in a caspase-independent manner.

Control of apoptosis

Apoptosis must be carefully controlled to ensure that cell death only occurs when and where neces-

sary. Apoptosis is therefore regulated in a complex manner involving both extracellular and intracellular mechanisms.

Extracellular controls

Death receptors provide the major mechanism for the extracellular control of apoptosis. They detect extracellular death signals and activate the cell's intrinsic apoptosis machinery. Death receptors belong to the tumour necrosis factor receptor (TNFR) superfamily and contain a cytosolic death domain (DD) which is able to engage intracellular apoptotic machinery or mediate other cellular functions.

Examples of death receptors are CD95 (also known as Fas or Apo-1) and TNFR1 (also known as p55 or CD120a) which are the best characterized, death receptor 3 (DR3, Apo-3, tyrosine-rich acidic matrix protein (TRAMP) or LARD), DR4, and DR5 (Apo-2, TNFR related apoptosis inducing ligand-receptor 2 (TRAIL-R2), TRICK2 or KILLER). In addition, the ligands that bind to these receptors

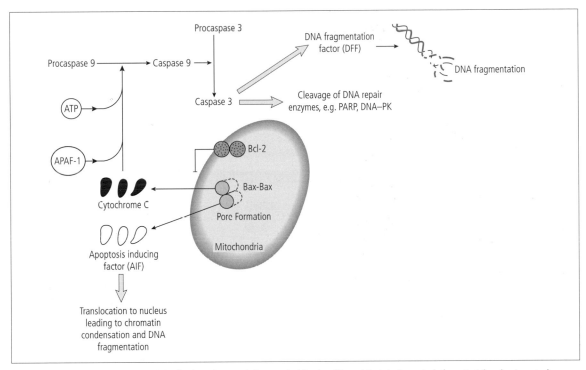

Fig. 4.10 Role of mitochondria and the bcl-2 family in the control of apoptosis. Mitochondria participate in the control of apoptosis by releasing cytochrome C, which together with APAF-1 and ATP activates caspase 9. Bax mediates the release of cytochrome C from mitochondria whereas Bcl-2 prevents its release. Caspase 9 activates caspase 3 which leads to DNA fragmentation and the cleavage of key DNA repair enzymes. AIF may act in a caspase-independent pathway to induce chromatin condensation and DNA fragmentation.

have also been identified. CD95 and TNFR1 are discussed below.

CD95 mediates cell death in a number of situations including the following.

• The peripheral deletion of mature T cells following an immune response.

• Killing of virus-infected or cancer cells by cytotoxic T lymphocytes (CTLs) or natural killer (NK) cells.

• Killing of inflammatory cells.

The ligand for CD95 (CD95L) exists as a trimer and binds to three CD95 receptor molecules resulting in clustering of the cytoplasmic DDs (Fig. 4.9). The FADD adapter protein then binds via its own DD to the clustered DDs of the CD95 receptor molecules. FADD possess a death effector domain (DED) which is able to recruit the precursor form of caspase 8 (also known as FADD-like interleukin 1β converting enzyme (FLICE) or MORT1-associated CED-3 homologue (MACH)). The resulting oligomerization of caspase 8 leads to its activation by self-cleavage. Caspase 8 then activates downstream caspases such as caspase 9 resulting in apoptotic cell death. The FLICE (caspase 8) inhibitory proteins (FLIPs) which prevent caspase 8 activation (Fig. 4.9) can inhibit this process. The Kaposi's sarcoma associated herpesvirus (KSHV, see Chapter 23) encodes a viral FLIP (v-FLIP) which is able to protect infected cells from apoptosis. Other cytoplasmic proteins, e.g. Daxx, can also bind to CD95. Daxx can induce the stress-activated c-JunNH$_2$ terminal kinase (JNK) pathway that can lead to potentiation of CD95-mediated apoptosis.

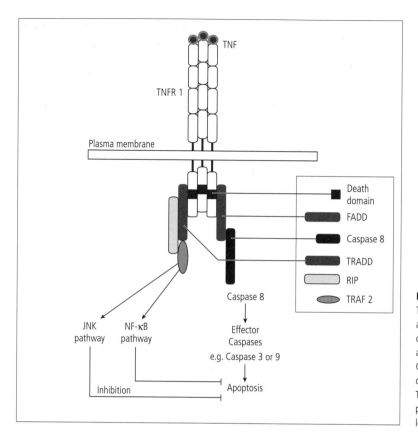

Fig. 4.11 TNFR1 signalling. TNF binding to TNFR1 causes trimerization of the receptors and aggregation of the cytoplasmic DDs. These can either recruit FADD, which leads to apoptosis via the mechanism outlined for CD95 or recruit TRADD. TRADD can recruit other signalling molecules, e.g. TRAFs or RIP. These signalling molecules activate other pathways (NF-κB and JNK, respectively) leading to the suppression of apoptosis.

TNF is a cytokine produced by activated macrophages and T cells in response to infection. It has many different effects on cells that are dependent on the cell type involved. In some cells TNF induces apoptosis. Thus, as with CD95, TNF binding to TNFR1 results in trimerization of the receptors and the aggregation of cytoplasmic DDs (Fig. 4.11). FADD may bind in a manner analogous to CD95 (see above) leading to apoptosis by the activation of caspase 8 and the subsequent effector caspases. The DDs may also bind an adapter protein known as TRADD (TNFR-associated DD protein) which recruits other signalling molecules to the activated receptor, including the TRAFs (TNFR-associated factors) and RIP (receptor-interacting protein). This initiates a very different signalling pathway leading to the activation of NF-κB and JNK/AP-1 and in turn the suppression of apoptosis. Thus, a single receptor may either induce or suppress apoptosis in different situations.

Another adapter protein is RAIDD (RIP-associated ICE-1/CED3 homologous protein with a DD) which like FADD has a DD allowing it to bind to TNFR1. However, the other end of RAIDD does not contain a DED but instead has a caspase recruitment domain (CARD). The CARD in RAIDD allows it to bind the CARD domain in procaspase 2 and thereby release active caspase 2. Other polypeptides associated with the cytoplasmic DD of TNFR1 include the SODD (silencer of DD) protein, which prevents the oligomerization of TNFR1.

Intracellular controls

Intracellular regulators, and in particular the Bcl-2 family of proteins play a major role in the control of apoptosis. The Bcl-2 family has been conserved throughout evolution. At the present time 15 members of the Bcl-2 family have been discovered in mammals. They all possess at least one of four

Table 4.2 The 15 mammalian members of the Bcl-2 protein family. Their effects upon apoptosis and homology with Bcl-2 are indicated. The proapoptosis family may be split further into the Bax and BH3 subfamilies.

Apoptotic effect	Protein	Homology with Bcl-2
Anti (pro-survival)	Bcl-2	
	Bcl-XL	BH1, BH2, BH3, BH4
	Bcl-W	BH1, BH2, BH3, BH4
	Mcl-1	BH1, BH2, BH3
	A1	BH1, BH2
Pro (pro-death)	Bax	BH1, BH2, BH3
	Bak	BH1, BH2, BH3
	Bok	BH1, BH2, BH3
	Bik	BH3
	Blk	BH3
	Hrk	BH3
	BNIP3	BH3
	Bim-L	BH3
	Bad	BH3
	Bid	BH3

conserved Bcl-2 homology domains (BH1 to BH4). This family of proteins can be split into those which suppress apoptosis and those which promote apoptosis (Table 4.2). Pro-survival members all contain at least BH1 and BH2 while proapoptotic members must contain the BH3 domain.

Pro- and antiapoptosis Bcl-2 family members can heterodimerize and block each other's function. The ratio of suppressors to promoters therefore determines the apoptotic susceptibility of the cell.

Some pro-survival proteins may bind to caspase activators and inhibit their function, e.g. Bcl-XL binds to APAF-1 preventing the activation of caspase 9. Proapoptotic proteins, e.g. Bik, may free APAF-1 from death inhibitors. The pro-survival proteins may also maintain organelle integrity. Many Bcl-2 family members have a hydrophobic tail and can bind to or insert into the membranes of mitochondria, endoplasmic reticulum and the nucleus. Some members of the Bcl-2 family can form pores in membranes, in a similar way to that caused by bacterial toxins, and thus alter membrane permeability, membrane potential or even puncture the membrane completely. Bcl-2 itself prevents mitochondrial cytochrome C release and subsequent activation of caspase 9. Conversely, Bax promotes apoptosis by binding to the mitochondria and causing the release of cytochrome C (Fig. 4.10). Additionally, Bax is induced by p53, providing a mechanism for the induction of apoptosis following cellular stress or DNA damage.

The Bcl-2 family are themselves regulated by cytokines and other death survival signals. The levels of particular proteins may be regulated by increased or decreased gene expression. Alternatively, regulation may occur via protein modification for example phosphorylation or protease cleavage. Bcl-2 can be activated by phosphorylation while the phosphorylation of Bad inhibits its ability to prevent the pro-survival role of Bcl-XL. Thus, the stimulation of the RAS pathway (see Chapter 22) leads the activation of phosphaditylinositol 3 kinase which in turn activates Akt. Akt is responsible for the phosphorylation of Bad. Bcl-2 cleavage by caspases inactivates its inhibitory function whilst Bid cleavage by caspases leads to the release of cytochrome C from mitochondria. Both of these lead to increased apoptosis.

Another family of intracellular apoptosis regulators, the inhibitors of apoptosis proteins (IAPs), has recently been discovered. IAPs directly inhibit caspases (primarily caspases 3 and 7) and are also able to induce NF-κB activation—ultimately leading to cell survival rather than apoptosis. A role for IAPs in cancer pathogenesis is suggested by the detection of an IAP known as *survivin* in many cancers but not in the normal counterpart tissues. Moreover, survivin levels correlate inversely with 5-year survival rates in colorectal cancer.

Summary

This chapter has described the important molecular events in cell reproduction, senescence and death. Disruption of these key cellular processes frequently leads to disease. In particular, abnormalities in each of these processes contribute to the development of neoplastic disease. This is considered more fully in Chapters 21 and 22.

Key points

1 The cell cycle is a sequence of events that leads to cell reproduction. It is controlled by the CDKs and their partner cyclins, which allow progress through the cell cycle by phosphorylating proteins such as pRb. The phosphorylation of pRb releases the E2F transcription factors which in turn allows DNA replication to proceed.

2 The CDK inhibitors comprise two families—the p21 family and the INK4 family. The CDK inhibitors act at specific parts of the cell cycle, known as 'checkpoints', to arrest progress through the cycle.

3 Cellular senescence occurs in most normal cells, usually after a finite number of cell divisions. Shortening of the telomeres may in part be responsible for the induction of cell senescence. Telomerase is an enzyme that can stabilize telomere length.

4 There are two forms of cell death: necrosis and apoptosis. Necrosis is usually initiated following noxious injury, whereas apoptosis is often physiological.

5 Apoptosis is controlled by a complex series of biochemical events involving both positive and negative regulators. The stimulus for apoptosis may be via extracellular signals, such as those delivered by CD95L or by intracellular signals.

Further reading

Gillett C.E. & Barnes D.M. (1998) Cell cycle. *Molecular Pathology* 51: 310–316.

Raff M. (1998) Cell suicide for beginners. *Nature* **396**: 119–122.

Miller L.J. & Marx J. (eds) (1998) Apoptosis; special section. *Science* **281**: 1301–1326.

The Inflammatory Response

Injury, trauma or infections induce a series of complex and interconnected reaction sequences, initiated at the site of tissue damage, which serve to contain and destroy the infection or damaging agent, prevent continued tissue damage and initiate repair processes to restore normal function.

This rapid response, employing a variety of components of the innate immune system, is known as *acute inflammation*. The toxic reactions, which are employed to destroy infectious organisms also, paradoxically, have the capacity to injure host tissues. There is therefore a delicate balance in this process. If these toxic responses are not tightly regulated then tissue injury may predominate over tissue protection and repair, leading to inflammatory disease. Similarly, if the infectious agent has evolved mechanisms to protect itself from attack by the immune system, it may persist giving rise to *chronic inflammation*.

The characteristics of the inflammatory response have long been identified and are part of everyday experience. The effects of even a minor wound such as a small splinter in the finger, allow us to confirm the observations of the Roman physician Celsus who described the four cardinal signs of inflammation: *rubor* (redness), *tumour* (swelling), *calor* (heat) and *dolor* (pain). The challenge is to explain the physiological events that generate this response.

Acute inflammation

The initial stimulus to the inflammatory response is tissue damage or the presence of infectious agents and their products. Within the damaged tissue a number of localized changes occur which include the following.

• The release of preformed inflammatory mediators from intracellular stores (e.g. the degranulation of mast cells).

• The initiation of reaction cascades through the activation of soluble plasma components produced initially by the liver.

• The new synthesis of inflammatory mediators ranging from membrane-derived eicosanoids to cytokines.

Release of preformed inflammatory mediators

The release of preformed inflammatory mediators from cells is one of the most rapid responses to tissue injury. The immediate response to damage of blood vessels is the aggregation of platelets, which adhere to exposed extracellular surface structures such as basement membrane, and collagen and elastic fibres. The release of *serotonin* from platelet stores is stimulated. This attracts further platelets and promotes aggregation. Serotonin causes *vasoconstriction*, reducing blood flow in muscular blood vessels such as arterioles and facilitating the formation of a platelet plug. Subsequently, in conjunction with products of the fibrin cascade (see below), a clot is formed.

Another important mediator, *histamine*, is released by the degranulation of mast cells. Histamine in contrast is a *vasodilator* that increases the volume of blood reaching the area of the damaged tissue. *Lysosomal enzymes* may also be released from damaged cells, and play a part in the breakdown of cell debris.

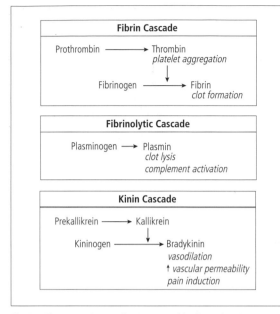

Fig. 5.1 Plasma protein cascades. Damage to blood vessels activates plasma clotting factor XII (Hageman factor), which in turn initiates the fibrin, fibrinolytic and kinin cascades that produce a range of plasma protein inflammatory mediators.

Initiation of plasma protein cascades generating inflammatory mediators

Damage to vascular endothelial cells results in the activation of the plasma clotting factor XII—*Hageman factor*. This in turn activates cascades of reactions that generate plasma mediators with a variety of roles in inflammation (Fig. 5.1).

Fibrin and fibrinolytic cascades

As described above, the release of serotonin stimulates the formation of a platelet plug. The activation of Hageman factor initiates a cascade of reactions that result in the conversion of prothrombin to *thrombin*. Thrombin also promotes platelet aggregation and converts fibrinogen to fibrin, which forms a mesh of fibres that trap a variety of circulating cells to form a clot. This not only prevents further loss of blood but also contains the damaged tissue and serves as a barrier to infection.

Another cascade of reactions triggered by activated Hageman factor brings about the conversion of plasminogen to the proteolytic enzyme *plasmin*, which breaks down clots releasing products that play a role in the inflammatory process. (Chapter 16 gives a fuller account of the arrest of bleeding and the coagulation cascade.)

Kinin cascade

Activated Hageman factor has a further role in triggering the kinin system. Here kallikrein is formed from its inactive precursor and is responsible for the conversion of kininogen to *bradykinin* that causes vasodilation, increases vascular permeability and induces pain.

Complement cascades

There are two complement pathways that interact through common intermediates and form a key part of the immune system. In addition to playing an important role as mediators of inflammation, components generated by the complement cascades:
• Bind to antigens and make them more amenable to phagocytosis (a process known as opsonization).
• Bind to viral antigens to neutralize their effects by causing aggregation or preventing attachment to and infection of host cells.
• Solubilize immune (antigen/antibody) complexes.
• Assemble the membrane attack complex within the surface membrane of target cells, resulting in their lysis.

Both pathways involve a cascade of reactions in which precursor proteins are cleaved to generate major and minor fragments. The major fragments decay rapidly unless they are able to bind to other components or surfaces and retain their activity. They in turn enzymically cleave and activate the next component in the pathway. The minor fragments frequently have functions that mediate the process of inflammation (see Fig. 5.2 for details of the complement pathways).

The assembly of complement components on antibody molecules that are complexed with one another or bound to target antigen surfaces initiates the *classical pathway*. This pathway is therefore principally dependent for its activation on the presence of antibody generated by an acquired immune response. It is not therefore involved in the early stages of the inflammatory response.

The *alternative pathway* is initiated by a variety of foreign cell surface components such as constituents

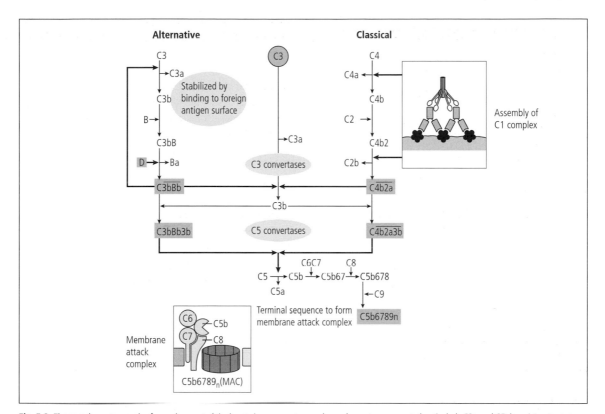

Fig. 5.2 The complement cascades form a key part of the innate immune system and complement components (particularly C3a and C5a) are important mediators of inflammation. The *alternative pathway* is initiated by a variety of foreign cell surface components such as constituents of bacterial or fungal cell walls. It is an essential element of the innate immune response. The complement component C3 undergoes spontaneous hydrolysis to C3a and C3b. Binding of C3b to foreign antigenic surfaces prevents its inactivation. In this environment, C3b binds to factor B, exposing a site that is cleaved by another component, factor D, releasing a small fragment Ba and leaving the active complex C3bBb, which has C3 convertase activity. The C3 convertase initiates the remaining stages of the complement cascade and is stabilized by properdin. The C3 convertase establishes a positive feedback loop converting further C3 molecules to C3a and C3b. This amplifies the response and leads to the production of C3bBb3b complexes. These have C5 convertase activity and, in turn, cleave C5 to generate C5a and C5b. C5b binds to antigenic surfaces, initiating the formation of a complex with C6, C7, C8 and C9—the membrane attack complex—a transmembrane channel that brings about cell lysis.

The *classical pathway* is initiated by the assembly of C1 complement components on antibody molecules bound to target antigenic surfaces. The active C1 complex cleaves C4 to release C4a and C4b. C4b is stabilized by binding to the antigenic surface and, in turn, acts as a binding site for C2, which is cleaved to release C2b. The remaining complex, C4b2a, has C3 convertase activity. The binding of C3b generates the C5 convertase of the classical pathway (C4b2a3b), which activates the formation of the membrane attack complex as described above.

of bacterial or fungal cell walls. It is an essential element of the innate immune response (Fig. 5.2).

The complement components C3a and C5a are formed as intermediates in both pathways and have a particularly important role in inflammation. Both stimulate platelet aggregation and the degranulation of mast cells, basophils and eosinophils (with concomitant release of histamine). C5a is important as a chemotactic factor for neutrophils and macro-

phages, plays a role in neutrophil activation, and increases the permeability of capillary endothelium to circulating leucocytes allowing their entry into the infected tissue (see below).

Both pathways terminate with the assembly of a complex of complement proteins that form a transmembrane channel—the membrane attack complex—in the underlying membrane of the target cell, resulting in lysis.

Synthesis of inflammatory mediators

Membrane phospholipid-derived eicosanoids

The disruption of cell membranes initiates the production of a family of compounds known as *eicosanoids*. These are synthesized from C20 poly-unsaturated fatty acids, most commonly from the tetraenoic acid *arachidonic acid*. Arachidonic acid is released from membrane phospholipids by the activity of phospholipase enzymes and is further metabolized by either the cyclooxygenase or lipoxygenase pathways. These reactions take place in a variety of cells involved in inflammation including monocytes/macrophages, neutrophils, mast cells, platelets and endothelial cells. The pattern of metabolites generated depends on the cell type.

The *cyclooxygenase pathway* converts arachidonic acid to *prostaglandins*, including *prostacyclin* (prostaglandin I_2 or PGI_2), and *thromboxanes*. These have a variety of functions. Platelets produce mainly thromboxane A_2 which causes vasoconstriction and platelet aggregation. Conversely, vascular endothelial cells produce mainly prostacyclin, which stimulates vasodilation and inhibits platelet aggregation.

The *lipoxygenase pathway* produces *leukotrienes* that are chemotactic, induce smooth muscle contraction (vasoconstriction or bronchoconstriction) and increase vascular permeability.

Cytokines and chemokines

Macrophages present in damaged tissues become activated to synthesize and secrete cytokines of which *interleukin 1* (IL-1) and *tumour necrosis factor* (TNF-α) are the most important. One of the effects of these cytokines is to induce the expression of adhesion molecules on the surface of cells of the vascular endothelium, which forms the barrier between blood and the damaged tissue. They also act on endothelial cells and other cells such as fibroblasts to induce the synthesis of cytokines such as *IL-8* and *monocyte chemotactic protein* (MCP). These molecules, which are also produced by monocytes and macrophages, are examples of a family of pro-inflammatory molecules known as *chemokines*. They attract particular types of leucocyte, regulate their expression of cell surface adhesion molecules, and facilitate their attachment to the vascular endothelial surface and their attraction towards localized concentrations of chemokine. These interactions have a very important role in bringing cells of the immune system such as neutrophils, and subsequently monocytes and lymphocytes to the site of injury and infection.

Effects of inflammatory mediators

The interconnected reaction sequences described above generate a wide range of inflammatory mediators (see Table 5.1 for a summary). The immediate responses are to isolate the area of tissue damage, and to restrict the loss of blood. This contains any infection to a localized area and forms a physical barrier to the entry of further infectious organisms. The flow of blood to the damaged tissue is then increased by vasodilation. The influx of plasma and plasma proteins to the area dilutes any toxic products from infectious agents, ensures a ready supply of the components of plasma protein cascades and also carries leucocytes to the site of injury. The increased permeability of vascular endothelium allows the damaged tissue to be flooded with fluid and plasma proteins. This fluid drains eventually via the afferent lymphatics to local lymph nodes. Foreign antigens carried to the lymph nodes will initiate an acquired immune response, which will in time generate antigen-specific effector lymphocytes that will return in the blood to the site of infection and supplement the activities of the innate immune system.

The exudate of plasma proteins 'leaking' into the damaged tissue causes localized *swelling* (oedema) and increased pressure. This pressure, along with the release of mediators such as bradykinin, triggers *pain* receptors in the tissue. The increased flow of blood to the wound causes *redness* and generates *heat*, the other cardinal signs of inflammation.

Cells of the innate immune system present at the site of injury will begin to attack any foreign microorganisms introduced. However, they may be few in numbers and an effective response will depend on the recruitment of many more leucocytes into the damaged tissue.

Table 5.1 The origin and functions of mediators of acute inflammation.

	Mediator	Origin	Functions
Released from intracellular stores	Serotonin	Platelets	Vasoconstriction, platelet aggregation
	Histamine	Mast cells	Vasodilation, increased permeability of vascular endothelium, smooth muscle contraction
Generated by plasma protein cascades	Thrombin	Plasma protein coagulation cascade	Promotion of platelet aggregation
	Fibrin and fibrinopeptides	Plasma protein coagulation cascade	Increased permeability of vascular endothelium, neutrophil chemotaxis
	Plasmin	Plasma protein fibrinolytic cascade	Proteolytic degradation of clots to release chemotactic factors, activation of classical complement pathway
	Kallikrein	Plasma protein kinin cascade	Cleavage of complement component C5 to generate C5a and C5b
	Bradykinin	Plasma protein kinin cascade	Vasodilation, increased permeability of vascular endothelium, smooth muscle contraction, stimulation of pain receptors
	C3a	Plasma protein complement pathway	Degranulation of mast cells, basophils and eosinophils, platelet aggregation
	C5a	Plasma protein complement pathway	Degranulation of mast cells, basophils and eosinophils, platelet aggregation, chemotaxis of leucocytes, neutrophil activation
Products of membrane phospholipid degradation	Prostaglandin	Cyclooxygenase breakdown of membrane phospholipids	Vasodilation, increased permeability of vascular endothelium, neutrophil chemotaxis
	Thromboxane	Cyclooxygenase breakdown of membrane phospholipids	Vasoconstriction, platelet aggregation
	Leukotriene B4	Lipoxygenase breakdown of membrane phospholipids	Neutrophil chemotaxis
	PAF	Conversion from lyso-PAF	Platelet aggregation, increased permeability of vascular endothelium, neutrophil activation, chemotaxis of eosinophils
Chemokines synthesized at the site of inflammation	IL-8	Monocytes, macrophages, fibroblasts, endothelial cells	Neutrophil chemotaxis, activation and degranulation of neutrophils
	MCAF	Monocytes, macrophages, fibroblasts, endothelial cells	Monocyte chemotaxis, macrophage activation

Systemic effects of cytokines

Systemic physiological responses are also associated with the release of cytokines during acute inflammation. IL-1 and TNF-α generated by activated macrophages at the site of infection act on other cells in the locality, such as fibroblasts, to stimulate their production of IL-6. IL-1, TNF-α and IL-6 bring about the alteration of the temperature set-point in the hypothalamus mediating fever through the stimulation of prostaglandin synthesis

(PGE$_2$). The same cytokines act on the adrenal pituitary axis to generate adrenocorticotropic hormone (ACTH) and induce production of glucocorticoids that act cooperatively with these cytokines to induce the synthesis of acute phase proteins in the liver. The acute phase proteins include a wide range of mediators including the following.
• Components of the coagulation and complement cascades.
• Proteinase inhibitors that control the effects of lysosomal hydrolases released at the site of infections.
• Metal binding proteins that prevent iron loss during injury and infection.
• The major acute phase proteins serum amyloid A, serum amyloid P and C-reactive protein, all of which show massive induction (1000-fold increase on normal levels).

Although glucocorticoids induce the synthesis of acute phase proteins, they provide a negative feedback loop by downregulating further synthesis of cytokines by macrophages at the site of infection.

Recruitment of leucocytes

Vascular endothelium separates the site of tissue injury from the circulating lymphocytes in the blood system. Vasodilation not only increases the volume of blood brought to the area but also reduces the rate of blood flow in capillaries adjacent to the site of inflammation. This increases the number of leucocytes arriving in the area and also provides a better microenvironment for their interaction with vascular endothelium. This interaction is initially of low affinity and is mediated by adhesion molecules that become expressed on the endothelial cell surfaces, and their ligands on leucocytes. The flow of blood within the vessel tends to detach the leucocytes, but new interactions may form to reattach the cell. This gives the appearance of the leucocyte 'rolling' along the endothelial surface (Fig. 5.3).

Attachment brings the leucocyte into contact with localized concentrations of chemokines secreted by the endothelial cells. The chemokines bind to specific chemokine receptors on the surface of leucocytes and trigger the *activation* of adhesion molecules. Cytokines induce the expression of additional adhesion molecules on endothelial cells. Interaction between these adhesion molecules brings about *firm adhesion* of leucocytes to the endothelial surface. The leucocytes then pass through the intercellular junction between endothelial cells and enter the damaged tissue. Concentration gradients of chemoattractants guide the migration of leucocytes into the site of infection. This process is termed *extravasation*.

Although the process of extravasation is similar in outline for all leucocytes, there are essential differences in the nature of the specific adhesion molecules and chemokines involved. In essence then, tissue damage triggers the generation of inflammatory mediators which cause changes at the vascular endothelial surface that provide the necessary signals for the recruitment of leucocytes.

The first cells to be recruited in significant numbers are neutrophils, followed by monocytes, which mature to form tissue macrophages. Antigen-specific lymphocytes arrive at a later stage. Naïve lymphocytes pass into lymph nodes by extravasation through high endothelial venules, in a similar manner to that described above. In lymph nodes proximal to the site of tissue injury, the lymphocytes encounter foreign antigen drained from the infected tissue in afferent lymphatics. Clonal selection and proliferation occur to generate effector lymphocytes that return in the blood to the site of injury. Whereas naïve lymphocytes express surface receptors that facilitate their adhesion to high endothelial venules and entry to lymph nodes, effector (including memory) lymphocytes have different combinations of receptors that enable them to bind preferentially to endothelial cells in specific tissues. This is described as *lymphocyte homing*.

Role of adhesion molecules in endothelial cell–leucocyte interactions

There are several families of adhesion molecules that play a role in inflammation including the following.
• Selectins.
• Immunoglobulin-like cell adhesion molecules.
• Integrins.
Selectins are glycoproteins that consist of a lectin-

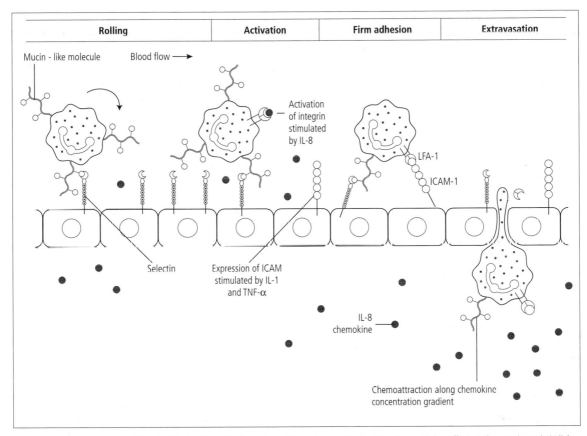

| Rolling | Activation | Firm adhesion | Extravasation |

Fig. 5.3 Leucocytes are recruited from the blood to fight infection at sites of tissue damage. Neutrophils adhere with low affinity to the vascular endothelial surface. The neutrophils are detached by the flow of blood within the vessel and appear to be *rolling* along the surface as they detach and re-adhere. Chemokines released from endothelial cells bind to receptors on the neutrophils and stimulate the *activation* of integrins on their surface. Cytokines (such as IL-1 and TNF-α) increase the expression of immunoglobulin-like intercellular adhesion molecules (ICAMs) on the surface of the vascular endothelium. Interaction between integrins (e.g. LFA-1) and ICAMs (e.g. ICAM-1) promotes *firm adhesion* of neutrophils to the vascular endothelial surface. The neutrophils pass between the intercellular junctions (*extravasation*) and are attracted along concentration gradients of chemokines within the damaged tissue.

like domain, an epidermal growth factor repeat, a variable number of domains resembling those found in complement binding proteins (containing approximately 60 amino acids), a transmembrane domain and a cytoplasmic tail. There are three main types—selectins P, E and L.

P-selectin is stored in granules in platelets and endothelial cells and is rapidly redistributed to the cell surface in response to histamine or components of the complement pathway. *E-selectin* is synthesized and expressed in endothelial cells in response to IL-1, TNF-α or bacterial endotoxins. Both P- and E-selectins bind to their appropriate ligands on the surface of neutrophils, monocytes and some

memory T lymphocytes. *L-selectin* is constitutively expressed on the surface of circulating lymphocytes, monocytes and neutrophils, and plays a role in their adhesion to vascular endothelium and to high endothelial venules.

Selectins bind to specific carbohydrate components including sialylated, sulphated and phosphated polysaccharides. Among these are another family of adhesion molecules, *mucins*, which are a group of glycoproteins rich in serine and threonine and displaying sialylated carbohydrate components.

Members of the *immunoglobulin supergene family* contain the characteristic immunoglobulin structural domain (consisting of approximately 110 amino acids in antiparallel β-pleated sheet conformation, with an intrachain disulphide bridge, see Chapter 6). Several of this family show adhesion properties such as the *intercellular* and *vascular cell adhesion molecules* ICAM-1, ICAM-2 and VCAM-1. ICAM-2 is expressed constitutively on the surface of endothelial cells. In contrast, although ICAM-1 is present at low densities on the surface of endothelial cells, its synthesis and expression are greatly increased by IL-1 and TNF-α. It is synthesized more slowly than E-selectin, but its expression is more prolonged. VCAM-1 expression is upregulated in a similar way, and supports the adhesion of monocytes rather than neutrophils.

The molecules of the immunoglobulin superfamily interact with a further group of adhesion molecules known as *integrins*. Integrins are protein heterodimers (consisting of α- and β-chains). The integrin leucocyte function-associated antigen-1 (LFA-1) ($\alpha_L\beta_2$) is present on the surface of neutrophils, monocytes and lymphocytes and binds to ICAM-1 and ICAM-2. Integrin molecules are stimulated by chemokines such as IL-8 and platelet-activating factor (PAF), secreted by vascular endothelial cells. Stimulation increases the affinity of integrins for ICAMs and promotes firm adhesion between leucocytes and the endothelial surface.

The importance of adhesion molecules in the recruitment of leucocytes is illustrated by immunodeficiency diseases such as *leucocyte adhesion deficiency* (LAD) where defective cell adhesion results in recurrent infections (see Chapter 12).

Leucocyte functions in inflammation

Neutrophils are the first cells to infiltrate the site of infection in significant numbers. Microbial products such as lipopolysaccharide (LPS) and *N*-formyl methionyl peptides and the products of other inflammatory cells such as PAF and TNF-α activate neutrophils. Activated neutrophils show increased expression of chemokine receptors and also secrete chemokines that attract monocytes and macrophages.

Both neutrophils and macrophages are phagocytic cells. Upon activation they show increased expression of complement receptors and Fc receptors which recognize complement components and antibodies, respectively. The increased receptor expression on neutrophils enhances the *phagocytosis* of microorganisms coated with complement and at a later stage with specific antibody (opsonization). Activation of neutrophils also increases the activity of the membrane-bound reduced nicotinamide adenine dinucleotide phosphate (NADPH) oxidase that generates *reactive oxygen intermediates* (the respiratory burst) including superoxide anions, hydroxyl radicals, hydrogen peroxide and hypochlorous acid, which are toxic to cells. Individuals with *chronic granulomatous disease* suffer from recurrent infections as a result of cellular defects in the generation of reactive oxygen intermediates (see Chapter 12). Cytoplasmic granules, including lysosomes, release *hydrolytic enzymes* such as proteases, elastases, collagenases and phospholipases that destroy invading microorganisms and digest cell debris.

Antigens carried to adjacent lymph nodes from the site of infection activate the clonal expansion of lymphocytes specific to foreign antigens. These lymphocytes return to the damaged tissue at a later stage in the inflammation process. They have a wide range of effector functions that contribute to the destruction of invading microorganisms. These are described in Chapter 6.

Resolution of the acute inflammatory response

Resolution of the acute inflammatory response is in part due to the short half-lives of the cytokines involved in the response. Glucocorticosteroids involved in the systemic response in the liver provide a negative feedback loop by inhibiting production of cytokines by tissue macrophages. In addition, naturally occurring antagonists interfere with the ongoing cascades of acute inflammation. These include IL-1 and TNF-α receptor antagonists, and cytokines such as IL-4 and IL-10. IL-4 and IL-10 are produced by helper T lymphocytes (Th2 cells) and downregulate IL-1, TNF-α and IL-8 production, and upregulate production of IL-1 receptor antagonist (IL-1RA). IL-4 also reduces the release of PGE_2 and superoxide anions. The release of IL-4 and IL-10 from cells close to the site of infection plays a large part in closing down the reactions of acute

Key points

1 Inflammation results from a complex and interconnected network of reactions, initiated at sites of tissue damage, that serve to contain and destroy infectious microorganisms, prevent continued tissue damage and initiate repair processes to restore normal function.

2 A wide range of inflammatory mediators, released or formed rapidly in response to infection or tissue damage, initiate acute inflammation. These mediators are released from granular stores within cells (e.g. histamine), generated by the activation of plasma protein reaction pathways (e.g. coagulation and complement cascades), derived from breakdown of membrane phospholipids (e.g. prostaglandins and leukotrienes) or synthesized *de novo* (e.g. cytokines).

3 The destruction of invading microorganisms depends on the recruitment of circulating leucocytes (particularly neutrophils, monocytes and lymphocytes), which is regulated by chemokines and adhesion molecules produced at the vascular endothelial surface separating blood from the site of tissue damage.

4 The effector functions of cells of the innate immune system, including phagocytosis, the generation of toxic reactive oxygen intermediates and the action of hydrolytic enzymes, provide the initial attack on invading microorganisms. These are later supplemented by an acquired immune response from lymphocytes specific for foreign antigens.

5 The toxic reactions employed to destroy infectious agents also have the capacity to damage host tissues. Chronic inflammation results when microorganisms or foreign bodies are resistant to destruction or where the inflammation process is inadequately regulated.

inflammation. Remaining inflammatory cells undergo apoptosis (see Chapter 4) and are phagocytosed by macrophages.

Chronic inflammation

Infectious agents that have evolved mechanisms to avoid or counteract the activities of the immune system (e.g. intracellular pathogens such as *Mycobacteria*) may persist at the site of infection. This induces *chronic inflammation* in which the mechanisms of inflammation, invoked in a vain attempt to destroy the invading microorganism, destroy the host tissue instead. Exposure to, and the intracellular accumulation of, foreign insoluble agents (e.g. silica or asbestos particles) can also have a similar effect. Chronic inflammation is characterized by the accumulation of macrophages that are activated by interferon γ (IFN-γ) and have increased cytokine production and microbicidal activities. Fibroblast proliferation and collagen synthesis lead to the formation of fibrous scar tissue. Often granulomata form (e.g. in *M. tuberculosis* infection) in which a mass of macrophages, many of which have changed their morphology to form epithelioid-like cells or have fused to form multi-nucleate giant cells, are surrounded by effector lymphocytes.

Chronic inflammation may also result from defective control or resolution of inflammatory reactions. Leucocyte-mediated tissue damage is a major component of a variety of disease processes including adult respiratory distress syndrome, autoimmune diseases and graft rejection. Many autoimmune diseases are characterized by altered endothelium with increased expression of adhesion molecules and increased leucocyte infiltration (e.g. Crohn's disease, diabetes mellitus, rheumatoid arthritis and ulcerative colitis).

Cells and tissues have different capacities for regeneration, which is dependent on the migration, proliferation and differentiation of nearby cells. Some cells no longer retain the capacity to divide (e.g. nerve cells). In such cases, fibrotic scar tissue is formed, consisting largely of connective tissue proteins such as collagen. Although this is adequate to maintain the structural integrity of the tissue it does not restore lost function.

Summary

Inflammation is the physiological response to tissue

injury and infection. It is a rapidly induced, complex network of molecular and cellular interactions that is carefully regulated and is normally resolved by the elimination of infection and tissue restoration. If inappropriately controlled, the toxic mechanisms that lead to the destruction of invading microorganisms can persist resulting in extensive damage to host tissues.

Further reading

Goldsby R.A., Kindt T.J. & Osborne B. (2000) *Kuby Immunology* (4th edn). W.H. Freeman, New York.

Janeway C.A., Travers P., Walport M. & Capra J.D. (1999) *Immunobiology: The Immune System in Health and Disease* (4th edn). Elsevier Science/Garland Publishing.

Roitt I., Male D. & Brostoff M.A. (1997) *Immunology* (5th edn). Mosby, St. Louis.

CHAPTER 6

The Immune System

The immune system functions as a network of cellular interactions which take place in a wide range of different microenvironments throughout the body. These interactions are facilitated by receptor molecules on the outer surface of cells which bind to molecules in the microenvironment, often on the surface of other cells. This can initiate biochemical changes within the cells, leading in turn to changes in gene expression and consequently in cell function. In this respect, the immune system is just a subset of the cellular interactions which take place within the body and determine its physiology. An understanding of the way in which cells of the immune system are influenced by, and interact with, other subsets (e.g. those which characterize the neuroendocrine or gastrointestinal systems) is only just beginning to emerge.

Lymphocytes and their receptors

The focus of attention for immunologists is on understanding the formation and function of cell surface receptors which recognize specific 'foreign' molecules, and as a result generate an immune response. There are two different types of receptor. The surface receptor of the *B lymphocytes* is a membrane bound form of the glycoprotein *immunoglobulin* (Ig). The counterpart on *T lymphocytes* is less imaginatively referred to as the *T-cell receptor*. These receptors recognize a diverse range of foreign molecules including the components or products of

microorganisms such as viruses, bacteria and fungi, other parasites such as helminth worms, and cells from unrelated human donors, as well as commonplace substances such as pollen or animal hair. Collectively these are referred to as *antigens* (Ag).

The B and T cells are central to *acquired* or *adaptive* immune responses, which in more highly evolved organisms complement and enhance *natural* or *innate immunity*. The latter consists of a variety of mechanisms to counteract infectious agents which include physical and chemical barriers to infection, or the synthesis of antimicrobial agents which interact in a non-specific way with infectious agents and their products, and often promote their lysis by cytotoxic cells, or their uptake and degradation by phagocytic cells. Some of these aspects of natural immunity are dealt with in more detail in Chapter 5.

Acquired immunity

Acquired or adaptive immunity has certain characteristics which are outlined below.

Specificity

The antigen receptors on the surface of any individual B or T cell are specific for a single molecular cluster or arrangement within the structure of an antigen. This molecular cluster or arrangement is referred to as an *antigenic determinant* or *epitope*.

49

Diversity

The body is able to mount responses against a wide range of antigenic determinants. Although each B or T cell has surface receptors with a single specificity, collectively these cells have a wide range of specificities facilitating the recognition of a similarly wide range of epitopes. This diversity is generated during B- and T-cell development, by random rearrangement of the genetic information encoding the polypeptides that make up the receptor molecules and is independent of the presence of antigen. The range of receptors (or *immunological repertoire*) produced will be unique to the individual, may alter with time and will contain receptors specific to epitopes that exist at present or which may by generated in the future as a consequence of evolutionary changes occurring in infectious organisms.

Memory

Once the immune system has encountered a particular antigen, it is able to make a quicker, more vigorous and more effective response to the same antigen on subsequent re-exposure, so the B and T cells have 'memory'. This is probably the most widely known property of the immune system—every parent knows that an infant contracting measles in childhood is protected from the disease in later life. It is the basis of vaccination, the first demonstration of which by E. Jenner in 1796 really marked the foundation of immunology as a discipline. Despite this, immunological memory is still relatively poorly understood at the molecular level.

Self and non-self discrimination

Under normal circumstances the immune system is able to mount an effective response against 'foreign' antigens, but does not attack other components of the body (i.e. self). In part, this is due to the removal or deletion of cells that carry receptors specific for 'self', before they become fully able to respond to antigen (i.e. before they become *immunocompetent*). Cells with self-reactive receptors are present however, and mechanisms exist which either prevent

their activation (*clonal anergy*), or actively suppress their function (*suppression*).

Generation of diversity in the immunological repertoire

Like other cells of the blood, B and T cells both originate from stem cells that are formed at first in the yolk sac, then in the fetal liver or spleen, and later in adult bone marrow. B cells complete their development in the bone marrow, but T-cell precursors migrate from the bone marrow to the thymus where they mature. The bone marrow and the thymus are responsible for the production of the repertoires of immunocompetent B and T cells, respectively, and are the *primary lymphoid organs* of humans.

The B- and T-cell receptors are both made up of two distinct types of polypeptide chain. These are the heavy and light chains of Igs on B cells, and the α- and β-chains in the most common form of the T-cell receptor (Fig. 6.1). In both cases, the polypeptides have a *non-polymorphic* or *constant* region, and a *polymorphic* or *variable* region which forms the antigen recognition site. Hypervariable amino acid residues within this region are involved in antigen recognition and binding.

In each individual, within each haploid set of chromosomes, there are a number of different versions of the gene segments (variable, joining and diversity gene segments) which carry the information for the synthesis of the polymorphic regions of the receptors, but usually only single versions of the gene segments which encode the constant regions. Rearrangement of the gene segments occurs to produce functional coding information for the diverse repertoire of B- and T-cell receptors (Fig. 6.2). The mechanisms by which this occurs show the same essential features in both B and T cells. The main features of this process are outlined below.

• The gene segments for a particular polypeptide are contained on a single chromosome. Although the gene segments can recombine in a large number of ways, a given chromosome in a particular cell can only make one rearrangement to produce a functional coding sequence. This is because the segments are brought together to form a functional

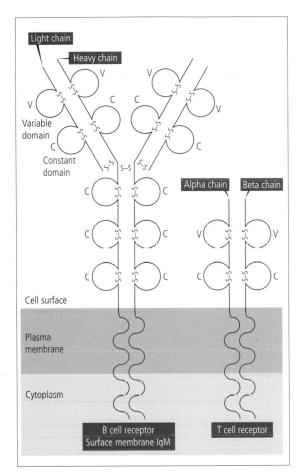

Fig. 6.1 Surface receptors of B and T lymphocytes. The specific antigen receptors of both B and T cells are composed of variable and constant region domains. These domains have a similar basic structure and are also found in a variety of other molecules which have an immunological function. They are members of the immunoglobulin (Ig) supergene family. Activated B cells can produce Igs with the same specificity, but with different heavy chain constant region domains. This allows them to be secreted from the cell as antibody molecules. Different heavy chain constant region domains also confer different effector functions on the antibody molecules. The subclasses of antibody IgM, IgD, IgG, IgA and IgE have μ, δ, γ, α, and ε heavy chains, respectively.

sequence by looping out of DNA, and the breakage and rejoining of the chromosome, which is an irreversible process. Even though the cells are diploid, and therefore contain two sets of gene segments on homologous chromosomes, successful rearrangement on one chromosome prevents rearrangement

of the other. This is termed *allellic exclusion*. It ensures that each cell has only a single receptor specificity.

• Gene rearrangement does not depend on the presence of antigen.

• Rearrangements occur at random, so that different precursor cells can rearrange in different ways to produce functional genes that encode receptors with different specificities.

• A functional gene is assembled from a single variable, joining, diversity (in some cases) and constant region segment. The more versions of the gene segments there are on the chromosome, the greater the number of possible combinations (combinatorial joining).

• When a junction between segments is formed, there is some variation in the precise point of joining (*junctional flexibility*), and extra coding information can be added at the junctions (*random nucleotide addition*).

• Functional receptors are formed by the pairing of the polypeptide products of two different types of rearranged gene (*heterodimer formation*). The number of possible receptor structures is therefore the product of the number of possible structures for each polypeptide.

Lymphocyte recirculation

Immunocompetent lymphocytes pass from the bone marrow or thymus into the lymphocyte circulation. They are transported around the body in the blood and the lymphatic system and reach the *lymph nodes* in arterial capillaries or *afferent lymphatics* (Fig. 6.3). They pass through the cuboidal endothelial cells of the venules (*high endothelial venules*) into the cortical tissues of the node. From here they are collected by *efferent lymphatics* draining the lymph nodes, and returned to the blood system via the thoracic ducts. Foreign antigens within the peripheral tissues are collected with other extracellular fluids, and drained to the nearest lymph node.

The lymph nodes, along with the other *secondary lymphoid organs* (the spleen and the mucosal-associated lymphoid tissues) provide a microenvironment which facilitates interaction between the

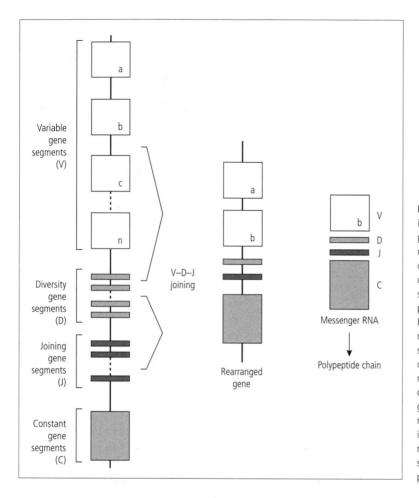

Fig. 6.2 Generation of diversity in the immunological repertoire. Each of the polypeptides making up the B- and T-cell receptors is encoded by a number of clusters of gene segments. There are a number of different versions of each of the gene segments in the variable, diversity (where present) and joining gene segment clusters. Functional genes are produced by rearrangements which bring together a gene segment from each of these clusters, with a constant region gene segment. The larger the number of gene segments in each of the clusters, the greater the number of functional gene combinations that can be produced by rearrangement. Additional variability is introduced through the random addition of nucleotides at the junctions between gene segments, and through flexibility in the precise point of joining.

lymphocyte surface receptors and foreign antigens. The secondary lymphoid organs are the location at which an immune response is initiated.

Lymphocyte activation

The immunological repertoire contains an enormous number of lymphocytes with receptors for different antigens. There is no reliable way to determine the size of the repertoire, but estimates suggest something like 10^{10} different B-cell receptors and rather more, maybe as many as 10^{15} αβ T-cell receptors. There are likely to be only a few cells with receptors of the same specificity. How then is the immune system able to counteract a particular infection effectively? This is explained by the *clonal selection*

theory, which is the central concept of immunology (Fig. 6.4).

When a B or T cell encounters an epitope for which its surface receptor is specific, it is in effect *selected*. Binding of epitope to the receptor triggers biochemical changes inside the cell which lead ultimately to proliferation and the production of a clone of cells all with the same receptor specificity. The antigen is therefore responsible for *clonal selection*, and receptor binding results in *clonal expansion*. Changes occur within the cells as they differentiate to form either *effector cells* or *memory cells*. The same process occurs in both B and T lymphocytes, but the details of receptor interaction are very different, as are the effector functions and the characteristics of the memory cells.

continued

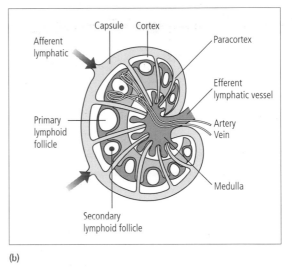

(b)

Fig. 6.3 (*continued*)

The role of MHC

B-cell receptors are able to recognize epitopes on the surface of complex antigens (e.g. components of the surface coat of bacteria). They recognize a particular three-dimensional arrangement of molecules on the antigen which interact with key amino acid residues in the receptor-binding site. These amino acids are the hypervariable residues, often described as *complementarity-determining regions*. The B-cell receptor therefore recognizes what is often described as a *conformational epitope*.

The situation in T cells is more complex. The T-cell receptor can only recognize short peptides displayed on the surface of cells by glycoproteins which are encoded by genes of the *major histocompatibility complex* (MHC; Fig. 6.5 and Table 6.1). These genes were first identified in the context of transplantation. A graft between genetically identical animals is usually successful, but if there are genetic differences between donor and recipient, the graft is rejected. The genes which are most important in this context are those of the MHC. In humans this gene region is referred to as the *human leucocyte antigen* (HLA) region. There are two sets of genes which produce two different types of protein (Table 6.1): the MHC class I genes (HLA-A, -B and -C in humans), and the MHC class II genes (HLA-DP, -DQ and -DR in humans).

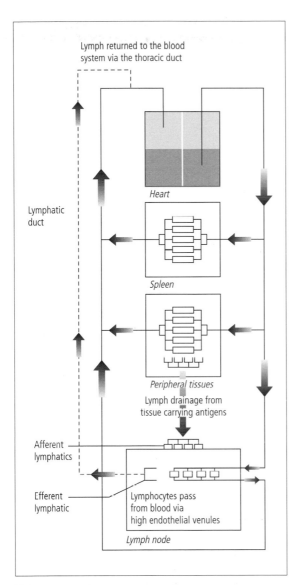

(a)

Fig. 6.3 (a) The routes of lymphocyte recirculation. Lymphocytes reach the lymph nodes in arterial capillaries or from afferent lymphatics draining the tissues. (b) The lymph node. This provides a site for the interaction between antigen and B cells carrying the appropriate surface receptor. B-cell stimulation occurs in primary follicles, leading to proliferation and differentiation, to form memory cells and antibody-secreting plasma cells in the secondary follicles.

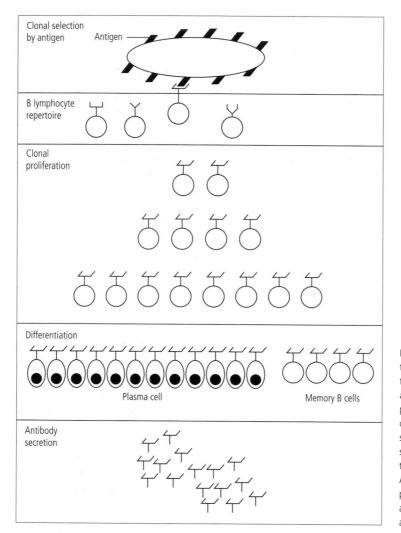

Fig. 6.4 Clonal selection. Lymphocytes from the B-cell repertoire, with surface receptors that can bind to surface epitopes on the antigen, are selected and triggered to proliferate and differentiate, forming plasma cells and memory cells. The plasma cells secrete antibody molecules of the same specificity, which are able to interact with the antigen to bring about its elimination. A similar process of clonal selection and proliferation operates on the T-cell repertoire, although the initial interaction between T cell and antigen is more complex.

In the population there are many different alleles for each of these genes, although more have been identified for some than for others. So there is a high level of polymorphism at the population level. Each individual carries only two alleles (one from each parent) for each of the three class I genes, and the same number for each of the class II genes. It is the nature of these alleles which characterizes a tissue type, a vitally important feature when considering the suitability of donors for transplantation.

Different alleles encode MHC molecules which have the same overall structure, but which differ in the structure of their peptide-binding sites, and are therefore specific for peptides with different structural motifs. Effective peptide binding is essential for effective presentation of antigens to T cells. The MHC therefore exerts a genetic influence on the ability to respond to particular antigens—it regulates *immune responsiveness*.

Antigen processing and presentation

As T cells can only recognize peptides presented by MHC molecules, there must be mechanisms by which antigens can be processed to produce peptides which are bound to MHC molecules and

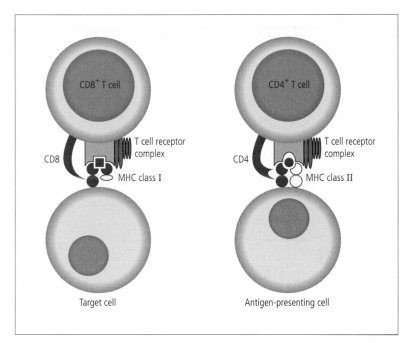

Fig. 6.5 Antigen recognition by T lymphocytes. T-cell receptors can only recognize short peptides, derived from antigens, and displayed on the surface of cells by the major histocompatibility complex (MHC) glycoproteins. There are two types of MHC molecule, MHC class I and II. They have different patterns of expression, bind peptides from different locations derived from separate pathways of antigen processing, and present peptides to different subclasses of T cell.

presented at the cell surface. There are separate mechanisms for MHC class I and II molecules.

MHC class I molecules are present on the surface of virtually all cells. They are produced in the endoplasmic reticulum and depend on peptide binding at this site for their assembly and transport to the cell surface (Fig. 6.6). They provide a mechanism for sampling the peptides available in the cytoplasm and endoplasmic reticulum.

Transporter proteins in the membrane of the endoplasmic reticulum bring about the import of peptides from the cytoplasm. In most cases the peptides presented will be derived from 'self' proteins. As T cells specific for 'self' are deleted in the thymus, this would not normally be expected to generate an immune response. However, if a cell is infected by a virus it may produce viral proteins which will be processed and presented at the cell surface where they will generate an immune response. In a similar way, tumour cells may produce antigens which are seen as 'non-self' (see Chapters 9 and 23). Peptides presented by MHC class I are only recognized by a subset of T cells which carry the surface glycoprotein CD8. The majority of these cells have a

Table 6.1 Genes of the major histocompatibility complex (MHC).

MHC class I	MHC class II
Presents peptides to CD8+ T cells (usually cytotoxic)	Presents peptides to CD4+ T cells (usually helper)
Encoded by HLA-A, -B and -C genes	Encoded by HLA-DP, -DQ and -DR genes
Expressed on the surface of virtually all cells	Expressed on the surface of antigen-presenting cells, e.g. B cells, dendritic cells, macrophages
Presents cytoplasmic peptides, e.g. from viruses or tumour antigens	Presents peptides from extracellular antigens, e.g. bacteria
Peptides complex with MHC by endogenous processing pathway	Peptides complex with MHC by exogenous processing pathway

cytotoxic function which brings about lysis of the target cell.

MHC class II molecules are restricted to the surface of particular cells, often referred to as antigen-presenting cells, which are associated with the

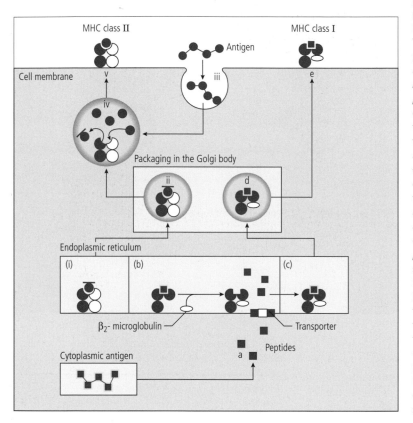

MHC class **II**   MHC class **I**

Fig. 6.6 Antigen processing and presentation. T cells only recognize peptides presented on the surface of cells by major histocompatibility complex (MHC) molecules. There are two discrete pathways of antigen processing by which peptides are produced and complexed with MHC molecules. *Presentation by MHC class I: endogenous pathway.* (a) Peptides generated from cytoplasmic antigens are transported into the endoplasmic reticulum by a peptide transporter. (b) MHC class I molecules are assembled in the endoplasmic reticulum and (c) bind peptides with appropriate structural characteristics. (d) Peptide binding facilitates the transport of the complex to the Golgi body and onwards to the cell surface. (e) Peptides are presented at the cell surface, to CD8+ T cells. *Presentation by MHC class II: exogenous pathway.* (i) MHC class II molecules are synthesized in the endoplasmic reticulum but in the presence of 'invariant chain', peptide binding is blocked. (ii) The molecules are transported to the Golgi body and on towards the cell surface. (iii) Extracellular antigen is taken into the cell by endocytosis in vesicles. (iv) In the endosomes, antigen is digested to produce peptides which may combine with MHC class II after the dissociation of invariant chain. (v) Peptides are presented at the cell surface, to CD4+ T cells.

immune system (e.g. dendritic cells, B lymphocytes and macrophages). Like MHC class I molecules they are produced in the endoplasmic reticulum, but are prevented from binding peptides at this site by the action of an additional polypeptide, referred to as the *invariant chain*. The molecules are eventually transported to the endosomal compartment where they are dissociated from the invariant chain and able to bind available peptides. These peptides are derived from proteins that have been taken up by endocytosis of exogenous antigens from the cell surface. MHC class II therefore samples and presents antigens from the extracellular compartment. In this case, the presented peptides are recognized by a subset of T cells which are defined by the presence of the glycoprotein CD4 on their surface. The majority of these CD4+ T cells have a *helper* function.

Effector functions

The role of lymphokines

The activation of helper T cells leads to the production and secretion of growth factors which are referred to as cytokines, or more specifically *lymphokines*. These interact with specific receptors on the surface of other cells and lead to changes in the cells which are associated with the processes of development, differentiation or activation (Fig. 6.7). The lymphokines usually act in a *paracrine* (on nearby cells) or *autocrine* (on the producing cell) manner, and are *pleiotropic* (i.e. they produce different effects in different cells).

Helper T cells have a central function in the immune response as the lymphokines that they produce have a role in the differentiation of other

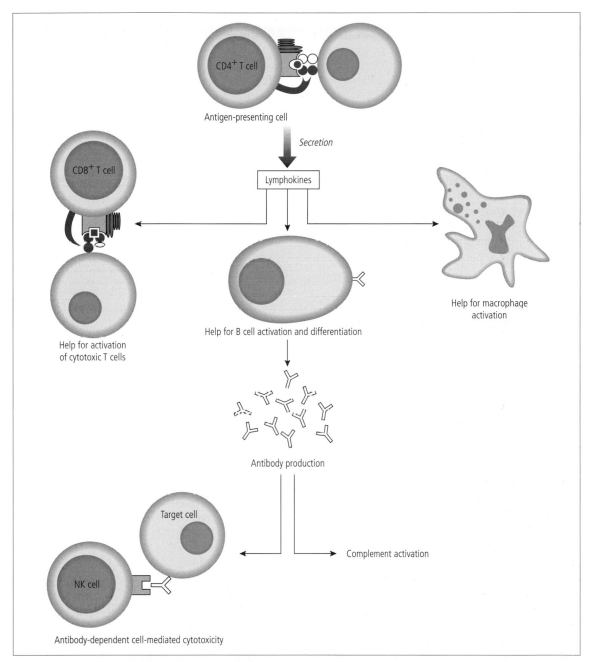

Fig. 6.7 The key role of helper T cells. Helper T cells have a central role in the regulation of the immune response. The lymphokines which they secrete on activation can provide 'help' in the activation, proliferation or differentiation of other cells. For example, lymphokines provide essential 'help' for the clonal proliferation and differentiation of B cells in the presence of antigen. The plasma cells produced secrete antibody which can stimulate additional components of the immune system such as complement activation or antibody-dependent cell-mediated cytotoxicity.

lymphocytes, and also play an important part in the activation of both B and T cells. They also link the acquired immune system to the innate immune system by activating non-specific effector cells such as macrophages and natural killer (NK) cells.

It now seems that there may be different subsets of helper T cells which produce different lymphokines. It may well be that different types of antigen activate different subsets of helper T cells which produce different 'cocktails' of lymphokines. Two subsets have been well characterized in mice. Helper Th1 cells secrete interleukin (IL) 2, interferon-γ and tumour necrosis factor β, in contrast to helper Th2 cells which secrete IL-4, -5, and -10. Different lymphokine secretions lead to the activation of different cellular components of the immune system, giving a bias to the response based on the nature of the antigen by which it was induced.

B- and T-cell interactions and antibody production

B cells display MHC class II molecules as well as specific antigen receptors on their surface. They are therefore able to recognize antigens, take them into the cell by endocytosis, and process them to produce peptides which can be combined with MHC class II molecules and presented on the surface. Helper T cells recognizing the presented peptide may be activated and produce lymphokines which provide 'help' to the B cell. B cells that have never been exposed to a particular antigen before are called *naïve* B cells. On activation, they proliferate and differentiate to produce plasma cells which secrete antibody. Other cells will differentiate to form memory cells. This is a *primary response*. Memory cells live longer, and on exposure to the same antigen on subsequent occasions, respond more rapidly and more vigorously to produce higher titres of antibody. This is referred to as a *secondary response*.

There are two further qualitative differences between primary and secondary responses. The antibody molecules produced in a primary response are usually IgM. Their heavy chains have a constant region encoded by the μ-gene segment. In the secondary response, antibody molecules are often produced from rearranged genes in which the information encoding the variable portion of the heavy chain is recombined with a different constant gene segment. The specificity of the antibody remains the same, but the portion of the molecule which is responsible for its effector function may be changed. This process is known as *class switching* and is regulated by lymphokines.

The antibodies generated in a secondary response also show an accumulation of changes in the amino acid residues which make up the antigen-binding site. These changes arise as a result of somatic mutation within B lymphocytes, and appear to be selected as they make the binding site of the antibody a better fit for its epitope. This increases the affinity of antibody for antigen and is called *affinity maturation*. Affinity maturation of B lymphocytes occurs within secondary lymphoid follicles (see Fig. 6.3).

Links with components of the innate immune system

There are many ways in which the antigen-specific cells of the acquired immune system interact with components of the innate immune system (see Fig. 6.7) some of which are detailed below.

• A subset of CD4+ helper T cells produces lymphokines including IL-2, interferon (IFN)-γ, and tumour necrosis factor (TNF)-β which attract and activate macrophages and lead to localized tissue destruction.

• Exposure to an antigen can generate plasma cells which secrete antibodies of the IgE subclass. These are able to bind to receptors on the surface of mast cells and basophils and sensitize them. Subsequent exposure of the cells to the same antigen results in degranulation of the sensitized cells, releasing chemicals which mediate a variety of physiological effects (see also Chapter 5).

• Antibody molecules complexed to antigen can initiate a cascade of reactions—the classical complement pathway—which generates biologically active molecules that can act as anaphylatoxins, promote phagocytosis or bring about cell lysis through the formation of a membrane attack complex (see Chapter 5).

Key points

1 Two forms of immunity may be recognized. Acquired or adaptive immunity and innate or natural immunity.

2 Acquired immunity has specificity, diversity and memory, and is able to discriminate between self and non-self.

3 Lymphocytes are of prime importance in acquired immunity. Lymphocytes have antigen receptors. The enormous repertoire of antigen receptor specificity is produced by rearrangement of the genes that encode the receptor proteins.

4 B lymphocytes have antigen receptors which are membrane-bound forms of the glycoprotein, immunoglobulin. Binding of antigen to the B-cell receptor leads to clonal expansion of B lymphocytes and the secretion of antibody by mature B lymphocytes, known as plasma cells.

5 T lymphocytes also have surface receptors for antigen. Unlike B lymphocytes, these receptors can only recognize processed antigen (usually in the form of short peptides) displayed on the surface of cells in association with MHC molecules. MHC class I molecules present intracellular antigens (e.g. virus proteins) to CD8+ T cells, whereas MHC class II molecules present extracellularly derived antigens to CD4+ T cells.

6 CD4+ cells have a 'helper' function and secrete lymphokines necessary for the activation and function of other effector cells (e.g. B lymphocytes). CD4+ T lymphocytes have a central role in the generation of effective immune responses.

• Antibody molecules binding cell surface antigens can attract cells such as NK cells which have receptors for the effector portion of the antibody molecule. The antibody thus forms a bridge between the two cells and facilitates the lytic killing of the target cell by the NK cell. This is *antibody-dependent cell-mediated cytotoxicity*.

Summary

This chapter has described the important features of acquired or adaptive immunity and how this relates to aspects of innate immunity. The importance of the immune system in the maintenance of health is well illustrated by the disorders of immunity. These may be grouped under three general headings: (a) hypersensitivity, characterized by abnormal or inappropriate responses to antigens; (b) autoimmunity, in which immune responses are directed against self antigens; (c) immunodeficiency, in which there is a deficiency in one or more components of the immune system. These disorders are the subject of Chapters 10–12.

Further reading

Goldsby R.A., Kindt T.J. & Osborne B. (2000) *Kuby Immunology* (4th edn). W.H. Freeman, New York.

Janeway C.A., Travers P., Walport M. & Capra J.D. (1999) *Immunobiology: The Immune System in Health and Disease* (4th edn). Elsevier Science/Garland Publishing.

Roitt I., Male D. & Brostoff M.A. (1997) *Immunology* (5th edn). Mosby, St. Louis.

Principles of Infectious Disease

Despite significant advances in the treatment and control of infectious diseases, they remain a major cause of morbidity and mortality in the modern world. The worldwide epidemic of acquired immunodeficiency syndrome (AIDS) and the re-emergence of serious diseases such as tuberculosis, caused by drug-resistant forms of mycobacteria, have highlighted the need for an extensive research effort in order to understand the nature of these important diseases and improve strategies for their control.

This chapter considers the delicate nature of the host–parasite relationship in infectious disease. Definitions and basic concepts are considered and features of the parasite and the host that are important in the establishment of disease are outlined.

Relationship between humans and their microbes

Humans are hosts to a variety of microorganisms and animals, not all of which cause disease. All associations in which one species lives in or on another are grouped under the general heading of symbiosis, which literally means 'living together'. A *parasite* may be defined as an organism which lives on or in another organism (the *host*), obtains nutrients directly from it, provides no benefit to the host and may also be harmful.

Humans support a wide range of microorganisms, mostly bacteria living on the skin, in the mouth and in the gastrointestinal tract. These are often referred to as *commensals* or 'normal flora' and are generally harmless. Commensals may also provide some benefit to the host, for example, the presence of gut commensals can prevent colonization from other, potentially harmful, organisms. However, if the host becomes immunosuppressed or if commensals colonize inappropriate sites then disease may result.

Parasites and pathogens

Some parasites are entirely dependent on the host for their reproduction and are therefore incapable of independent existence. These are termed *obligate parasites*. Viruses are examples of obligate parasites.

Those organisms that are capable of existing outside the host are called *facultative parasites*. Most bacterial parasites belong to this latter group.

Intracellular parasites (e.g. *Mycobacterium tuberculosis*, viruses), are adapted for life within cells, whereas those that exist outside cells are *extracellular* parasites (e.g. *Streptococcus mutans*).

Parasites are aerobic if they have a strict requirement for oxygen (e.g. *Pseudomonas aeruginosa*) or anaerobic where oxygen is not required and for some organisms may be toxic (e.g. *Clostridium tetani*). *Facultative anaerobes* are microorganisms that can survive whether oxygen is present or not (e.g. *Escherichia coli*).

A parasite growing in or on a host can cause an infection but when the infection leads to a disease state the parasite is referred to as a *pathogen*. Pathogenicity therefore is defined as the ability to cause disease.

While infectious diseases are responsible for significant morbidity and mortality, in biological terms it is not in the best interests of the parasite to kill the host. Survival of the host enables the maintenance of a reservoir of potentially infectious organisms, which may be transmitted to other susceptible hosts.

The adaptation of parasite and host goes through several stages. A pathogenic organism entering a new population previously not exposed to it often causes acute disease in people of all ages—this represents the classic picture of an *epidemic*. Over generations, the population develops some resistance to the organism and the disease will become *endemic*. This is characterized by widespread lower grade disease or routine childhood illness. With further adaptation by host and parasite a symbiotic relationship may develop and the host may not be harmed.

Syphilis is a good example of the effect of a new disease on a population. When the causative organism of syphilis, *Treponema pallidum*, first appeared in Europe in the fifteenth century it caused very severe disease. Half a century later, symptoms were generally limited to the genitals, face and nervous system and death was a less frequent outcome.

Koch's postulates

The nineteenth century microbiologist, Robert Koch, devised a set of postulates that should be satisfied before a particular organism can be named as the aetiological agent for a given disease. These are outlined below.

• The pathogen must always be present when there is disease and absent when there is no disease.
• The pathogen must be isolated from an infected host and grown in pure culture.
• Disease must result from reintroduction of the pathogen into a healthy host.
• Subsequently, the same pathogen must be isolated from the second host.

These postulates are not always easily satisfied. For example, the presence of specific antibodies to a given microorganism is often the only indicator that infection has occurred. In addition, for pathogens which only infect human hosts, the third and fourth postulates cannot be satisfied for ethical reasons.

Transmission of infectious disease

In order to produce infectious disease pathogens must be transmitted to the host. The following are several ways in which transmission can take place.
• Transmission through air: pathogens can be transmitted in droplets or droplet nuclei in air to susceptible hosts (e.g. *M. tuberculosis*).
• Transmission by water and food: ingestion of contaminated water or food can lead to infection. Examples of organisms transmitted in this way include *Vibrio cholerae* and *Salmonella typhi*.
• Transmission by contact: pathogens can be passed on by direct contact, for instance through sexual contact (e.g. *T. pallidum*, human immunodeficiency virus), or be inoculated through the skin by animal (e.g. rabies virus) or insect bites (e.g. *Plasmodium falciparum*). Some infections can be transmitted by *fomites* (i.e. inanimate objects or materials on which pathogens may be conveyed) such as dust particles (e.g. *M. tuberculosis*).

Where and in which groups infection occurs may be determined by factors including environmental conditions (e.g. housing, water supply and sanitation) and climate (e.g. rainfall and temperature).

Factors contributing to the establishment of an infectious disease

Features of the pathogen

• *Virulence* is the degree of pathogenicity and refers to the ability of the pathogen to invade and multiply within the host and cause damage, for instance by the production of toxins. Pathogens have many different types of virulence factors or *determinants* and these are dealt with in more detail in Chapter 8.
• *Evasion of host immunity.* Some pathogens have developed ways of evading the host's immune system. For example, African trypanosomes (Fig. 7.1) can rapidly change their surface antigens thereby evading attack by specific antibodies and T cells. Other pathogens have devised mechanisms that allow intracellular survival. An example of this is the survival of *M. tuberculosis* within phagocytic cells.
• *The number of infectious organisms* to which an individual is exposed is important in determining

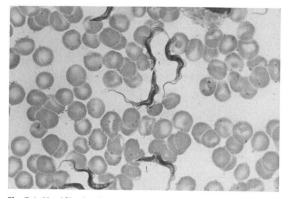

Fig. 7.1 Blood film showing typical *Trypanosoma brucei gambiense* organisms with characteristic flagellae.

whether or not disease will result. In general, the larger the infective dose, the greater the probability of disease. The *minimum infective dose* refers to the minimum number of organisms required for infection and varies for different pathogens. In this context, the ID_{50} (*infective dose 50*) and the LD_{50} (*lethal dose 50*) are important laboratory measures of the virulence of the pathogen. They refer to the numbers of organisms required to cause an infection in (ID_{50}), or kill (LD_{50}) 50% of test host animals within a specified time period.

Features of the host

Host factors, such as age, nutritional status and genetic constitution are important in determining whether infection will occur following exposure to a potential pathogen. The very young and the very old are more susceptible to infection—a reflection of developing and gradually failing immune systems, respectively. Malnutrition also increases disease susceptibility. Some populations are more susceptible to certain types of infection as a result of genetic differences.

The status of the host's immune system is a crucial determinant. An alteration in any of the natural barriers to infection may enable entry of potential pathogens. For example, breaks in the integrity of the skin or decreased levels of mucosal antimicrobial proteins, such as immunoglobulin A (IgA), can predispose individuals to infection. Immunodeficiency, whether *inherited* (see Chapter 12) or *acquired*

(e.g. by certain drug treatments or virus infections) can have devastating effects on the host, often allowing disease to occur as a result of opportunistic infection by those organisms not normally regarded as pathogenic.

Types of infectious disease

Infectious diseases are *acute* when they are of short duration. The signs and symptoms of acute infections are often severe and usually appear suddenly. In contrast, a *chronic* infection usually develops slowly and is long lasting. There may also be periods of *latency* when overt symptoms are absent. This is often the case with viral infections, particularly of the *herpesvirus* family. *Systemic* infections involve the whole body, whereas *localized* infections are restricted to a particular body site. *Opportunistic* infections are those caused by organisms that are non-pathogenic under normal circumstances. However, they can cause disease when there is impaired immunity or loss of normal flora.

Many different types of organisms can cause disease. The most important groups are *bacteria*, *viruses*, *fungi*, *protozoa* and higher *eukaryotic* organisms such as *helminths*. In addition, very simple agents such as *prions* (*proteinaceous infective particles*) can cause important diseases such as scrapie in sheep but are yet to be fully characterized. Bacteria and viruses are the subject of Chapters 8 and 9. Fungi, parasites and other medically important infectious agents are considered below.

Medically important fungi

Fungi are microorganisms that obtain nutrients from the dead remains of animals or plants, or occur as parasites on living hosts. Of the thousands of species known, the vast majority do not cause disease in humans or other mammals. Those which do, commonly cause disease by invading the tissue or by eliciting an allergic response. Another type of disease (*toxicosis*) occurs when the metabolic products of fungi, present in spoiled food, cause poisoning on ingestion.

The fungi responsible for human disease can be divided into two major groups, on the basis of either

Table 7.1 Selected examples of superficial and deep mycoses. Organisms that can produce deep mycoses may also cause infections which remain localized to the skin and mucous membranes (e.g. *Candida albicans*).

Superficial mycoses	Deep mycoses
Ringworm	Candidosis
	Aspergillosis
	Histoplasmosis
	Cryptococcosis

the type of infection they produce or their growth characteristics.

Type of infection

Two types of fungal infection (*mycoses*) are recognized (Table 7.1): (a) *superficial mycoses*, where fungus growth is confined to body surfaces, including skin, hair and nails; and (b) *deep mycoses*, when infection of internal organs occurs.

Growth characteristics

Pathogenic fungi may exist as *branched filamentous forms* or as *yeasts*. Some fungi show both growth forms depending on the environmental conditions and are often referred to as *dimorphic* fungi. The filamentous forms (often referred to as *moulds*) produce branching *hyphae* (Fig. 7.2a) which can extend as a result of transverse divisions forming a network of hyphae, or *mycelium*. Asexual reproduction results in the formation of spores known as *conidia*. Dispersal of the spores is the means by which the fungus is spread. Yeasts are single cells (Fig. 7.2b) that can reproduce by simple division. Budding of yeast cells may occur resulting in the formation of *pseudohyphae*.

Among fungi causing human infection, many are normally free-living saprophytes or plant parasites and infection follows their accidental introduction into the host tissues. Many of these species have an optimum growth temperature close to blood heat, resulting from saprophytic adaptation to other warm habitats such as self-heating accumulations of decomposing vegetation. The following section gives examples of medically important fungi and are used to illustrate the general features of fungal infections.

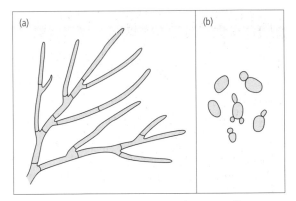

Fig. 7.2 Growth characteristics of fungi. Some fungi exist as filamentous forms, producing branched hyphae (a). Others exist as single cells and are known as yeasts (b). A third group, known as dimorphic fungi, can exist in both filamentous and yeast forms. Their transition from one form to another is dependent on the prevailing environmental conditions.

Candida albicans

C. albicans is a commensal organism, found in the gut of many species of mammals and birds, particularly those which habitually have a diet high in sugar and other carbohydrates. Approximately 60–70% of healthy people carry the species in the intestine and probably 40–50% also in the mouth. In addition, some 40% of women have *C. albicans* in the vaginal mucosa. In most healthy people *C. albicans* is harmless. However, under certain circumstances, such as during immunosuppression, it may cause serious disease.

Infections by *C. albicans* (and, less commonly, by other species of *Candida* such as *C. tropicalis*, *C. krusei* and *C. parapsilosis*) can take many forms depending upon the part of the body involved. These range from fatal infection of deep organs to superficial skin rashes and diseases of mucous membranes of the alimentary and genitourinary system.

Deep infections

Serious, often fatal, deep infection occurs in two main groups of hospitalized patients. Firstly, among patients undergoing immunosuppressive therapy for organ transplantation, *Candida* infections of deep organs such as liver, kidney and brain represent a common cause of morbidity and mortality. A second major group of cases occurs among surgical patients, often without severe immunosuppression

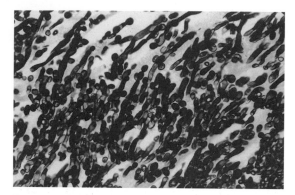

Fig 7.3 Growth of *Candida albicans* in the tissue of a heart valve (from a case of *Candida* endocarditis).

but in whom physical barriers to infection have been removed. A smaller third group is represented by intravenous drug abusers who may inject *Candida* organisms directly into the blood stream.

Candida septicaemia (the presence of *Candida* organisms in the blood stream) is a serious complication in immunosuppressed patients. Clinical indicators of systematically spread *Candida* are the development of discrete cutaneous lesions and *endophthalmitis* (infection within the eye). *Candida* septicaemia in immunocompetent individuals may result in colonization of the endocardium (Fig. 7.3) leading to endocarditis, particularly if there is already some abnormality of heart structure.

Superficial infections

Candida infection of the skin of the napkin area is a common problem in infants, producing *macular erythema* (discrete patches of redness especially in the skin folds and inguinal fold). Smaller 'satellite' lesions also occur outside the main area of reddening. Similar changes are seen in adults, especially in diabetics who are particularly prone to skin infections.

Candida infection of the mouth and vagina (often referred to as 'thrush') represents another common form of superficial infection. White plaque-like lesions are produced on the epithelia which are seen to be reddened if the plaque is removed. The plaque consists of a mixture of keratinized epithelial cells and fungal hyphae and yeast cells.

Oral thrush is common in infants, in diabetic patients and under denture plates. It is also commonly encountered in patients with AIDS (see case study 4). Vaginal thrush causes itching and burning sensations and a discharge is common. Women with diabetes, and those in advanced pregnancy are particularly prone to vaginal thrush.

Chronic mucocutaneous candidosis is a special type of superficial infection that occurs in children, at least some of whom have been shown to have inherited defects of the immune system. It is characterized by the development of extensive and persistent skin infection and oral thrush at a very early age. As the child grows, the infection causes disfiguring scaly swellings.

Aspergillosis

Aspergillosis is the clinical term given to disease produced by members of the genus *Aspergillus*. These saprophytic filamentous fungi are ubiquitous in the environment where they are commonly isolated from decaying organic debris. *A. fumigatus* is the most common pathogen in this genus, although *A. flavus*, *A. terreus*, *A. nidulans* and *A. niger* may occasionally cause disease.

Asexual spores (conidia) are produced in vast numbers from the heads of maturing conidiophores (Fig. 7.4) from which they are liberated into the environment. *Aspergillus* species are opportunistic pathogens that are unable to invade or colonize healthy lungs but can cause devastating systemic infection in immunocompromised patients. The two most common forms of aspergillosis in non-immunocompromised patients are allergic aspergillosis and aspergilloma; in neither of these is the fungus invasive.

Allergic aspergillosis

This is a localized reaction to inhaled spores and the mycelium produced by their subsequent germination in the bronchi. It is primarily a type 1 (IgE-mediated) hypersensitivity response (see Chapter 10) and may be particularly severe in atopic individuals. In addition, the production of circulating *Aspergillus*-specific IgG antibody results in the formation of antibody–antigen complexes leading to complement activation (see Chapter 5) and localized tissue damage.

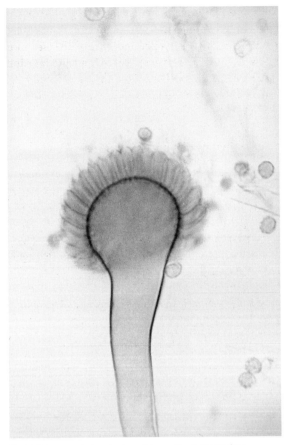

Fig. 7.4 Spore-producing structure of *Aspergillus fumigatus* from *in vitro* culture.

Aspergilloma

Aspergilloma is the name given to the fungus ball that can colonize old tuberculosis or other pre-existing lung cavities (see case study 7). The fungus grows as a compact mass of mycelium and normally does not invade adjacent tissue. This infection is only serious if the patient becomes immunosuppressed or if the fungus ball impinges on a blood vessel. Damage to the blood vessel can lead to bleeding in the lungs which is often clinically apparent as *haemoptysis* (the coughing up of blood).

Invasive aspergillosis

The most serious form of the disease is invasive aspergillosis. This is seen in immunocompromised patients, especially those with low neutrophil counts. In these patients, inhalation of spores may be followed by extensive growth of fungal forms within the lungs and frequent dissemination to other organs, especially the brain. Invasive aspergillosis is rapidly fatal and is often only diagnosed *postmortem*.

Dermatophytosis (ringworm)

Ringworm is caused by a group of fungi known as dermatophytes. These fungi live on the keratinized tissue of the skin, hair and nails and although closely related to certain soil fungi, many have become adapted to a purely parasitic existence.

Human infections can be caused by *anthropophilic*, *zoophilic* or *geophilic* species. Anthropophilic dermatophytes are entirely dependent on passage from one human host to another and infections can occur in any body site. They are passed on to susceptible hosts by direct contact or by contact with shed infected skin cells in which the fungus can lie dormant for several years. Zoophilic species have become adapted to life on animal hosts. When they are passed to humans infection most often occurs in the exposed sites of the head, neck, trunk and limbs. Infections with geophilic species are rare. These dermatophytes are more suited to a saprophytic existence in the soil but can cause infection following contact with contaminated soil.

There are three main genera of dermatophyte fungi: *Trichophyton*, *Microsporum* and *Epidermophyton*. The three genera are indistinguishable in tissue. In culture, all three genera produce distinctive multicellular macroconidia or large spores. In addition, *Trichophyton* and *Microsporum* species produce unicellular macroconidia. Hair infections are characterized by the production of large numbers of athroconidia (spores formed from fragmentation of hyphae). These may be *ectothrix*, forming a sheath around the hair, or, *endothrix* in which hair penetration is followed by spore production within the hair shaft.

Probably the most common and therefore the best known anthropophilic dermatophytosis is athlete's foot or *Tinea pedis*, caused most often by *Trich. rubrum* or *Tin. interdigitale*. Athlete's foot is common in affluent countries where there is ready access to swimming baths and sports facilities where use of communal changing rooms facilitates transfer from host to host. Occlusive footwear also provides the warm, moist conditions in which the fungus thrives. Athlete's foot is characterized by itching, skin peeling, maceration and fissuring of the toe webs often with concomitant nail infection in which the nails may become discoloured and crumbly. Lesions on smooth skin are itchy, *erythematous* (red) and flaky and may take on the circular appearance from which the term 'ringworm' was derived.

Infections with zoophilic species often induces a more marked inflammatory response. Occasionally, suppurating highly inflammatory lesions known as *kerions* may be produced.

Mycetoma

This exemplifies a range of mycoses which are mainly subcutaneous in nature, resulting from traumatic inoculation of a saprophytic fungus through the skin. Many fungal species and aerobic actinomycetes (bacteria capable of forming hyphal forms) are able to cause mycetoma and whilst they show minor differences in histological appearance there are several unifying features. The inoculated fungus grows slowly in the presence of a massive and intense host inflammatory response. The resulting mycelial microcolonies appear as tightly packed 'grains' just visible to the naked eye. These microcolonies break apart and reform, enabling a slowly progressive, localized infection to develop. There is often massive swelling of the affected area, which may penetrate and erode underlying bone. Sinus tracts filled with pus develop around the grains and

these may drain out onto the surface of the skin. Left untreated, many mycetomas will continue an inexorable spread further and further from the original site and cause death if vital viscera become involved. Initial infections most often occur on the feet and render amputation a possible form of treatment.

Medically important parasites

Earlier in this chapter, a parasite was defined as an organism which lives on or in another organism (the host), takes nutriment directly from it and which, under certain circumstances, may be harmful. However, in the study of microbiology, the term 'parasite' is often used to designate protozoa and members of the animal kingdom that infect and cause disease in other animals including humans. Three main groups are recognized. These are the *protozoa*, *helminths* and *arthropods*.

Protozoa

Protozoa are single-celled organisms that are larger than bacteria and whose DNA is organized in a nucleus. Protozoa are further subdivided into *amoebae*, *flagellates*, *ciliates* and *sporozoa* (Table 7.2).

Helminths

These are the parasitic worms. They are large multicellular organism and are divided into three groups: the tapeworms (Cestoda), flukes (Trematoda) and roundworms (Nematoda). Examples of important disease-causing helminths are given in Table 7.3.

Table 7.2 Important classes of pathogenic protozoa.

Group	Features	Example	Disease produced
Amoebae	Move by extending pseudopodia	*Entamoeba histolytica*	Amoebiasis
Flagellates	Move by beating of one or more flagella	*Trypanosoma* spp.	Trypanosomiasis
		T. cruzi	Chagas' disease
		T. brucei gambiense,	African trypanosomiasis
		T. brucei rhodesiense	or sleeping sickness
		Giardia lamblia	Giardiasis
Ciliates	Move by beating of cilia	*Balantidium coli*	Balantidiasis
Sporozoa	All are intracellular parasites	*Plasmodium* spp.	Malaria
		P. falciparum, *P. vivax*,	
		P. ovale, *P. malariae*	

Table 7.3 Examples of medically important helminths.

Group	Examples	Comments
Tapeworms	Human tapeworms (e.g. *Taenia solium* and *T. saginata*)	Human infection follows ingestion of larvae in pork (*T. solium*) or beef (*T. saginata*). Adult tapeworms found in gut of humans but larvae develop in other tissues of pig and occasionally humans (*T. solium*) and cattle (*T. saginata*)
	Dog tapeworm (*Echinococcus granulosus*)	Hydatid disease is acquired by ingestion of eggs from faeces of infected canines. Embryos migrate through gut to form hydatid cysts, especially in the liver of sheep, other herbivores and occasionally of humans
Flukes	*Schistosoma haematobium, S. japonicum, S. mansoni*	Larvae released by aquatic snails penetrate human skin and pass through blood to liver where they mature to form adults. Adults migrate to final site (*S. haematobium* to veins surrounding bladder, *S. japonicum* and *S. mansoni* to veins around the small intestine)
	Human liver fluke (*Clonorchis sinensis*)	Organism acquired by ingestion of fish containing larval stages. Young flukes released in the intestine move up the bile duct and attach to bile duct epithelium
	Common liver fluke of sheep (*Fasciola hepatica*)	Infection follows ingestion of vegetation contaminated by larvae
	Oriental lung fluke (*Paragonimus westermanii*)	Human infection acquired by ingestion of crustacea containing larvae. Larvae migrate from the intestine across the diaphragm and penetrate the lungs. Normally, the adult flukes develop within fibrous cysts that connect with the airways allowing an exit route for the eggs produced by these organisms
Nematodes	*Ascaris lumbricoides*	Human infection acquired by ingestion of eggs. Larvae hatch in intestine, penetrate bowel wall and migrate to lungs. From the lungs the worms are swallowed once again reaching the intestine. Adult worms live freely in gut lumen. Female worm lays eggs which are passed in faeces
	Hookworms (e.g. *Ancylostoma duodenale*)	Human infection acquired when larvae present in faeces penetrate the skin and migrate to the lungs and bronchi where they are swallowed. Adult worms live in gut and attach to the intestinal mucosa using their specialized mouth parts. Female hookworms lay eggs that hatch in the faeces shortly after defaecation
	Filaria (e.g. *Wuchereria bancrofti*)	Larvae are introduced through the skin by mosquitoes and develop slowly into long, thin, adult worms located in lymphoid tissues and lymphatic vessels. Blockage of lymphatic vessels can lead to gross enlargement of affected tissues ('elephantiasis')
	Toxocara canis	Eggs from dog are ingested and hatch in the intestine. Larvae migrate from the gut to many tissues including lung, liver, eyes and CNS

Arthropods

Most arthropods which attack humans are blood-feeders (e.g. mosquitoes, ticks and fleas) and reside only briefly on the host. Many of these arthropods are vectors for the transmission of other infectious agents (Table 7.4).

Some arthropods, notably the louse, *Pediculus humanus,* and the crab louse, *Phthirus pubis,* can reproduce on humans and produce inflammatory reactions following penetration of the skin during feeding. The scabies mite, *Sarcoptes scabiei,* lives permanently on humans, burrowing into the skin to feed and lay eggs.

Summary

Infectious diseases are caused by pathogens—parasitic organisms that are capable of causing disease. Subsequent chapters of the book consider the diverse range of bacterial and viral pathogens

Table 7.4 Examples of vector-borne disease transmitted by arthropods.

Infectious agent	Disease	Arthropod vector
Arboviruses	Dengue fever	Mosquitoes
	Yellow fever	Mosquitoes
Bacteria		
Yersinia pestis	Plague	Fleas
Borrelia burgdorferi	Lyme disease	Ticks
Protozoa		
Trypanosoma cruzi	Chagas' disease	Reduviid bugs
T. brucei gabiense,	Sleeping sickness	Tsetse flies
T. brucei rhodesiense		
Plasmodium spp.	Malaria	Mosquitoes
Helminths		
Wuchereria bancrofti	Filariasis	Mosquitoes

Key points

1 Pathogens are parasites that are capable of causing disease.
2 In general, Koch's postulates have to be satisfied before an organism can be identified as the aetiological agent for a given disease.
3 Parasite and host factors determine whether infectious disease will occur.
4 Parasite factors include the effect of virulence factors, the ability of the parasite to evade host immunity and the size of the infective dose.
5 Major host factors are age, nutritional status, genetic constitution and the integrity of the immune system.

and the infinite variety of strategies that enable them to survive in or on the human host. An understanding of the mechanisms by which infectious agents cause disease should enable the development of more rational approaches to the treatment and prevention of infectious disease.

Further reading

Barrett J.T. (1998) *Microbiology and Immunology Concepts.* Lippincott–Raven, Philadelphia.
Brooks G.F., Butel J.S. & Morse S.A. (eds) (1998) *Jawetz, Melnick and Adelberg's Medical Microbiology* (21st edn). Appleton & Lange, Stanford.

CHAPTER 8

Bacterial Infection

Bacteria are amongst the most successful living organisms. Their ubiquity ensures that humans are obliged to live in constant and intimate contact with a wide variety of species and to encounter, if briefly, many more. Fortunately, relatively few species routinely cause disease (the so-called pathogenic bacteria) but many others have the potential to do so, given appropriate conditions.

Whether or not a bacterial encounter leads to disease is determined by the balance of two principal factors—host factors, including the state of the individual's immune system and features of the bacterium that enable it to cause disease. These bacterial features are termed *virulence determinants*. Virulence determinants enable bacteria to: compete successfully with the normal microflora; survive in adverse conditions; adhere to or enter their targeted cells; and evade defence mechanisms.

This chapter examines some general characteristics of bacteria and considers in detail the structure of the cell wall of the major groups of bacteria. The classification of bacteria is briefly considered and routes of entry and modes of transmission are outlined. Finally, the important bacterial virulence factors are considered in detail.

General features of bacteria

Bacteria are *prokaryotes*, that is they lack an organized nucleus. Their genetic information is carried in a double-stranded, circular molecule of DNA which is often referred to as a chromosome although it differs from eukaryotic chromosomes in that no introns (non-coding sequences of DNA) are present.

Some bacteria possess small circular extrachromosomal DNA fragments known as *plasmids* which replicate independently of the chromosomal DNA. Plasmids may contain important genes coding for virulence factors or antibiotic resistance and may be transferred from one bacterium to another. The cytoplasm of bacteria contains many ribosomes but no mitochondria or other organelles.

In all bacteria, the cell is surrounded by a complex cell wall. The nature of the cell wall is important in the classification of bacteria (see below) and in determining virulence.

The importance of the bacterial cell wall

In 1884, Christian Gram observed that the majority of bacteria could be classified into two broad groups, depending upon their ability to retain crystal violet dye after decolorization. Those retaining dye were termed Gram-positive and those failing to do so Gram-negative. This staining phenomenon, which is still of great importance in the initial laboratory identification of bacteria, results from fundamental differences in the cell walls of the two types of organism (Fig. 8.1).

All bacteria are bounded by a cytoplasmic membrane, composed of a typical phospholipid bilayer, the function of which is to supply the cell with energy via its associated enzyme systems and to regulate the passage of metabolites into and out of the cell.

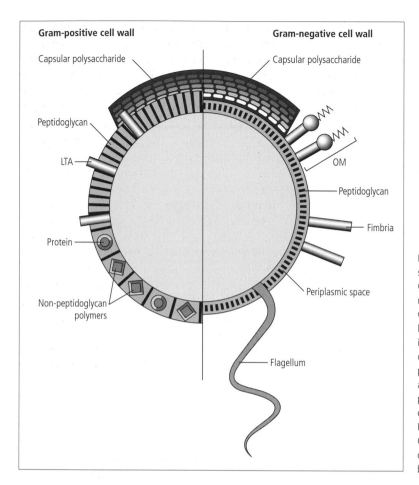

Gram-positive cell wall

Gram-negative cell wall

Capsular polysaccharide

Capsular polysaccharide

Peptidoglycan

LTA

OM

Peptidoglycan

Protein

Fimbria

Non-peptidoglycan polymers

Periplasmic space

Flagellum

Fig. 8.1 Schematic illustration of the structure of the cell wall of Gram-positive and Gram-negative bacteria. The cytoplasmic membrane (CM) in both Gram-positive and Gram-negative organisms is surrounded by a layer of peptidoglycan which is much thicker in Gram-positive cells. In Gram-positive organisms numerous surface proteins and polymers, including lipoteichoic acid (LTA), are also present. Gram-negative organisms possess a second outer membrane (OM) containing lipopolysaccharide and protein. Flagella and fimbriae are also present in some Gram-negative cells. An external layer of capsular polysaccharide is common to both types.

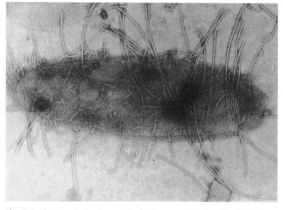

Fig. 8.2 Electron photomicrograph of a Gram-negative bacillus showing the presence of both fimbriae and flagella. Flagella are longer than fimbriae and enable the bacterium to move in a fluid medium. Conversely, fimbriae are mainly involved in the adherence of bacterial cells to other bacteria and to host tissues.

Surrounding the cytoplasmic membrane is a layer of *peptidoglycan*, a complex polymer of polysaccharide chains linked by short peptides. This layer gives the cell its strength and shape and is much thicker in Gram-positive cells (accounting for more than 40% of the dry weight of the cell wall) than in Gram-negative cells (where it accounts for around 10%). In Gram-positive organisms, numerous surface proteins and polymeric molecules other than peptidoglycan are also found closely associated with the peptidoglycan layer. A second outer membrane is present in Gram-negative organisms which contains lipopolysaccharide and protein molecules.

Flagella and *fimbriae* are cell appendages, composed of tubular filaments of polymerized protein that project from the cell wall of some Gram-negative bacterial cells (Fig. 8.2). Flagella are much longer than most fimbriae and generate propulsive forces which enable the bacterium to move within a fluid medium. Fimbriae, often also referred to as *pili*, are mainly involved in the adherence of bacterial cells to other bacteria and to host tissues. The notable exceptions are the sex pili which are important in the transfer of bacterial DNA, usually plasmids, from one bacterium to another.

Finally, external to the cell wall, most pathogenic bacteria, whether Gram-positive or -negative, are covered with a protective layer of carbohydrate known as *capsular polysaccharide*.

Classification of bacteria

It is beyond the scope of this book to consider in detail the classification systems in use for separating the major groups of bacteria. However, it is useful to acknowledge, in general terms, how this classification is achieved.

The simplest classification is based entirely on *staining characteristics* (e.g. Gram-positive or Gram-negative) and *morphology* (Fig. 8.3). However, this method alone will not differentiate significant pathogens from other organisms. Descriptions of the colony types produced when bacteria are grown on simple artificial media will improve differentiation considerably in experienced hands, but this is not reliable enough for routine diagnostic use. For this reason, a range of biochemical properties, e.g. the ability to ferment certain sugars, is normally examined; the wider the range, the more accurate the designation.

In practice, a combination of all these methods is used, thereby allowing bacteria to be characterized into families, genera, species and strains (Fig. 8.4). For example, a Gram-negative *diplococcus* (spherical bacteria in pairs), which grows aerobically on serum-enriched media, and ferments maltose and glucose, might be identified as *Neisseria* (genus) *meningitidis* (species) the causative agent of *meningococcal meningitis*.

Perhaps the most definitive method of classification is the examination of bacterial DNA sequence

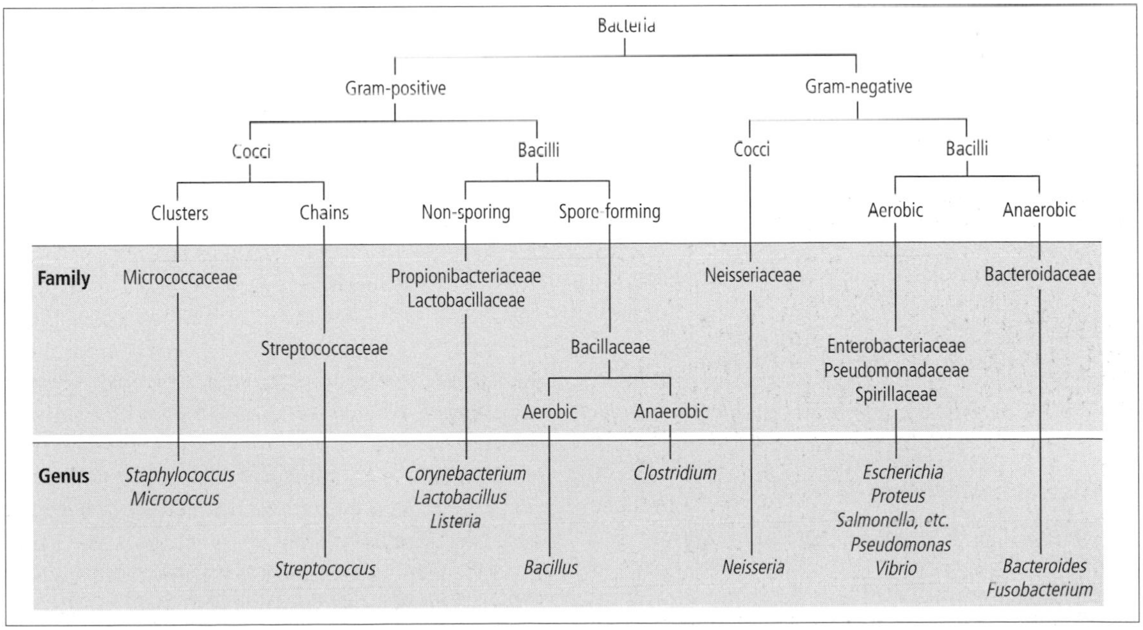

Fig. 8.3 Simple classification of Gram-stainable bacteria of clinical significance. A number of properties of bacterial cells may be exploited in order to classify bacteria into specific groups. Bacteria may be classified into broad groups depending upon their ability to retain crystal violet dye after decolorization. Those retaining dye are termed Gram-positive and those failing to do so, Gram-negative. Other characteristics including morphology (see also Fig. 8.4) and biochemical properties may be used to further subdivide bacteria.

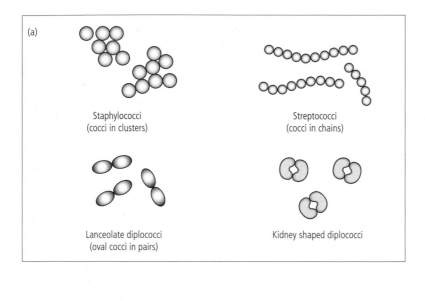

Staphylococci
(cocci in clusters)

Streptococci
(cocci in chains)

Lanceolate diplococci
(oval cocci in pairs)

Kidney shaped diplococci

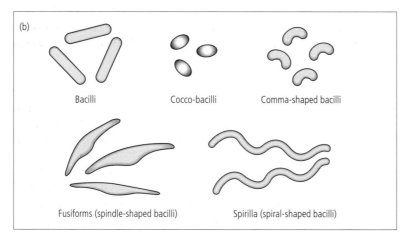

Bacilli

Cocco-bacilli

Comma-shaped bacilli

Fusiforms (spindle-shaped bacilli)

Spirilla (spiral-shaped bacilli)

Fig. 8.4 Basic bacterial forms. Microscopic examination of the morphology of bacteria in stained preparations is useful in classifying bacteria. Two major morphology types are recognized: cocci (a) which are roughly spherical in shape, and bacilli (b) which are rod-shaped. Within each major group certain variations exist, e.g. cocci are identified as streptococci if they are arranged in chains or diplococci if they are organized into pairs.

homology, although this is not a method which is routinely used in the laboratory identification of bacteria.

Routes of acquisition

Bacteria causing infection are acquired from two principal sources: either from amongst the patient's own normal flora (*endogenous infection*) or from external sources, e.g. from food (*exogenous infection*).

Exogenous infections may be acquired by one of the four principal routes detailed below.

• *Ingestion*, e.g. food poisoning associated with the consumption of foods contaminated with *Salmonella* species.
• *Inhalation*, e.g. inhalation of airborne droplets containing *Mycobacterium tuberculosis*, leading to pulmonary tuberculosis.
• *Inoculation*, e.g. rose-thorn punctures introducing *Clostridium tetani* and leading to clinical tetanus.
• *Direct contact*, e.g. *Neisseria gonorrhoeae*, acquired by intimate person-to-person contact.

Transmission of infection

The transmission of a bacterial infection is dependent upon several factors including the characteristics of the 'host' population at risk, the bacterium concerned and the nature of the environment.

Important *host factors* include the degree of immunity to a particular pathogen within the population, the proximity of individuals to each other and the general state of health and hygiene. It is worth mentioning here that some individuals, while apparently healthy, may harbour and transmit pathogenic bacteria—these individuals are often referred to as *carriers*. For example, healthy individuals can excrete *Salmonella* species for prolonged periods, causing outbreaks of food poisoning if they are involved in the preparation of food.

Bacterial factors include: the general properties of the organism, in particular, its virulence; its ability to survive in the environment; the size of the infecting dose; and the route by which the bacterium is acquired.

Environmental factors affecting transmission include: climate (bacterial growth generally being favoured by warm humid conditions); the standard of sanitation; and the presence of non-human 'vectors', e.g. ticks, which transmit bacteria whilst feeding on human or animal blood.

Bacteria can be transmitted between individuals of the same generation (horizontally, e.g. *M. tuberculosis* spread by respiratory droplets) or from mother to baby (vertically). An example here is *Listeria monocytogenes*, which may be transmitted from mother to child *in utero* and cause generalized sepsis in the fetus or newborn child.

Virulence determinants

As alluded to earlier, pathogenic bacteria possess so-called 'virulence determinants', which are responsible for their ability to cause disease. Many of these virulence determinants are cell wall constituents. An understanding of the nature and mode of action of virulence determinants is essential if we are to appreciate the mechanisms which underlie the pathogenesis of bacterial diseases.

Virulence determinants specific to Gram-positive bacteria

Non-peptidoglycan polymers

These are a heterogeneous group of *teichoic acid-like polymers* containing sugar alcohols and phosphodiester linkages, which are found on the surface of Gram-positive cells, bound covalently to peptidoglycan. Their precise role in the pathogenesis of disease is unclear, but they are thought to be involved in the stimulation of the inflammatory response (see Chapter 5). They are strongly immunogenic and form the identifying group antigens of many species of streptococci.

Unlike these 'secondary' cell wall polymers, the closely related molecule, *lipoteichoic acid*, lies in contact with the cytoplasmic membrane and protrudes through the peptidoglycan layer (see Fig. 8.1). It is thought to be important in the adherence of bacteria to surfaces, in particular, the binding of decay-causing organisms, such as *Streptococcus mutans*, to tooth enamel.

Surface proteins

Many different cell surface proteins have been identified, the majority of which do not appear to be virulence factors. One notable exception, however, is the 'M' protein of group A β-haemolytic streptococci (e.g. *Streptococcus pyogenes*). By binding to various serum proteins, bacteria expressing M proteins are able to avoid recognition and ingestion by phagocytic cells and inhibit neutrophil chemotaxis (see Chapter 5).

Virulence determinants specific to Gram-negative bacteria

Lipopolysaccharide

Lipopolysaccharide (LPS) is one of the most important bacterial virulence factors and is often referred to as *endotoxin*. It is an integral part of the outer surface of the outer membrane of Gram-negative cell walls and consists of an *inner glycolipid* (lipid A) attached to a 'core' *oligosaccharide*, with or without a variable length, outer, *'O' polysaccharide*.

Lipid A is a very potent toxin and is responsible

for all the toxic properties attributed to endo-toxin, although these are enhanced when the lipid molecule is associated with an *O* polysaccharide. Although incompletely understood, endotoxin exerts a profound effect when introduced into the host, producing widespread stimulation of the immune system and activation of the complement and the clotting cascades (see Chapter 16). This results in generalized damage to the host manifested in features collectively referred to as *endotoxic shock*, which may result in death.

The *O* polysaccharide chain of LPS addition-ally confers resistance to the bacteriolytic effects of serum and protects the bacterial cell from phagocytosis.

Outer membrane proteins

Numerous protein molecules can be found within the outer bacterial membrane. They are closely asso-ciated with LPS and often difficult to purify, but do appear to have functions in cell transport and ion binding. In some bacterial species, however, these proteins are also major virulence factors, enabling bacterial cells to adhere to their target tissues. Par-ticular examples are found in enteropathogenic forms of *Escherichia coli* (EPEC) which cause diarrhoea in young children.

In other species, such as entero-invasive *E. coli* (EIEC) and *Shigella* species, which cause a dysentery-like illness, the outer membrane proteins not only help the bacteria to adhere to the gut epithelium, but also enable them to enter the host cell where they multiply and subsequently kill the cell. The precise mechanisms of this invasive process are not yet fully understood.

Flagella and fimbriae

Flagellar proteins are strong immunogens and represent the 'H' antigens used in typing many Gram-negative bacteria, notably the Salmonellae. However, apart from conferring active motility, which may be a useful attribute in certain circum-stances, it is not thought that flagella are of major importance as far as virulence is concerned.

Conversely, fimbriae are very significant viru-lence factors. Their presence is dependent upon the conditions under which the bacteria are growing but they are often present in the majority of Gram-negative bacteria. Traditionally, fimbriae have been divided into two groups, depending on whether or not their ability to agglutinate erythrocytes of sev-eral animal species can be blocked by the presence of D-mannose. The *mannose-sensitive* (MS) variants are commonly encountered and are referred to as 'common fimbriae'. They facilitate binding to a num-ber of cells and proteins, but their precise role remains unclear.

The role of *mannose-resistant* (MR) fimbriae, how-ever, is better understood, at least in certain species. The fimbriae of *N. gonorrhoeae*, for example, adhere to a number of host cell types. In addition, the fimbriae also prevent binding of the bacterium to leucocytes, thereby inhibiting phagocytosis. Certain strains of *E. coli* isolated from patients with infec-tions of the kidney (*pyelonephritis*), possess fimbriae that bind to glycolipids present on the lining epithe-lium of the upper urinary tract. Bacteria possessing such fimbriae are less likely to be flushed away by the normal flow of urine and therefore more likely to produce clinical infection.

Another example of fimbrial adherence is seen in enterotoxin-producing *E. coli* which cause diar-rhoeal disease, including the verotoxin-producing *E. coli* (VTEC) which can give rise to haemorrhagic colitis and renal failure. The fimbriae of these organ-isms adhere to the colonic epithelium allowing direct interaction between the potent toxins pro-duced by the bacteria and the epithelial cells.

Virulence determinants common to Gram-negative and Gram-positive bacteria

Capsular polysaccharides

The polysaccharide matrix surrounding many bac-teria is highly variable in structure and is often derived from either the non-peptidoglycan poly-mers in the case of Gram-positive organisms or the *O* polysaccharide chains of Gram-negative organ-isms, and is termed the 'K' antigen in enterobacteria.

Capsular polysaccharides enable the bacterium to adhere by forming a sticky layer on surfaces and are important, for example, in the formation of dental plaque and the colonization of implanted medical devices and intravenous cannulae. They also render the bacterial cell wall inaccessible to the action of complement and to phagocytosis. Some capsular polysaccharides have the added advantage of mimicking host tissue antigens and so are not recognized as foreign by the immune system. For example, certain strains of *E. coli* are able to cause meningitis in newborn infants. These organisms possess the so-called K1 capsule, which is structurally similar to proteins found in the central nervous system of newborn infants. The immune system sees the K1 capsule as 'self' and the bacteria are therefore not destroyed.

Toxins and enzymes

Large numbers of toxins are known to be produced by bacteria. They are usually proteins of varying molecular weight and are traditionally referred to as *exotoxins* to differentiate them from the endotoxin of Gram-negative bacteria. They are numerous and wide ranging in their effects and are conveniently grouped on the basis of the following three main characteristics.

• *Site of action of the toxin*. Some exotoxins act only at the site at which they are released. For example, the enterotoxin of *C. perfringens* acts locally on intestinal epithelial cells to cause diarrhoea. Conversely, certain toxins may have more generalized systemic effects. Diphtheria toxin, for example, acts systemically, inhibiting host cell protein synthesis and resulting in damage to most major organs.

• *Mode of action*. Exotoxins may either act directly to cause their effects or their effect may be mediated through other agents. Tetanus toxin, for example, acts directly by blocking the release of neurotransmitters, leading to paralysis, whereas *staphylococcal toxic shock syndrome toxin* causes the release of immune mediators from macrophages, resulting in widespread tissue damage.

• *Structure of the toxin*. The toxin of *Strep. pyogenes*, streptolysin O, is a single molecule which binds to cell membranes causing lysis, whereas diphtheria toxin, after binding to a cell, requires cleavage by proteolytic enzymes before its active component can enter the cytoplasm.

Some toxins are enzymes but many other enzymes not regarded as toxins are produced by bacteria of all types. Their role as virulence factors is unclear, although some are able to lyse molecules of immunoglobulin A (IgA), which may enable them to become more easily established on mucous membranes, while others may assist in the local spread of bacteria once infection has occurred.

Other important enzymes, which cannot be classed as true virulence factors but are nevertheless important in human disease, are the enzymes produced by bacteria to counter the effects of antibiotics used to treat infections. Examples of this are the β-lactamase enzymes produced by bacteria that are capable of inactivating penicillin-like compounds.

Factors influencing bacterial virulence

Many bacteria do not have the potential to express virulence factors and are only able to do so if they acquire the necessary genetic material from plasmids or bacteriophages. Plasmid-mediated virulence factors are important in infections caused by several Gram-negative species. As transmissible units of genetic material, plasmids offer enormous potential for the exchange and recombination of gene sequences coding for virulence.

Bacteriophages are viruses capable of infecting bacterial cells and may also mediate the transfer of genetic material from one bacterial cell to another. The best example of bacteriophage-mediated virulence is *Corynebacterium diphtheriae* which requires the β-phage genome in order to produce its toxin. In some bacteria, genetic material coding for virulence factors is confined to a single region of the genome. However, other strains may acquire numerous virulence genes distributed around the chromosome, known as pathogenicity islands.

Successful pathogens must have the ability to activate and repress these genes in order to obtain maximum advantage in a given situation. It is now known that expression of virulence factors depends upon a complex interaction between bacterial and host cells and their immediate environment, i.e. environmental sensing. Environmental signals are many and varied, examples being temperature, nutrient availability, pH and presence of antibiotics. These signals may act directly on the gene, or indirectly through an intermediate response regulator.

Closely related to these mechanisms are the effects of cellular communication processes, both between bacteria and between host cells and bacteria. The former are mediated principally by diffusible molecules within bacterial populations; the latter involve cellular interactions subsequent to binding of bacteria to host cells.

Key points

1 Bacteria are prokaryotes that may be classified on the basis of staining properties, morphology and biochemical characteristics.

2 Bacterial infections may be acquired from two principal sources: (a) from amongst the patients' own flora (endogenous infection); and (b) from external sources (exogenous infection).

3 Bacteria capable of causing disease (so-called 'pathogenic bacteria') possess virulence determinants that are responsible for their ability to cause disease.

4 Most virulence determinants are associated with the cell wall of pathogenic bacteria.

Summary

There remains much to learn about the nature of bacterial pathogenicity, a task hindered by the diversity and adaptability of bacteria. By endeavouring to understand the basic mechanisms of bacterial infection it should be possible to devise new and more effective methods for their prevention and treatment.

Further reading

Hewlett E.L., Petri W.A., Mann B.J., Relman D.A. & Falkow S. (1995) Microbial virulence factors. In: Mandell G.L., Bennet J.E. & Dolinu R. (eds) *Mandell Douglas and Bennett's: Principles and Practice of Infectious Diseases* (4th edn) pp. 2–30. Churchill Livingstone, New York.

Kolenbrander P.E. (1998) Environmental sensing mechanisms and virulence factors of bacterial pathogens. In: Collier L., Balows A. & Sussman M. (eds) *Topley and Wilson's Microbiology and Microbial Infections* (9th edn) volume 2, pp. 307–325. Arnold, London.

Parker M.T. (1998) Bacteria as pathogens: historical introduction. In Collier L., Balows A. & Sussman M. (eds) *Topley and Wilson's Microbiology and Microbial Infections* (9th edn) volume 3, pp. 1–10. Arnold, London.

CHAPTER 9

Virus Infections

Viruses are resistant to antibiotics, are smaller than bacteria (30–200 nm), and are composed of a single type of nucleic acid (either DNA or RNA) surrounded by a protein coat (*capsid*) which may be further enclosed in an *envelope*. They are *obligate intracellular parasites*, i.e. they can only replicate within a living host cell. Virus replication is a stepwise series of metabolic events involving both virus-encoded proteins and the metabolic machinery of the cell. During evolution viruses have developed exquisite molecular features which allow them to replicate at the expense of the cell. It is virus replication, resulting in the release of new virus particles (*virions*) and the subsequent cell death which normally follows, that is responsible for virus disease. In most cases the specific pathology and disease syndrome is a result of the killing of specific cell types (virus cell tropism) and/or the immune response to the virus. In some cases the immune system is itself a target for virus infection. This can lead to the destruction of important immune cells, which in turn can lead to immunosuppression. An example of this is the immunosuppression that results from human immunodeficiency virus (HIV) infection of CD4+ T lymphocytes. In some cases virus infection may also contribute to the development of neoplasia (see Chapter 23).

In this chapter, virus structure and replication are briefly discussed. Modes of virus spread are then considered in relation to the important routes of transmission. The remainder of the chapter discusses in detail the effects of virus infections on the host, ranging from asymptomatic infection through to severe debilitating disease and death.

Virus structure and replication

Viruses are classified into a number of families based upon differences in their structure and modes of replication. Table 9.1 summarizes the properties of some virus families and Fig. 9.1 shows a diagrammatic representation of four selected virus particles.

During replication, viruses undergo a series of steps that ultimately lead to the successful release of several hundred progeny virions. In *step 1* (attachment and penetration) the virus attaches, via the viral capsid or envelope, to a specific receptor on the surface of a target cell, triggering off a series of events which allows the virus to penetrate the cell. It is this initial interaction which accounts for the predisposition of certain viruses to infect particular species or tissue types. For example, HIV attaches to one main receptor, the CD4 receptor found on certain cell types (T-helper cells, see Chapter 6) and one of two coreceptors. Attachment to CD4 occurs via a 120-kDa envelope protein (gp120) and fusion/penetration is achieved via a 41-kDa envelope protein (gp41). Absence of the coreceptor on some individuals appears to make them genetically unsusceptible to HIV. Following penetration of the cell the virus is uncoated releasing the virus genome. In the case of many viruses, the genome migrates rapidly to the host cell nucleus where it may integrate within the host cell DNA or exist as a separate

Table 9.1 Taxonomic chart of selected virus families.

Family	Characteristics	Typical members	Diseases caused
Poxvirus	Double-stranded DNA, 'brick'-shaped particles; largest virus	Vaccinia Variola	Laboratory virus Smallpox (now eradicated)
Herpesvirus	Double-stranded DNA, icosahedron capsid enclosed in an envelope, latency in host common	Herpes simplex Varicella-zoster Cytomegalovirus Epstein–Barr virus	'Cold' sores, genital infections Chicken pox, shingles Febrile illness or disseminated disease in immunosuppression Glandular fever. Virus is also associated with certain malignancies, e.g. Burkitt's lymphoma
Adenovirus	Double-stranded DNA, icosahedron with fibre structures, non-enveloped	Adenoviruses (many types)	Respiratory and eye infections, tumours in experimental animals
Papovavirus	Double-stranded circular DNA, 72 capsomeres in capsid, non-enveloped	Human papillomaviruses	Warts, association with some cancers (e.g. cervical cancer)
Hepadnavirus	One complete DNA minus strand with 5' terminal protein, DNA circularized by an incomplete plus strand, 42 nm enveloped particle	Hepatitis B virus	Serum hepatitis, association with hepatocellular carcinoma
Paramyxovirus	Single-stranded RNA, enveloped particles with 'spikes'	Parainfluenza virus Measles virus Respiratory syncytial virus	Respiratory tract infection ('croup') Measles Bronchiolitis
Orthomyxovirus	Eight segments of single-stranded RNA, enveloped particles with 'spikes', helical nucleocapsid	Influenza virus	Influenza
Reovirus	Ten to twelve segments of double-stranded RNA, icosahedron, non-enveloped	Rotavirus	Infantile diarrhoea
Picornavirus	Single-stranded RNA, 22–30 nm particle of cubic symmetry, non-enveloped	Poliovirus Coxsackie virus Rhinovirus Hepatitis A virus	Poliomyelitis Myocarditis Common cold Infectious hepatitis
Togavirus	Single-stranded RNA, enveloped particles, icosahedron nucleocapsid	Rubella virus Arbovirus	German measles Yellow fever
Rhabdovirus	Single-stranded RNA, bullet-shaped, enveloped particle	Rabies virus	Rabies
Retrovirus	Single-stranded RNA, enveloped particles with icosahedral nucleocapsid, employ reverse transcriptase enzyme to make DNA copy of genome on infection	Human T-lymphotropic virus 1 Human immunodeficiency virus (HIV)	Adult T-cell leukaemia and lymphoma Acquired immunodeficiency syndrome (AIDS)

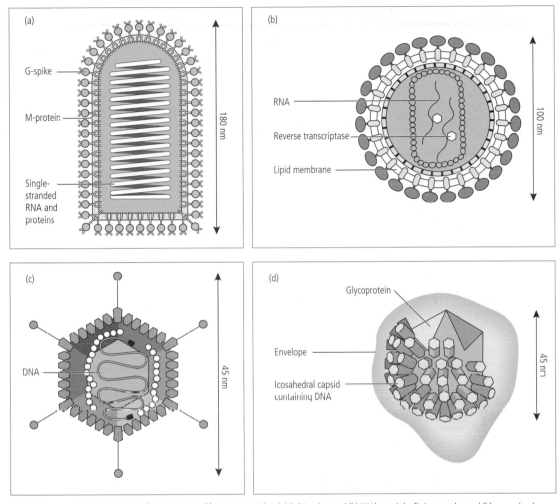

Fig. 9.1 Diagrammatic representation of the structure of four virus particles. (a) Rabies virus and (b) HIV have tight-fitting envelopes; (d) herpes simplex has a loose-fitting envelope whereas (c) adenovirus is non-enveloped. The diagrams are based on electron microscopic observation and molecular configuration exercises.

extrachromosomal entity (episome). In others the genome remains within the cytoplasm. Integration is often only achieved with the help of a virus-encoded protein. With respect to HIV, where integration is essential for virus replication, the virus uses its own 'integrase' enzyme.

In *step 2* (macromolecular synthesis) viral nucleic acid is used for the synthesis of virus structural proteins (those proteins that will make up new virions) or non-structural proteins (i.e. the virus enzymes required for the manufacture of the structural proteins). The nucleic acid also replicates to provide the

genome for progeny virions. The complexity of the different mechanisms used by viruses to reproduce themselves is well illustrated by the RNA viruses. In the case of 'positive-strand' RNA viruses the viral RNA is the mRNA and is translated directly the virus enters the cell. The 'negative strand' RNA viruses firstly make mirror image copies of their genome, which acts as the mRNA. The retroviruses have a more complex replication mechanism (Fig. 9.2) which involves the use of a viral reverse transcriptase enzyme, which makes a DNA copy of the viral RNA. This DNA copy is integrated into the

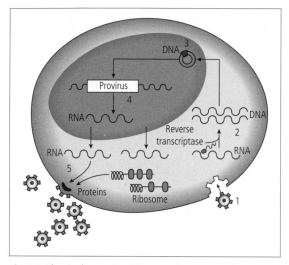

Fig. 9.2 Lifecycle of a retrovirus: (1) retrovirus binds to a specific receptor on the cell surface and enters the cell; (2) the virus is uncoated and reverse transcriptase employed to make a double-stranded DNA copy of the RNA genome; (3) the DNA copy is transported to the nucleus and integrated into the cellular genome where it is known as a provirus; (4) viral DNA is transcribed to produce genomic RNA and mRNA for the synthesis of structural virus proteins and enzymes; (5) the new virus particles are assembled and leave the cell by budding at the cell membrane.

host cell DNA where it is referred to as a provirus. The provirus is then transcribed to generate the early viral proteins required for replication. Generation of these proteins requires a virus-encoded 'protease' enzyme. The reverse transcriptase and protease enzymes are targets for chemotherapy and at the time of writing are inhibited by the use of combination therapy, which has been successful in severely limiting the replication of HIV.

In *step 3* (assembly) the newly formed viral proteins enclose the viral nucleic acid to form mature virus particles.

In *step 4* (release) these particles leave either by lysing the infected cell or by budding from the host cell plasma membrane. In some cases host-derived membrane proteins may form part of the virus envelope. Virus release usually leads to cell death.

In many cases the early steps of virus infection trigger a series of events within the cell resulting in cell death by apoptosis (Chapter 4). This cell death means that virus replication and the production of progeny virions is totally or severely inhibited.

However, several viral genes have been identified whose actions delay the onset of apoptosis. Cowpox virus, for example, expresses an inhibitor of an enzyme involved in the apoptotic pathway, the interleukin 1β-converting enzyme (ICE, also known as caspase 1) and thereby blocks apoptosis and inflammation. Similar antiapoptosis genes are found in many other virus types, including the Kaposi's sarcoma associated herpesvirus (KSHV) and the Epstein–Barr virus (EBV) (see Chapter 23).

During infection, virus proteins are often processed by the host cell into peptides and presented on the surface of the cell in association with major histocompatibility complex (MHC) class I molecules (see Chapter 6). Infected cells therefore can be recognized and destroyed by cytotoxic T lymphocytes carrying the CD8 surface receptor. Although an effective immune response against a virus-infected cell often depends upon an efficient cytotoxic T-cell response, other immune effector systems may also be important. The immune responses to virus infection are summarized in Fig. 9.3. It is important to emphasize that while replication of viruses can cause cell death and therefore tissue damage, in many cases this is further exacerbated by the immune response to the infection which will also lead to significant tissue destruction.

During coevolution with their hosts, viruses have adopted several measures to counteract the various host defence mechanisms. These include inhibition of peptide processing, resistance to serum inhibitors, resistance to or poor inducers of interferon, inhibition of phagocytes, suppression of immune responses, low capacity to evoke an immune response, alteration of lymphocyte traffic, effects on cellular modulators, depression of complement activity, resistance to the immune response and antigenic variation. Thus, the high mutation rate of many RNA viruses, e.g. HIV, creates mutants that are no longer recognized by antibody molecules. Influenza virus undergoes constant change in the environment (so-called antigenic 'drift' of its haemagglutinin molecule) leading to the appearance of different strains of virus, capable of replication in previously immune hosts. Most of the herpesviruses escape the immune system whilst latent in their host and many during replication (e.g. EBV)

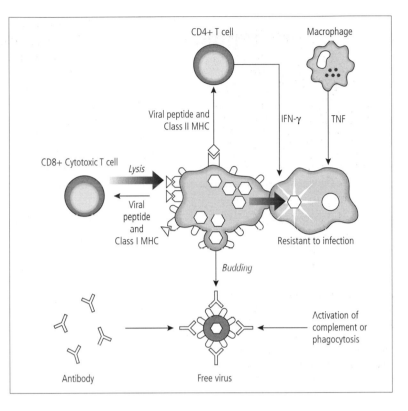

Fig. 9.3 Summary of immune responses to viral infection. A virus-infected cell is able to process viral peptides and present these on the surface of the cell in association with MHC class I molecules. This complex is recognized by CD8+ T cells which are able to lyse the infected cell. CD4+ T cells recognize viral antigens associated with MHC class II molecules and these cells, together with macrophages, release cytokines that act on other cells making them resistant to further viral infection. Free viruses released by infected cells may be bound by specific antibodies. Subsequent activation of complement may lead to lysis of viral particles or promote their phagocytosis.

may specifically inhibit the intracellular transport mechanism by which viral peptide fragments are presented to the cell-mediated immune system. Adenovirus, poxvirus and cytomegalovirus (CMV) interfere with peptide presentation by downregulating the expression of the MHC class I protein. Vaccinia virus, reovirus, adenoviruses and EBV are examples of viruses capable of inhibiting the action of interferon, usually by interfering with the action of a cellular protein kinase enzyme. Both herpes simplex virus (HSV) and EBV structural proteins interfere with the complement cascade mechanism. Herpes simplex virus, in addition, has a structural protein, present on infected cell surfaces, which has Fc-receptor activity, thus preventing complement fixation or opsonization by phagocytes.

The ability of viruses to evolve more rapidly than their host means that virus replication and its subsequent disease will continue to threaten the health of the world's population. The evolutionary process has also led to the emergence of new viruses capable of replicating in different species, including humans.

Virus spread

In order to persist and evolve in nature, viruses need a large population of susceptible hosts and an efficient means of spread between these hosts.

The *respiratory route* is the most common pathway for virus entry and exit. Following inhalation, viruses can infect and replicate within epithelial cells of the upper or lower respiratory tract. Following release from these cells, progeny virions enter surrounding airways and exit via sneezing and coughing. Examples of viruses that are transmitted in this way include the influenza and parainfluenza viruses, the common cold viruses, adenoviruses and the respiratory syncytial virus (RSV).

Although the entry and exit of many viruses is via the respiratory tract, some viruses do not remain within the respiratory tract but may enter the blood stream causing viraemia (defined as the presence of infectious virions in the blood stream) and subsequent infection of other target organs. Examples of such viruses include the varicella-zoster virus, which is responsible for chicken pox, the measles virus and the rubella virus, the causative agent of German measles.

The *oral–gastrointestinal* route is used mainly by those viruses responsible for gut infections (rotavirus, Norwalk virus, and the enteroviruses, including echo, polio and coxsackie viruses). Again many of these viruses (e.g. polio and coxsackie viruses) leave the gastrointestinal tract and cause serious debilitating diseases elsewhere, in many cases within the central nervous system (CNS). Vast numbers of infectious virus particles can be excreted in faecal material (e.g. of the order of 10^{12} particles/g) facilitating the easy spread of these viruses in conditions of poor sanitation. The drinking of faecally contaminated water, and consumption of contaminated shellfish and food prepared by unhygienic food handlers are ways in which these viruses are spread between susceptible hosts. Infections caused by these viruses are widespread in developing countries where poor sanitation is a particular problem.

Whilst the *skin* normally provides an impenetrable barrier to virus invasion, infectious viruses can enter following trauma to the skin. This may be a bite from an animal vector (e.g. transmission of the rabies virus from the bite of an infected canine), or an arthropod vector (e.g. the transmission of the yellow fever virus by mosquitoes). HIV, hepatitis B or hepatitis C virus may be transmitted by the injection of blood or blood products either in the form of a blood transfusion, a needle-stick injury or by intravenous drug abuse.

Sexual transmission of viruses is an important route for the spread of HSV (genital herpes) and the papillomaviruses (genital warts). However, the advent of the acquired immunodeficiency syndrome (AIDS) highlighted the ease with which viruses, in this case HIV, can be transmitted during unprotected sexual intercourse. Unprotected penetrative anal intercourse among homosexuals has been the main route by which HIV has been transmitted in the Western World. In Sub-Saharan Africa and the Caribbean, where the virus is endemic in the heterosexual population, transmission during vaginal intercourse is the most important route for viral spread. Heterosexual spread is now also common in Asian and Far Eastern countries.

Viruses may also be transmitted *vertically* that is from mother to offspring, via the placenta, during childbirth, or in breast milk. For example, rubella virus and CMV infections acquired by the mother during pregnancy may be transmitted to the developing embryo and can lead to severe congenital abnormalities and/or spontaneous abortion. Some virus infections, e.g. HSV infections, if acquired *in utero* or during birth can present as an acute disease syndrome at birth. Alternatively, the child may be born without any overt signs of infection but carries the virus as an asymptomatic infection. The development of this 'carrier state' follows congenital infections with viruses like HIV or the hepatitis B virus. The developing fetus of an HIV-positive mother has an estimated 40–60% chance of becoming infected with HIV but the risk is reduced if prophylactic chemotherapy is given during pregnancy.

Some of the routes for virus spread within the host are summarized in Fig. 9.4.

Virus pathogenesis and the clinical results of virus infections

The outcome of a virus infection is dependent on several factors. These include various host-related factors including age, immune status, nutritional state, route of infection, viral load and viral strain. Thus, HSV is usually fatal in a neonate but may cause inapparent infections or minor epithelial lesions (e.g. 'cold sores') in older children and adults. EBV causes a very mild febrile illness in infants but infectious mononucleosis (glandular fever) in teenagers; the same virus in parts of tropical Africa and in China is believed to contribute to the development of Burkitt's lymphoma and nasopharyngeal carcinoma, respectively. CMV in a healthy individual may cause a mild febrile illness, but in immunosuppressed individuals can lead to fatal pneumonia. Measles only rarely has side-effects in healthy well-nourished children, but kills around 900 000 children per year in developing countries. There are also many 'unknowns' in studies on virus infections. Why, for example, even in the absence of vaccination, do most people infected with poliovirus show no signs of ill health, and in those with symptoms why do only about 10%

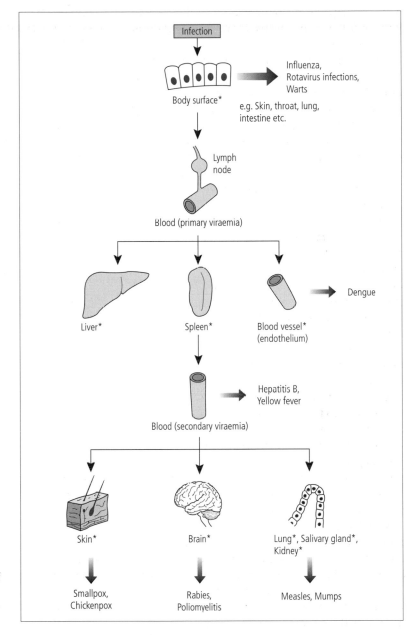

Fig. 9.4 Virus spread within the host. Different viruses have different modes of spread within the host. Some viruses remain localized at the site of entry, whereas others may spread to involve other tissues. Routes of infection are shown, together with examples of possible clinical outcomes. *, Possible sites of replication.

suffer CNS damage? Likewise, why do a very small proportion of cold sore sufferers develop fatal HSV encephalitis?

Those viruses that cause disease are termed 'pathogenic'. To be pathogenic, viruses must be capable of spreading from host to host, invading tissues (often mucous membranes), replicating inside cells, interfering with host defences and damaging the host. Cellular changes are both biochemical and morphological (cytopathic effect of viruses) with a shutdown of host cell macromolecular synthesis, chromosome alterations, inclusion body formation, resulting in direct cytotoxicity. The resultant disease syndrome is often a combination of cell damage and host response to infection. Influenza virus, which kills endothelial cells lining the respiratory tract, induces very high levels of interferon which itself gives rise to severe symptoms (overall lethargy, depression, etc.). Pathogenesis is therefore a multifactorial phenomenon with a number of viral genes contributing to the process.

For the purpose of the foregoing discussion the clinical outcome of a virus infection will be considered under several general headings. It will be seen that the distinction between these clinical groups is not always clear cut and in some cases there may be considerable overlap between them.

Inapparent (asymptomatic) infection

Many virus infections are subclinical, there being no apparent outward symptoms of disease. This is virtually always true in the immune host, where recovery from a previous infection or vaccination protects the host from virus growth following reinfection by the wild-type virus. However, several viruses, including some respiratory viruses and enteroviruses, do not produce clinical symptoms even in non-immune individuals. Thus, the poliovirus, in 80% of infected individuals, replicates in the epithelial cells of the gastrointestinal tract, is excreted in the faeces, but causes no symptoms. After a few days the virus is eradicated and the host acquires life-long immunity.

Disease syndrome, virus eradication and recovery

The pattern we expect following most virus infections in otherwise healthy individuals, is that of clinical symptoms of varying degrees of severity, i.e. disease syndrome, followed by virus eradication by the immune system, recovery and often lifelong immunity. This is true of most childhood virus in-fections, e.g. measles, mumps and German measles, most respiratory infections, of which there are a huge number of viruses responsible, and a vast spectrum of other virus infections including those resulting from hepatitis A virus (infectious jaundice), rotavirus (gut infections) and coxsackie virus (myocarditis, pericarditis, conjunctivitis). The

following section outlines the typical patterns of infection seen with both a local and a systemic virus infection.

Local virus infection

RSV infections are confined to the respiratory tract and are responsible for severe respiratory distress in children less than 12 months old. RSV infection causes necrosis of the bronchiolar epithelium, which sloughs off, blocking the small airways. This in turn leads to obstruction of airflow and respiratory distress. Obstruction is compounded by the increased secretion of mucus and the presence of inflammatory exudates within the airways. This bronchiolitis may progress to pneumonia, when oedema and necrosis of the lung parenchyma result in the filling and collapse of the alveoli. Children recovering from acute RSV bronchiolitis are often left with a weakened and vulnerable respiratory system, predisposing them to a lifetime of chronic lung disease. Figure 9.5 illustrates the possible outcomes of respiratory invasion by viruses.

Systemic virus infection

Following respiratory infection with measles, the virus replicates in the lymph nodes that drain from the infected tissue. The virus spreads to the rest of the lymphoid system and respiratory tract through the blood in a primary viraemia. Giant cells (multinucleated virus-infected cells) are formed in lymphoid tissue and on epithelial surfaces, these giving rise to free virus which again enters the blood stream in a secondary viraemia. These viruses subsequently infect the skin and viscera, kidneys and bladder. At this stage the patient is highly infectious and may present with fever, malaise, sneezing, rhinitis, congestion, conjunctivitis and a cough. The distinctive measles rash appears about 14 days postinfection. The rash is characterized by vascular congestion, oedema and epithelial necrosis. The primary events of a measles infection are summarized in Fig. 9.6.

Latency

A restricted range of viruses, most being in the herpesvirus family (HSV, varicella-zoster, EBV and

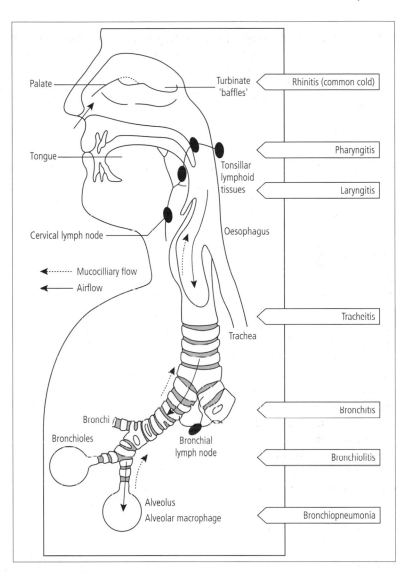

Fig. 9.5 Routes of infection in the respiratory tract. Virus infections can produce a variety of respiratory disorders depending on the area of the respiratory tract infected.

CMV) are not eradicated from the body following recovery, but instead become 'latent' within the host. Virus replication may be initiated some time later (reactivation) and cause clinical symptoms which are similar to those observed in primary infection.

Thus, HSV can reactivate many times during the life of an individual and produces the typical painful 'cold-sore' lesions on the mouth or genitals. Following primary infection, HSV travels via the nerve axon to the CNS where it lays dormant in the trigeminal or sacral ganglia. During this dormancy there is no viral replication, indeed no proteins are produced. One mRNA species, the LAT (latency) transcript, is produced but is not translated. HSV may remain dormant for the lifetime of the patient, for several years or occasionally only for a few months before reactivating. A variety of stimuli including menstruation, exposure to ultraviolet light and stress induce the virus to reactivate and to travel back down the axon to the periphery, where it causes the characteristic lesions. HSV can spread by

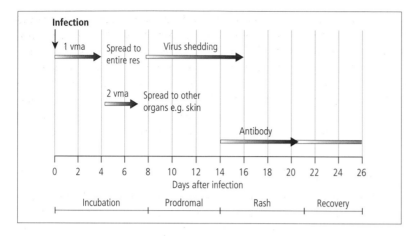

Infection

1 vma → Spread to entire res

Virus shedding →

2 vma → Spread to other organs e.g. skin

Antibody →

| 0 | 2 | 4 | 6 | 8 | 10 | 12 | 14 | 16 | 18 | 20 | 22 | 24 | 26 |

Days after infection

Incubation — Prodromal — Rash — Recovery

Fig. 9.6 The course of clinical measles. Measles is characterized by a primary viraemia (1 vma) followed by a secondary viraemia (2 vma). Virus shedding occurs, at which point the patient is highly infectious. A prodromal phase is followed by the typical symptoms and signs of measles, including rash. The appearance of antibody is usually followed by complete recovery and life-long immunity. res, Reticuloendothelial system.

cell-to-cell fusion, thus protecting it from the high concentrations of HSV antibody found in the sera of infected patients. Cytotoxic T cells are eventually responsible for abrogating clinical infection.

Alternatively, a very different clinical syndrome may result following virus reactivation. Thus, primary infection with the varicella-zoster virus produces chicken pox, whereas reactivation is associated with the development of shingles. Shingles is characterized by a localized area of extremely painful vesicles from which the varicella-zoster virus can be isolated. The lesions may clear after 1–2 weeks but often result in an aftermath of severe neuralgia, which may persist for months or years. It is, however, unusual for patients to present with further attacks of shingles unless they are immuno-compromised.

It is important to make the distinction here between clinical latency and microbiological latency. Microbiological latency defines a situation where the virus exists within a cell but does not replicate, usually producing only those virus proteins required to maintain the virus within the cell. Microbiological latency usually also results in clinical latency, there being no outward signs of infection. The difficulty in accurately defining latency is well illustrated in the case of EBV. Following primary infection, EBV persists in the host within B lymphocytes where the virus is usually latent. This latent state is characterized by the production of only those viral proteins required for the maintenance of the viral genome within the cell and there is

no viral replication. However, free virus can be isolated from the saliva of normal individuals during this clinically latent infection, implying that virus is replicated at low levels in the oropharynx. Reactivation of EBV often occurs during immuno-suppression and is characterized by the onset of the typical symptoms of infectious mononucleosis with or without the development of lymphoproliferative disease (see case study 12).

Carrier/persistent state

Although a rare event after virus infection, the virus carrier state is often seen following hepatitis B virus, hepatitis C virus or HIV infection. Around 5–10% of individuals infected with hepatitis B virus will carry the infective particles in their blood for months or years. Estimates suggest that 300 million individuals worldwide carry the virus in their blood and body fluids. However, this figure is rapidly increasing. One reason for this is that in addition to being transmitted horizontally the virus is also passed from mother to offspring. Unfortunately, chronic hepatitis B carriers have a greatly increased risk of developing hepatocellular carcinoma (see Chapter 23). The immediate clinical consequences of infection with hepatitis C virus are usually very mild; 70–80% of infected individuals are asymptomatic. However, the majority of primary infections become established as long-term, usually life-long, chronic persistent infections. The mechanism that allows this virus to remain persistent and the ease with which it overcomes the immune system is one of its most intriguing features. Some 200 million carriers exist worldwide, and, as with hepatitis B, they have an increased risk of developing liver cirrhosis and hepatocellular carcinoma. Hepatitis C infections are at present the single predominant reason for liver transplants in the USA.

Following exposure to HIV, the virus nucleic acid becomes integrated into the chromosome of host cells (see Fig. 9.2). The primary infection results in a significant viraemia, which usually subsides to extremely low levels. However, HIV continues to replicate at a low level. During this time the virus undergoes a series of mutations, some of which result in more pathogenic and less immunogenic forms. The infected individual (who is antibody positive) will carry infectious virus and virus-infected cells in their blood, semen, vaginal fluid and saliva. If untreated a majority (70–80%) of HIV carriers will progress to develop AIDS in a 7–12-year period. A small percentage (5–10%) are termed rapid progressors and will develop AIDS within a year, whereas another group, the long-term progressors (5–10%) will not have progressed over 20 years postinfection. This latter group forms the basis of much experimentation at present.

Host immunosuppression

Although mild immunosuppression can often result from virus infections such as measles and glandular fever, the advent of AIDS has highlighted how dramatic virus invasion of the immune system can be. HIV infects and grows best in cells which express CD4 receptors (i.e. T-helper cells). The progression from HIV positivity to a pre-AIDS syndrome and ultimately to AIDS is usually best indicated by a rise in viral load (the number of viruses present within an infected individual) and a dramatic drop in the CD4+ cell count, extremely low levels demonstrating the extent to which the patient may become immunosuppressed. This drop in CD4+ cells is brought about by the virus, which lyses the cell in which it is harboured, releasing hundreds of progeny virions, which infect and kill other CD4+ cells. The T-helper cell is of central importance in the immune system (see Chapter 6) and

depletion rapidly leads to invasion by opportunistic pathogens including HSV, CMV, *Pneumocystis carinii* and *Candida albicans* (see case study 4). The appearance of widespread lesions of Kaposi's sarcoma is also typical of a person with AIDS (see Chapter 23). Whilst there is still no vaccine against HIV, triple agent chemotherapy is proving effective in raising CD4 counts and reducing viral load.

Neoplastic growth

Introduction of genetic material and the rearrangement or switching on of cellular genes are events that can be mediated by viruses. In some situations this can contribute to the development of neoplastic disease. This area is discussed in detail in Chapter 22.

Death

Whilst many virus infections are fatal in distinct circumstances and others in a percentage of victims, some are almost always fatal. Rabies, HIV infection leading to AIDS, and a range of neurological conditions resulting from virus infections, including subacute sclerosing panencephalitis (SSPE), are examples. SSPE is a very rare condition, which occurs some months or years after a primary measles infection and is the result of the slow and persistent growth of the measles virus within brain cells.

Whilst the incubation period of rabies is 30–90 days, patients with initial symptoms of the disease die within 7–12 days. Following a bite, the virus may enter the peripheral nerves and moves centripetally to the spinal cord and brain where it replicates. Virus then leaves the CNS and spreads centrifugally to virtually all tissues of the body, including the salivary glands where it is excreted in saliva. The patient develops a variety of abnormalities including hydrophobia (aversion to water), rigidity, photophobia (aversion to light), fasciculations (muscle twitches) and paresis (motor weakness), cerebellar signs, cranial nerve palsies, hypo- or hyperreflexia, focal or generalized convulsions and a variety of autonomic disturbances. Development of a flaccid paralysis and onset of coma precede fatal complications.

Key points

1 Viruses are small intracellular parasites that are composed of a single type of nucleic acid (either DNA or RNA) surrounded by a protein coat (capsid) and in some cases by an outer envelope.

2 Viruses can only survive and replicate inside host cells. Distinct stages in virus replication can be recognized: (a) attachment and penetration; (b) macromolecular synthesis; (c) assembly; and (d) release, which often results in cell death.

3 The tissue damage caused by virus infections is the result of the direct cytopathic effects of the virus or the immune response to the virus, or a combination of both.

4 Viruses can gain access to the host through the skin and mucous membranes, via the respiratory or gastrointestinal tracts, or through sexual contact. Viruses may also be transmitted vertically from the mother to her offspring.

5 Infections caused by viruses are either localized at or near the site of virus entry or systemic where the virus spreads from its point of entry to involve one or more target organs.

6 In humans the outcome of a virus infection follows basic patterns: (a) inapparent infection; (b) disease syndrome, virus eradication and recovery; (c) latency; (d) carrier state; (e) immunosuppression; (f) neoplasia; and (g) death.

Summary

Virus infections are responsible for more visits to general practitioners than any other single disease condition and yet to date most remain untreatable. Whilst a handful of vaccines are available, for several the efficacy is poor and their cost is prohibitive to countries with poor economies. Viral infections will therefore continue to cause severe morbidity and mortality until such a time as technical advances and a favourable economic climate allows the development of effective vaccines and non-toxic chemotherapeutic agents.

Further reading

Heritage J., Evans E.G.V. & Killington R.A. (1999) *Microbiology in Action.* Cambridge University Press, Cambridge.

Mahy B.W.J. & Collier L. (1998) *Topley and Wilson's Microbiology and Microbial Infections*, volume 1. *Virology.* Arnold, London.

Nicklin J., Graeme-Cook K., Paget T. & Killington R.A. (1999) *Instant Notes in Microbiology.* Bios, Oxford.

Hypersensitivity

The term *hypersensitivity* is used to describe situations in which the immune system reacts inappropriately or excessively to antigens, which otherwise appear to be relatively harmless. Gell and Coombs classified hypersensitivity reactions into four different types based on their underlying immunological mechanisms and clinical manifestations.

Substances that induce an immune response are usually foreign to the individual and are termed *antigens*, those which elicit a hypersensitive response may also be described as *allergens*. The term 'hypersensitivity' is often used interchangeably with allergy (meaning altered reactivity); however, the latter term is probably best restricted to type 1 hypersensitivity. Hypersensitive reactions may also be directed against 'self-antigens' in the context of autoimmune diseases (see Chapter 11).

Multiple factors determine whether a hypersensitive rather than a normal immunological response occurs, including the genetic make up of the individual, the physical and chemical properties of the antigen and its mode of delivery into the individual.

A particular disease may involve more than one hypersensitivity mechanism, and an understanding of the four types of hypersensitivity helps to explain the immunopathogenesis of many conditions.

Type 1 hypersensitivity

In humans there are five classes of immunoglobulin: *IgG, IgM, IgA, IgD* and *IgE* which differ in their structure and function. Type 1 hypersensitivity reactions appear within minutes of exposure to allergen,

and involve the interaction of *allergen*, *allergen specific IgE* and tissue *mast cells*. IgE is normally present in very low concentrations in the serum but levels are increased in patients with parasitic infections, in most atopic patients, as well as in many apparently healthy individuals. Atopic patients are defined as suffering from a combination of three clinical conditions: *allergic rhinitis, eczema and asthma*. One of the key physiological roles of IgE is thought to be the eradication of parasitic infections and type 1 hypersensitivity appears to be a particular problem in areas of the world where such infections are no longer endemic.

In order to mount a type 1 response, an individual's immune system must previously have encountered the antigen/allergen and have stimulated B cells to produce antigen/allergen-specific IgE. A high total serum IgE is insufficient to cause an allergic response, the IgE must be produced in response to an allergen and therefore bind to it specifically. Mast cells, found in the mucosae of the airways and gut as well as in connective tissues, bind this IgE via specialized surface receptors for the Fc portion of IgE molecules (Fig. 10.1).

On re-exposure to allergen, IgE molecules on the surface of the mast cells bind allergen via their available antigen-binding (Fab) portions and become cross-linked. This initiates a series of intracellular signals, which results in the release of the mast cells' cytosolic granular contents into the surrounding microenvironment. These consist of a series of preformed mediators including histamine, heparin, lysosomal enzymes and proteases, neutrophil

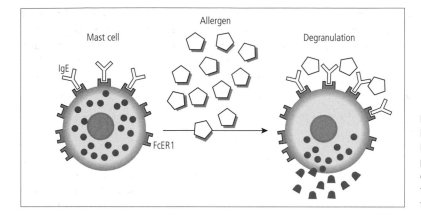

Fig. 10.1 Type 1 (immediate) hypersensitivity involves the interaction of allergen-specific IgE, Mast cells bearing receptors for the Fc portion of IgE (FcER1), and allergen. Release of preformed mediators shown here is followed 4–6 h later by release of newly formed mediators.

Table 10.1 The physiological effects of early and late phase mediators in type 1 hypersensitivity reactions.

Mediators	Effect
Preformed (early)	
Histamine	Vasodilatation, increased vascular permeability, bronchoconstriction
Heparin	Anticoagulation
Lysosomal enzymes	Proteolysis
Neutrophil chemotactic factor	Chemotaxis of neutrophils
Eosinophil chemotactic factor	Chemotaxis of eosinophils
Newly synthesized (late)	
Leukotrienes (LTC4, LTD4, LTB4)	Vasodilatation, bronchoconstriction, chemotaxis
Prostaglandins, thromboxanes	Vasodilatation, platelet activation, bronchoconstriction
Platelet-activating factor	Platelet activation

chemotactic factor (NCF) and eosinophil chemotactic factor (ECF). These mediators have an effect on surrounding blood vessels and smooth muscle, and the attraction of certain types of white blood cells to the area, is responsible for the early clinical manifestations of type 1 hypersensitivity.

In addition to this *immediate response*, *allergen* exposure activates the metabolism of arachidonic acid within the mast cell via the lipooxygenase and cyclooxygenase pathways (see Chapter 10).

These pathways result in the synthesis of leukotrienes, prostaglandin, thromboxanes and chemotactic and activating factors (the previously

described 'slow-reactive substance of anaphylaxis' is a mixture of leukotrienes (LTC4 and LTD4). This second group of mediators, which are released late (usually 4–6 h after allergen exposure) have important clinical consequences in exacerbating disease. The physiological effects of early and late phase mediators are summarized in Table 10.1.

The clinical manifestations of type 1 hypersensitivity include allergic rhinitis, asthma, eczema and urticaria. Individuals predisposed to this group of conditions are referred to as 'atopic', and an atopic tendency can often be traced back through families. The effects of the mediators described (see Table 10.1) directly accounts for the clinical features of these conditions.

Allergic rhinitis is characterized by facial flushing, itching of the nose, mouth and eyes and watery nasal discharge (rhinorrhoea), following exposure to allergens such as pollens (hay fever) or dust mite (perennial rhinitis). Vasodilatation and transudation of vascular fluid cause the flushing and rhinorrhoea and the intense itching which is typical of the conditions caused by local histamine release, stimulating sensory nerve endings.

Allergens which penetrate further into the respiratory tree and lodge in the bronchi cause the features of *asthma* (see case study 9), with narrowing of the airways being caused both by constriction of smooth muscle and accumulation of fluid within the mucosa.

The most severe form of type 1 hypersensitivity is called an *anaphylactic reaction* and is a life-threatening condition. Generalized vasodilatation causes a fall in blood pressure and the patient often collapses with loss of consciousness. There may be other features such as skin rash, abdominal pain, vomiting, diarrhoea and breathing difficulty due either to bronchoconstriction or swelling (angiodema) affecting the throat. The clinical features result from the widespread activation of mast cells and circulating basophils releasing their mediators throughout the body. Basophils are a small subset of polymorphonuclear granulocytes which, like mast cells, bind IgE molecules and when these are cross-linked, release their mediators into the systemic circulation. This may occur in particularly sensitive individuals in response to any allergen, but until recently the most common cause was in response to parenterally administered protein antigens such as insect (e.g. bee/wasp) venom, or drugs (e.g. penicillin allergy). The recent rapid increase in the recognition of peanut allergy has resulted in this allergy now being the most common cause of anaphylactic reactions occurring outside hospital in the UK.

The most important aspect of the long-term management of a patient with type 1 hypersensitivity is the identification of the likely precipitating allergen and its careful avoidance where possible. However, complete allergen avoidance is not always possible and an understanding of the underlying mechanisms of the condition have led to rational approaches to drug therapy both in the acute stage and in long-term prevention.

Disodium cromoglycate is a mast cell stabilizer, which prevents mast cell degranulation and therefore release of mediators. Its use is confined to the prevention of allergic attacks and in order to be effective, it must be taken on a daily basis whether or not the patient is currently symptomatic.

Antihistamine preparations directly antagonize the action of the major mast cell mediator, histamine, and provide excellent symptomatic relief in a wide range of clinical conditions.

Corticosteroid preparations are useful in long-term management and may be given locally (e.g. via nasal spray) or systemically. Their appropriate use during acute severe attacks will prevent the occurrence of late-phase reactions.

Adrenaline (*epinephrine*) is the drug of choice for acute anaphylactic reactions. It will rapidly relieve airway obstruction and restore blood pressure. Many patients with a tendency to develop anaphylactic reactions carry self-administration systems containing adrenaline for emergency treatment.

Type 2 hypersensitivity

Type 2 hypersensitivity reactions are also mediated by antibody, but in contrast to type 1 reactions the antibodies involved are either of the IgG or IgM class. A characteristic of type 2 reactions is that the antibody response is directed against antigens that are expressed on cell surfaces and therefore the damage that results from these responses tends to be limited to a particular organ or cell type. The pathogenic antibodies in these reactions bind to cells via their Fab portion.

There are several possible consequences of antibody binding to cell surface antigens (Fig. 10.2). These are explained in detail in the sections below.

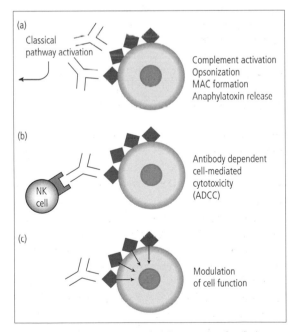

Fig. 10.2 Type 2 hypersensitivity involves the interaction of antibody with cell-bound antigen. This may have several consequences including (a) activation of the complement cascade; (b) recruitment of cytotoxic cells; or (c) modulation of cellular function.

Activation of complement system

Activation of the complement cascade at the surface of the cell leads to the production of the anaphylatoxins C3a and C5a, with recruitment of inflammatory cells to the area (see Chapter 5). Ultimately, the assembly of the terminal complement pathway components C5–C9 into the membrane attack complex (MAC) causes pore formation in the cell wall. Cellular damage is enhanced via the deposition of C3b on the cell wall (opsonization) which allows phagocytes to bind and release their lysosomal enzymes.

Antibody-dependent cell-mediated cytotoxicity

The direct interaction of the Fc portion of the bound antibody with Fc receptor-bearing cells (natural killer or NK cells, platelets, phagocytes) allows these cells to engage the target tissues, focusing their damaging effects onto the antigen-expressing cellular membrane. This is antibody-dependent cell-mediated cytotoxicity (ADCC, see also Chapter 6).

These two mechanisms, complement activation and ADCC, are part of the immune system's normal armamentarium for fighting infection. A normal response causes damage to cells bearing foreign (e.g. microbial or tumour) antigens. These responses may be considered to be abnormal or hypersensitive in two situations: when they are directed against an individual's own cellular antigens, or when the scale of the response to a foreign antigen is such that it causes damage to the individual's own cells disproportionately to the potential hazard of the antigen(s) concerned.

Typical examples of type 2 hypersensitivity include transfusion reactions, autoimmune haemolytic anaemia, hyperacute graft rejection, Goodpasture's syndrome and Graves' disease. Transfusion reactions and hyperacute graft rejections involve the recognition of truly foreign antigens and ought to be preventable in conditions with adequate blood grouping, tissue typing and cross-matching. In autoimmune haemolytic anaemia, the antibody is directed against 'self' blood group antigens, e.g. the rhesus system (see also Chapter 11).

Goodpasture's syndrome is characterized by autoantibodies to glomerular basement membrane (GBM) which can cause acute renal failure but the autoantibodies also react with pulmonary basement membranes causing severe pulmonary haemorrhage (see case study 8).

Antibody-mediated modulation of cellular function

Graves' disease is a good illustration of how antibody recognition of a cell surface antigen may result in modulation of the cell's function. The autoantibodies in this case are directed against the thyroid-stimulating hormone (TSH) receptor. The result is that the antibody mimics the effect of TSH and causes the gland to secrete an excess of thyroxine, causing clinical hyperthyroidism. In this condition, treatment is directed towards reducing the thyroid gland response using either antithyroid drugs or surgical resection.

Type 3 hypersensitivity

Type 3 reactions are also antibody mediated but in contrast to type 2 reactions, the antigenic targets of type 3 reactions are soluble and not cell membrane bound. The combination of soluble antigen and specific antibody, of IgG or IgM class, results in the formation of circulating *immune complexes*. These immune complexes circulate in the blood stream and as a consequence, the damage caused is not limited to one particular cell type or organ, but may occur at remote sites throughout the body.

Immune complexes are formed during normal antibody responses, as a means of assisting antigen disposal, but in the normal response are quickly cleared by the monocyte/macrophage system, in particular by the phagocytes of the liver, the Kupffer cells. When immune complexes are allowed to persist, either in the circulation or as deposits within tissues, they activate a number of inflammatory pathways and the response becomes hypersensitive. Antigens that cause immune complex formation may be either *exogenous* (infectious or environmental agents) or *endogenous* (self-antigens in autoimmune responses). Two classic examples of type 3 reactions demonstrate the effector mechanisms involved.

The *Arthus reaction* occurs in animals that have been repeatedly immunized with antigen, resulting in high levels of antigen-specific IgG. An intradermal injection of antigen causes the rapid local accumulation of immune complexes and a reaction, which peaks approximately 6–24 h later. The immune complexes cause local complement activation, with recruitment of polymorphonuclear phagocytes to the perivascular area. The release of lysosomal enzymes causes vascular damage resulting in oedema and haemorrhage which is seen as raised reddened areas on the skin.

Serum sickness is a condition that was seen in the preantibiotic era when patients were treated with large doses of antibody made in other animal species, e.g. horses. The 'foreign' immunoglobulin protein is antigenic and stimulates the production of antibodies and the formation of immune complexes. Serum sickness is minimized in modern antibody therapy by the use of monoclonal antibodies that have had their constant antigens modified to resemble the human antibody molecules (humanized antibody). It was characterized by urticaria, arthralgia (joint pain) and glomerulonephritis (inflammation of the renal glomeruli) and the reaction is reproduced by the injection of foreign antigen into experimental animals. Approximately 1 week after injection, antibody is formed which reacts with the persisting antigen to form immune complexes in the circulation (Fig. 10.3); this causes complement activation and the appearance of clinical features. Immunofluorescent examination demonstrates deposition of immune complexes and complement components within glomeruli and small blood vessels, and symptoms persist as long as immune complexes are detectable in the circulation. Repeated injections of antigen cause persistence of the immune complexes and the serum sickness syndrome.

A number of factors including complex size, duration of antigen exposure, host response and local tissue factors, determine when immune complexes persist and cause hypersensitive reactions.

Complex size

Large immune complexes generally activate complement efficiently and become coated with complement fragments (e.g. C3b). This enables blood cells, which bear the CR1 receptor to bind the immune complexes via C3b and transport them to the liver for degradation by Kupffer cells. Small immune complexes are also cleared by the reticuloendothelial system, whereas this pathway less efficiently deals with intermediate-sized immune complexes. Therefore, intermediate-sized immune complexes are most likely to persist and cause hypersensitivity reactions.

Duration of antigen exposure

Chronic antigen exposure allows continuous immune complex formation, analogous to the serum sickness model where repeated injections of antigen were administered. Clinical examples of conditions in which chronic antigen exposure is believed to be important in generating a type 3 response include infections (e.g. hepatitis B virus infection, bacterial endocarditis), or autoimmune conditions (e.g. systemic lupus erythematosus or SLE).

Host response

Host responses are considered important in both the production of immune complexes and in the failure to remove them from the circulation. Individuals

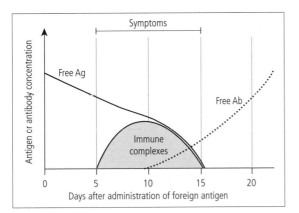

Fig. 10.3 Experimental serum sickness demonstrates the formation of immune complexes typical of type 3 reactions. Ab, antibody; Ag, antigen.

who preferentially produce low affinity antibody favour the production of small/intermediate immune complexes that are difficult to clear. In addition, individuals deficient in the early components of the classical pathway, C2 and C4, have an increased incidence of immune complex-mediated diseases (see Chapter 12). This is due to their reduced ability to cleave C3 via the classical pathway and therefore their diminished ability to coat circulating immune complexes effectively with C3b and so facilitate their disposal.

Local tissue factors

Local tissue factors are also important in determining where immune complexes are deposited and hence at which anatomical sites inflammation is focused. Haemodynamic factors such as *blood pressure, turbulence and filtration* affect immune complex deposition. High blood pressure and increased filtration rate contribute to immune complex accumulation in the renal glomerulus. Turbulence occurs particularly at sites of vessel bifurcation and increases immune complex deposition at these sites. Furthermore, physicochemical properties of the antigen or immune complex, including particle size, electrostatic charge and degree of glycosylation of complexes will also influence their ultimate tissue destination.

Classical examples of human disease involving type 3 hypersensitivity are immune complex-mediated glomerulonephritis, SLE and extrinsic allergic alveolitis. In immune complex-mediated glomerulonephritis (see also case study 11) the nature of the glomerular damage is greatly influenced by the type of immune complex involved and its rate of deposition. With rapidly deposited immune complexes, a proliferative response is likely (e.g. poststreptococcal glomerulonephritis), whereas with slower deposition, membranous glomerulonephritis occurs.

In extrinsic allergic alveolitis (e.g. allergic aspergillosis, see Chapter 7), the patient has preformed IgG antibody to inhaled allergen and develops an Arthus-type reaction in the alveoli upon exposure. The clinical features of acute alveolitis usually occur about 6 h after exposure, corresponding to immune complex formation and recruitment

of the damaging effector mechanisms, including complement and polymorphonuclear phagocytes.

Type 4 hypersensitivity

Type 4 hypersensitivity reactions are cell mediated and therefore differ from types 1–3 in that they cannot be transmitted from animal to animal by injection of serum. Type 4 responses are also referred to as 'delayed-type hypersensitivity' as the reactions occur 12 h or more following exposure to antigen. They are further classified into three subtypes based on the time of peak response, their clinical manifestations, and the cell types and sites of the body involved (Table 10.2). The common feature is the involvement of T lymphocytes (particularly the CD4+ T-helper subset), and antigen-presenting cells (APCs).

Contact hypersensitivity

This phenomenon is caused by low molecular weight antigens, which alone are incapable of eliciting an immune response. They act as *haptens* by binding to normal body proteins and in this form are capable of stimulating the immune system. The most common example is nickel hypersensitivity where affected individuals develop a hyperreactivity to nickel (which may be contained in costume jewellery, watches, trouser buttons, etc.). The rash that appears is red, itchy and eczematous but is usually limited to areas of skin which have been in direct contact with the metal. The immunological mechanism of the reaction is well defined and is divided into *sensitization* and *elicitation* phases. Nickel (or another low molecular weight hapten) is absorbed directly through the skin and is taken up

Table 10.2 Peak response times for the three forms of type 4 hypersensitivity reactions.

Type 4 reaction	Peak response
Contact	48–72 h
Tuberculin	48–72 h
Granulomatous	21–28 days

in the epidermis by *Langerhans' cells*. These are related to interdigitating dendritic cells and are APCs. They migrate from the skin to the paracortical regions of local lymph nodes where the antigen is presented to T cells, stimulating the development of memory T cells. This results in the sensitization of the individual to the allergen. In the elicitation phase, cutaneously absorbed antigen is presented to the memory T cells in the dermis causing the secretion of cytokines such as interferon γ (IFN-γ) and tumour necrosis factor α (TNF-α). These soluble mediators induce keratinocytes to express major histocompatibility complex (MHC) class II molecules and the intercellular adhesion molecule type 1 (ICAM-1) which is also induced on dermal endothelial cells. These two factors contribute to the recruitment of further lymphocytes and macrophages to the inflamed area and within 24 h, lymphocytes are entering the epidermis. By 48 h, the epidermis contains lymphocytes and macrophages and is oedematous, causing the clinical appearance of an eczematous rash. This sequence of events explains the mechanism of the patch test used in the clinical diagnosis of contact hypersensitivity.

Tuberculin hypersensitivity

In contrast to contact hypersensitivity, tuberculin hypersensitivity is a phenomenon chiefly involving the dermis (Fig. 10.4). Koch observed that when patients suffering from tuberculosis were administered an intradermal injection of tuberculin (an antigen derived from *Mycobacterium tuberculosis*) they suffered both a local and a systemic reaction. The local skin reaction is characterized by an area of induration and swelling and this response is now recognized as being mediated by sensitized lymphocytes.

This type 4 reaction is used clinically as a means of determining the sensitization status of individuals in tests for tuberculosis and leprosy. The *Mantoux test* and *Lepromin test* involve the intradermal injection of *M. tuberculosis* and *M. leprae* extracts, respectively. Following the intradermal injection of antigen, lymphocytes begin to accumulate around blood vessels at about 12 h and peak at approximately 48 h. There is a predominance of CD4+ cells, with a CD4+ : CD8+ ratio of 2 : 1. Macrophages accumulate in the dermis simultaneously with

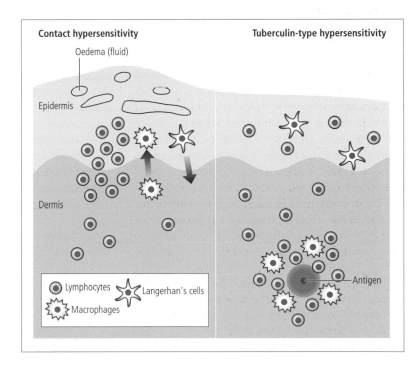

Fig. 10.4 The anatomical sites of contact (epidermal) and tuberculin-type (dermal) hypersensitivity (see text).

lymphocytes and there is migration of some Langerhans' cells from the epidermis. These cells are focused at the site of foreign antigen in the dermis; however, the response is usually self-limiting, as antigen is progressively removed by the immune system. Both contact sensitivity and tuberculous reactions may be contrasted with a type 3 Arthus reaction in that they do not involve antibody, complement activation or recruitment of neutrophils and other polymorphonuclear cells.

Granulomatous hypersensitivity

Where antigen persists, however, the initial tuberculin response may develop into a granulomatous hypersensitivity which is the most severe form of type 4 hypersensitivity and clinically the most important. Granulomas are collections of macrophages, some of which coalesce to form giant cells, surrounded by a cuff of small lymphocytes (see Chapter 5). The macrophages often have the appearance of epithelial cells, and are known as *epithelioid* cells. Granulomas are formed when the immune system fails to remove foreign antigen, which is then allowed to persist, usually within macrophages. Granuloma formation is not confined to skin reactions but occurs in many organs.

Studies of granulomatous conditions in experimental situations have focused attention on the factors involved in the initiation and persistence of type 4 lesions. Antigen presentation is associated with production of the cytokine interleukin 1 (IL-1) by APC, causing the activation of T cells, which in turn produce IL-2 and express the IL-2 receptor on their cell membrane. These events contribute to the proliferation of T cells and induction of the cellular response. High levels of IL-1 have been demonstrated in early experimental lesions, suggesting that macrophage production of this cytokine is an important early event in recruitment of cells for granuloma formation.

The activated T cells are predominantly of the T-helper 1 (Th1) phenotype, i.e. they preferentially produce IFN-γ and IL-2. They are therefore potent activators of monocytes/macrophages and of other T cells and hence contribute to the accumulation of the cells necessary for granuloma formation. In the

later stages of experimental lesions, TNF-α production appears to predominate over IL-1 production suggesting that there may be initial cellular recruitment followed by a maintenance phase which may be partially defined in terms of local cytokine production. The Th1/Th2 model, which was developed from the murine system has been helpfully applied to the understanding of some human disease; however, the human system has some important differences. Whilst T cells in mice clearly differentiate into either Th1 or Th2 cells, in humans it appears that T cells will express a bias towards one or other pole of this spectrum, but retain some heterogeneity in terms of cytokine secretion. Much has been learnt recently from newly recognized disorders of IFN-γ receptor expression. One must therefore be cautious in drawing simplistic analogies; however, there are some useful clinical examples to consider. The human conditions associated with significant immunological granuloma formation include *tuberculosis, leprosy, schistosomiasis* (see Chapter 7), *leishmaniasis* and *sarcoidosis*.

In pulmonary tuberculosis, much of the lung damage is due to granuloma formation. Reactivation of the disease, which is often seen in later life, is associated with an age-related reduction in memory T-cell function, allowing renewed mycobacterial growth.

Leprosy is an excellent example of how the immune status of an individual determines the clinical manifestation of disease. There are two major forms of leprosy, *tuberculoid* and *lepromatous leprosy*. Tuberculoid disease is largely asymptomatic and is characterized by hypopigmented (pale) areas of the skin which histologically appear as typical granulomatous lesions with few detectable mycobacteria. These patients have potent type 4 hypersensitivity responses to *M. leprae*, the CD4+ T-cell population being predominantly of the Th1 phenotype. This results in the more effective clearance of organisms. In lepromatous leprosy, there are widespread skin lesions containing numerous bacilli but few lymphocytes. These patients have a predominant Th2 phenotypic response to the organism (Th2 cells secrete IL-4, IL-5 and IL-10) and no clear granuloma formation. Consequently *M. leprae* are able to proliferate and disseminate more freely in lepromatous

Key points

1 Hypersensitivity defines situations where the immune system responds inappropriately or excessively to antigens which often appear harmless. The term hypersensitivity is often used interchangeably with allergy which literally means 'altered reactivity'.

2 Hypersensitivity responses are classified into four types based upon their different underlying mechanisms and clinical manifestations.

3 Type 1 hypersensitivity reactions are immediate and involve allergen, allergen-specific IgE and mast cells. In its most severe form, a type 1 hypersensitivity reaction leads to the development of systemic anaphylaxis which is a life-threatening condition.

4 Type 2 hypersensitivity reactions are also antibody mediated but, in contrast to type 1 reactions, the antibodies involved are either IgG or IgM. Type 2 reactions are directed against antigens expressed on the surface of the cell.

5 Type 3 hypersensitivity reactions are also antibody mediated but the antigenic targets of type 3 reactions are soluble and not cell membrane bound. The combination of soluble antigen and specific antibody results in the formation of circulating immune complexes.

6 In contrast to types 1–3, type 4 hypersensitivity reactions are cell mediated, commonly involving the participation of T lymphocytes and APCs.

leprosy and the patient suffers the systemic effects of the infection. Host response in the form of hypersensitivity may therefore be advantageous under certain circumstances.

Summary

A knowledge of the mechanisms of hypersensitivity reactions is important for the understanding of many disease processes. Different hypersensitivity responses may occur in a single disease process and they are best understood as physiological responses which happen either out of context or to an abnormally severe degree, resulting in deleterious effects to the host. Increased understanding of the cellular interactions involved in hypersensitivity is increasingly assisting us in the design of new therapeutic strategies.

Further reading

Chapel H., Haeney M., Misbah S. & Snowden N. (1999) *Essentials of Clinical Immunology* (4th edn). Blackwell Science Ltd., Oxford.

Janeway C.A., Travers P., Walport M. & Capra J.D. (1999) *Immunobiology: The Immune System in Health and Disease* (4th edn). Elsevier Science/Garland Publishing, Oxford.

Reeves W.G. & Todd I. (2000) *Lecture Notes in Immunology* (4th edn). Blackwell Science Ltd., Oxford.

CHAPTER 11

Autoimmunity

The role of the immune system is to protect the host against invading pathogens and to mount responses to them leading to their elimination. The immune response involves complex interactions between a variety of cell types. These include T lymphocytes, whose role is recognition of a pathogen and control of the immune response to it; B lymphocytes, which produce specific antibodies capable of recognizing and binding to the pathogen; and phagocytic and cytotoxic cells which destroy the pathogen.

The immune system is highly specific in the recognition of antigens and a critical feature is its ability to discriminate between self and foreign antigens. Self-reactivity is prevented by a number of processes which occur early during lymphocyte development. Under certain circumstances, these mechanisms break down and the body reacts against itself. This concept is known as *autoimmunity* and was first proposed by Paul Ehrlich in 1899 who gave it the name 'horror autotoxicus'. The earliest evidence for the existence of *autoimmune disease* was the identification of *autoantibodies* to red blood cells in a haematological complication of syphilis. It is now recognized that almost every organ and system of the body can be affected by autoimmune disease.

This chapter introduces the concept of *self-tolerance* and examines how its breakdown leads to the development of autoimmunity both at the cellular and humoral level. The spectrum of auto-immune diseases is described and factors pre-disposing individuals to autoimmune disease are discussed. Current and potential treatments for autoimmune conditions are considered.

Immunological tolerance

Immunological self-tolerance is the failure to respond to self-antigens. Tolerance occurs predomin-antly at the T-cell level and the thymus gland plays a critical role in 'educating' T cells to discriminate between self and non-self. Immature T cells arise in the bone marrow and migrate to the thymus for fur-ther development. T cells possess surface receptors which enable them to recognize antigens and an early event in T-cell maturation in the thymus is the rearrangement of the genes which code for these receptors (see Chapter 6). This gives rise to a vast repertoire of receptors able to bind to a wide range of antigens. Inevitably, some of these receptors will recognize self-antigens and the T cells which bear them are eliminated by a process called *apoptosis* in which the cells degrade their own DNA (see Chapter 4).

Some T cells which are reactive against self-antigens escape elimination in the thymus and are released into the general circulation. In this situation *peripheral tolerance* plays a role in protecting against self-reactivity, in which T cells are 'switched off' when they interact with antigen in the absence of other signals necessary for activation. Also, other regulatory T cells may suppress self-reactive T cells.

Autoimmune B cells can exist in the general circulation but they are prevented from mounting an antibody response by lack of appropriate T-cell help. Some B cells need to be tolerized directly and these are either deleted in the bone marrow or are rendered unresponsive.

As discussed later in this chapter, breakdown in tolerance is central to the development of autoimmunity. However, it should be emphasized that although many individuals mount autoreactive responses, only a few develop autoimmune diseases. This is probably because normal individuals can control the activity of autoreactive cells.

The spectrum of autoimmune diseases

Autoimmune diseases may be classified as either *organ-specific* where the autoantigen is localized in one organ only (e.g. thyroid peroxidase and thyroglobulin in Hashimoto's thyroiditis) or *systemic* where the autoantigen is widespread (e.g. components of the cell nucleus in systemic lupus erythematosus). The more common autoimmune

diseases together with their target antigens are shown in Table 11.1.

There is considerable overlap between the autoimmune diseases at either end of the spectrum. For example, patients with systemic lupus erythematosus (SLE) may have the clinical features of scleroderma and rheumatoid arthritis (RA), and patients with autoimmune thyroid disease quite often have gastric autoimmune disease. Such patients are said to have 'overlap syndrome'. However, there is usually little overlap between organ-specific and systemic diseases.

Different autoimmune processes may occur in the same tissue, leading to different clinical outcomes. For example, Hashimoto's thyroiditis involves the destruction of the thyroid cells resulting in hypothyroidism and is associated with immune recognition of thyroid peroxidase and thyroglobulin. Graves' disease involves the opposite effect of hyperthyroidism due to autoantibodies triggering the thyroid-stimulating hormone receptor. Conversely, different autoimmune processes affecting the same tissues may have similar clinical effects. Thus, Goodpasture's

Table 11.1 Autoimmune diseases, target autoantigens and HLA associations.

Diseases	Autoantigen	HLA type
Organ-specific		
Hashimoto's thyroiditis	Thyroid peroxidase and thyroglobulin	DR3, B8
Graves' disease	Thyroid-stimulating hormone receptor	DR3, B8
Pernicious anaemia	Intrinsic factor	DR4, DR2, DR3
Addison's disease	Secretory cells of adrenal cortex	DR3, B8
Type 1 (insulin-dependent) diabetes mellitus	Pancreatic islet cells	DR3, DR4, B8, B15
Goodpasture's syndrome	Glomerular and alveolar basement membrane	DR2, B7
Myasthenia gravis	Acetylcholine receptor	DR3, A1, B8
Pemphigus vulgaris	Intercellular component of epidermis	DR4, DR6
Bullous pemphigoid	Epidermal basement membrane	No known associations
Primary biliary cirrhosis	Bile ducts of liver	DR3, B8
Systemic		
Autoimmune haemolytic anaemia	Red blood cells, rhesus antigen	B8
Sjögren's syndrome	Extractable nuclear antigens	DR3, DR4, DR1, A1, B8
Rheumatoid arthritis	IgG rheumatoid factor	B44, B15
Dermatomyositis	Soluble nuclear proteins	DR3, B8, B14
Scleroderma	Nucleoli	DR5, B8
Mixed connective tissue disease	Ribonucleoprotein	DR4
Systemic lupus erythematosus	Double-stranded DNA	DR3, DR2, B5, B8

syndrome and SLE can both cause glomerulone-phritis, but through type II and III hypersensitivity mechanisms, respectively (see Chapter 10).

Much of what we know about autoimmune diseases comes from studies of animal models. Such models are disease-specific and exhibit some clinical and immunological features with similarities to the human conditions. Some disease models may occur spontaneously. For example, the BB rat and NOD mouse are models of type 1 (insulin-dependent) diabetes mellitus and spontaneously develop diabetes. The islets of Langerhans in the pancreas become infiltrated with lymphocytes and complete loss of the insulin-producing β-cells follows. Onset of the disease is associated with the presence of autoantibodies reacting with islet cell components. These features are similar to events occurring in the pancreas of diabetic human patients.

Another spontaneous model is the obese strain (OS) chicken which develops thyroiditis and auto-antibodies to thyroid components. Neonatal bursec-tomy (surgical resection of the bursa of fabricus to remove maturing B cells) dramatically reduces thyroiditis which suggests an important role for antibodies in the pathogenesis. Other animal models for autoimmunity can be induced experimentally. For example, injection of thyroglobulin produces thyroiditis in some susceptible mouse strains.

T lymphocytes and cytokines in autoimmunity

T helper (Th) cells are central to the generation of an immune response to both foreign and self-antigens. They recognize antigens on the surface of antigen-presenting cells (APC) in association with class II human leucocyte antigen (HLA) molecules, and are thus activated to produce a cascade of cytokines which control the immune response at various levels. Th cells can be classified according to the profile of cytokines they secrete. Th1 cells produce primarily interleukin 2 (IL-2) and interferon γ (IFN-γ) and are associated predominantly with cell-mediated immunity whereas Th2 cells produce IL-4, IL-5 and IL-10 and are implicated mainly in the control of antibody responses.

Th1 cytokines, although beneficial in the clearance of some pathogens, also produce deleterious

Table 11.2 Examples of aberrant HLA class II expression by epithelial cells in autoimmune diseases

Disease	Cells expressing class II
Autoimmune thyroid diseases	Thyroid epithelium
Type 1 diabetes mellitus	Pancreatic β-cells
Inflammatory bowel disease	Gut epithelium
Autoimmune protracted diarrhoea of infancy	Immature jejunal enterocytes
Alopecia areata	Hair follicular cells
Primary biliary cirrhosis	Bile duct epithelium
Sjögren's syndrome	Salivary ducts

effects in a number of models of autoimmunity. For example, mice manipulated experimentally to express IFN-γ in the islets of Langerhans spontaneously develop type 1 diabetes. In contrast, the systemic administration of IL-4 and IL-10 inhibits the onset of diabetes in the NOD mouse model. This would suggest a role for Th2 cells in the prevention of diabetes and a role for Th1 cells in disease pathogenesis.

A wide range of cytokines have been isolated from the joints of patients with RA. These include IL-1α, IL-1β, IL-6, tumour necrosis factor α (TNF-α), IL-8 and transforming growth factor (TGF). TNF is central to the production of other cytokines and in RA the cytokine network operates in series with TNF, promoting the secretion of IL-1 followed by IL-6. Blocking TNF action suppresses the production of most of the other proinflammatory cytokines, these effects being more profound than just blocking IL-1 alone.

Cytokines play an important role in regulating the expression of class II HLA molecules, which in turn may contribute to autoimmune pathogenesis. The aberrant expression of class II molecules by target epithelial cells was first reported in autoimmune thyroiditis but there is now a growing list of autoimmune diseases where abnormal epithelial expression has been observed (Table 11.2). It has been hypothesized that expression of class II on these cells enables them to present their own surface molecules to activated autoreactive T cells, thus bypassing the need for conventional APCs. IFN-γ is a strong inducer of class II expression. In auto-

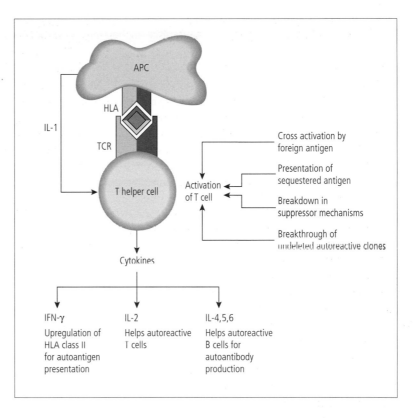

Fig. 11.1 Activation of autoreactive cells and the role of cytokines in autoimmunity.

immune thyroiditis, for example, it has been suggested that autoreactive T cells infiltrating the thyroid gland produce IFN-γ which causes the spread of class II expression through the gland, thus potentiating the autoimmune process. Figure 11.1 summarizes the role of activated Th cells and cytokines in the induction of autoimmunity.

Autoreactive T cytotoxic (Tc) cells are likely to contribute significantly to the tissue damage in some autoimmune diseases, e.g. type 1 diabetes and autoimmune thyroiditis.

B lymphocytes and antibodies in autoimmunity

B lymphocytes capable of producing autoantibodies are present in the normal human B-cell repertoire. Normal human serum contains natural autoantibodies of the immunoglobulin M (IgM) and IgG classes that can recognize a wide range of self-antigens including nuclear antigens and membrane

components. These natural autoantibodies are produced by a subset of B lymphocytes expressing a molecule called CD5, and are usually *polyreactive*, i.e. they recognize bacterial antigens and also show cross-reactivity with self components. However, in normal individuals these antibodies are thought not to be autoaggressive and may be beneficial in providing an early form of natural immunity to bacterial infections. Furthermore, natural autoantibodies may actually prevent pathological autoimmunity by binding to microbial epitopes that are similar or identical to epitopes of self antigens.

The production of autoantibodies by B cells is normally only possible when T lymphocytes recognize the self-antigen and produce the appropriate cytokines necessary for B-cell triggering. However the CD5+ B cells do not require T-cell help and these cells are found in increased numbers in SLE, multiple sclerosis, Hashimoto's thyroiditis and RA.

In contrast to natural polyreactive autoantibodies, specific disease-associated autoantibodies in the serum are helpful markers for diagnostic purposes and may be particularly useful for predicting disease onset. For example, autoantibodies to islet cell components are found several years prior to the onset of type 1 diabetes. Studies of first-degree relatives of type 1 diabetic patients have established that there is an increased risk for disease development in individuals who have antibodies to islet cell antigens, especially if the titre of the antibodies is high. Autoantibodies that are associated with the disease may or may not be directly pathogenic. The autoantibodies to cytoplasmic islet cell antigens are probably produced as a consequence of islet cell destruction and may not cause islet damage themselves. By contrast, other autoantibodies are directly involved in producing clinical disease, e.g. antibodies to the thyroid-stimulating hormone receptor in Graves' disease and antibodies to the glomerular and alveolar basement membrane in Goodpasture's syndrome (see case study 8).

Contributory factors in the aetiology of the autoimmune diseases

Genetics

Family studies

Much evidence for the role of genetic factors in autoimmune diseases has come from family studies. Familial tendencies have been seen in type 1 diabetes, autoimmune thyroid disease and RA. For example, relatives of patients with type 1 diabetes have a greater chance of developing the disease than age-matched controls. The genetic associations are complex with, for example, at least 15 genetic loci contributing to the susceptibility to type 1 diabetes.

Studies with identical and non-identical twins are useful for identifying genetic susceptibility. The disease concordance rate is higher in identical twins. For example, in type 1 diabetes disease concordance is up to 50% in identical twins compared to 5% in non-identical twins. However, the disease concordance rate in identical twins is never 100% which would suggest that environmental factors are also important in triggering the development of autoimmunity.

HLA associations

The genes of the HLA system are major determinants of the susceptibility to autoimmune disease. These genes code for cell surface molecules which serve as identity markers and play a major role in antigen recognition. The HLA system is the human form of the major histocompatibility complex (MHC) and comprises a set of tightly linked genes located on chromosome number 6. Autoimmune diseases are usually associated with the HLA class II alleles DP, DQ and DR. For example, 80–90% of patients with RA carry either the DR1 haplotype or one of three variants of the DR4 haplotype (Dw4, Dw14 or Dw15). Similarly, for type 1 diabetes, DR3 and DR4 lead to increased susceptibility, compared to DR2 and DR5 which are protective. Further details of HLA associations are given in Table 11.1.

The population of HLA genes characteristically displays the phenomenon of linkage disequilibrium —specific pairs of alleles of different HLA genes that are inherited together with a much higher frequency than expected by chance. It now appears that the HLA association of type 1 diabetes is not with DR3 and DR4 but with specific DQ alleles that are commonly inherited together with (in linkage disequilibrium with) DR3 or DR4.

It has been shown that HLA-DQ alleles that encode aspartic acid at position 57 of the β-chain in the peptide-binding site of the HLA molecule confer protection against type 1 diabetes, whereas alleles that encode valine, serine or threonine at this position are associated with susceptibility to IDDM.

Analyses of HLA disease associations are complex. Multiple gene loci may be involved in determining susceptibility. In many cases the gene(s) responsible may, as yet, be unidentified but in linkage disequilibrium with HLA alleles that are currently observed to be associated with disease susceptibility. Full elucidation requires an understanding of the molecular mechanisms that link the products of susceptibility genes, and their functions, to the disease process.

Hormone effects

The sex hormones have a major effect on the functioning of the immune system. Generally autoimmune diseases are more common in females and this has been demonstrated in animal models of SLE where the female sex hormones accelerate the disease process. Oestrogens can increase the level of antibody production by inhibiting suppression by T cells.

Environmental factors

Infectious agents
Autoimmune diseases can occur following chronic infection. An example is the development of rheumatic heart disease following infection with group A streptococci. Patients with leprosy or tuberculosis often have rheumatoid factors circulating in the blood.

Drugs and chemicals
Administration of L-dopa has been implicated in some cases of SLE and penicillamine can cause a variety of autoimmune diseases such as scleroderma and pemphigus vulgaris. Toxins such as silicon and vinyl chloride have also been associated with scleroderma and cigarette smoking, and exposure to hydrocarbon solvents has been linked to the development of Goodpasture's syndrome (see case study 8). Possible mechanisms whereby environmental agents may trigger autoimmunity are considered in the following section.

Mechanisms of autoimmunity

The stimulation of self-reactive lymphocytes is under tight control of the individual. Precisely how autoimmune disease develops is still uncertain in most instances, but a number of mechanisms have been proposed to explain how these controls might be bypassed either at the level of the T cells (see Fig. 11.1) or B cells.

Molecular mimicry

Some viral and bacterial proteins share antigenic epitopes with proteins of the host. In this way they may 'fool' the immune system into granting them free access because of the maintenance of self-tolerance. Conversely, an immune response mounted by the host against the epitope of the infectious

agent may cross-react with the mimicked host protein sequence leading to autoimmunity (Fig. 11.2a). An example is provided by the association of group A streptococci with rheumatic heart disease, in which cross-reactivity of anti-streptococcal antibodies with cardiac muscle has been demonstrated.

Provision of foreign T-cell epitopes

Another mechanism whereby T-cell help may be given to autoreactive B cells is by the linking of foreign antigens containing T-cell epitopes to host proteins (Fig. 11.2b). Some drugs and chemicals mentioned in the previous section may exert their effects in this way.

Release of sequestered antigens and exposure of cryptic epitopes

Some self-antigens are not normally exposed to the cells of the immune system and if released during adult life will be seen as 'foreign'. For example autoimmune responses to proteins released from a damaged eye can give rise to sympathetic ophthalmia (i.e. damage to the other eye).

APCs are constantly degrading antigens into peptide fragments for presentation. However, some self-epitopes are never normally exposed to thymic T cells to induce tolerance. These are referred to as *cryptic epitopes* and are essentially recognized as 'foreign', but are usually present at low densities and are therefore unable to activate autoreactive T cells. Responses to cellular stress, poorly controlled apoptosis, infection of APCs and activation of APCs by cytokines might alter the pattern of peptides presented so that cryptic epitopes become dominant and induce autoreactivity.

Failure of suppressive mechanisms

Failure to control autoreactive Th cells may be of major importance in the development of some autoimmune diseases. Controlling factors include the suppressive action of T cells and their lymphokine products, and of other cytokines and hormones. Breakdown in one or more of these factors may lead to an autoimmune response. For example,

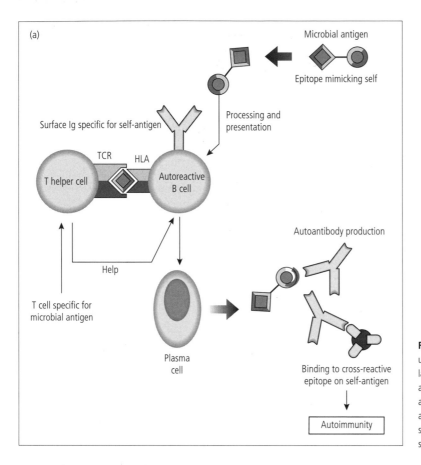

(a)

Microbial antigen

Epitope mimicking self

Surface Ig specific for self-antigen

Processing and presentation

TCR   HLA

T helper cell   Autoreactive B cell

Autoantibody production

Help

T cell specific for microbial antigen

Plasma cell

Binding to cross-reactive epitope on self-antigen

Autoimmunity

Fig. 11.2(a) Autoreactive B cells are usually unable to produce autoantibodies due to lack of appropriate T-cell help. Microbial antigens which share similar structures to self-antigens can prime T cells to provide help for autoreactive B cells. These cells are induced to secrete antibodies which can cross-react with self and microbial antigens.

removal of the thymus at birth from OS chickens exacerbates the development of thyroiditis, presumably due to the removal of T-cell control.

Anti-idiotype reactivity

During an immune response, antibodies produced against foreign antigens may stimulate the production of a second wave of antibodies directed against their antigen-binding sites (*idiotypes*). The *anti-idiotypes* may have binding sites which resemble the original epitope. In the case of viral infection, if an antibody is directed at a cell-binding virus component then an anti-idiotype antibody could itself combine with the host cell surface receptor for the virus. Such an anti-idiotype would then be classed as an autoantibody (Fig. 11.3). For example, it has been shown experimentally that anti-idiotypes to anti-

bodies directed against neuron-binding component of reovirus type 3 can themselves bind to neurons.

Immunotherapy of autoimmune diseases

The metabolic defects resulting from some organ-specific autoimmune diseases can be corrected by replacing the missing products of the defective organ. For example type 1 diabetes can be controlled by administration of insulin, and pernicious anaemia (see Chapter 14) by administration of vitamin B_{12}. Immunosuppressive and cytotoxic drugs are used to dampen down the autoimmune response but, because of the side-effects, tend only to be used in progressive or life-threatening disorders.

Newly emerging forms of therapy involve methods for re-establishing tolerance and manipulating T-cell recognition of autoantigens. Orally induced

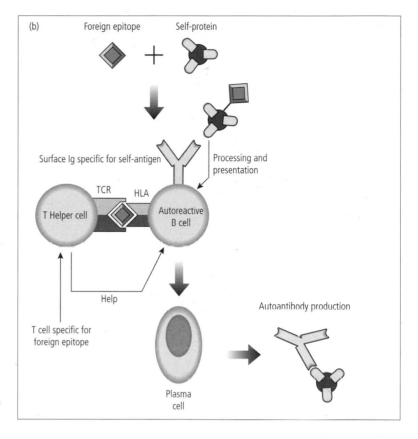

Fig. 11.2(b) Foreign antigens which link to self-antigens may be recognized by T cells which can therefore help the B cells to produce autoantibodies.

tolerance has proved effective in reducing the symptoms of autoimmune disease in animal models. Feeding myelin basic protein to animals with experimental allergic encephalomyelitis can prevent or reverse paralysis, and type II collagen is effective in delaying the onset of experimental RA. Small-scale clinical trials on humans have already shown promising results. Peptide epitopes of autoantigens administered experimentally can induce peptide-specific tolerance in neonates and can modify autoimmune responses in adults.

More direct approaches aim to remove the subsets of T cells or cytokines involved in the pathogenesis of autoimmune disease. Monoclonal antibodies against the CD4 molecule of T cells have been used in clinical trials of patients with RA and multiple sclerosis (MS). Unfortunately, anti-CD4 therapy is non-specific and might produce general immune suppression if administered over prolonged periods of time. Monoclonal antibodies against cytokines are showing promising results as immunotherapeutic agents. Anti-IFN-γ can prevent experimental autoimmune thyroiditis and diabetes in NOD mice. Collagen-induced arthritis in mice may be prevented by the administration of anti-TNF-α monoclonal antibodies.

Anti-TNF antibodies have proven effective in clinical trials of patients with RA by helping to block the inflammatory cytokine network. Patients showed a reduction in joint swelling, stiffness and other clinical symptoms, and a decline in serum levels of rheumatoid factors and markers of inflammation. The antibody was well tolerated by the patients, and repeated therapy following relapse was successful.

Summary

Autoimmune disease is the end result of a number of highly complex interconnecting immune reactions.

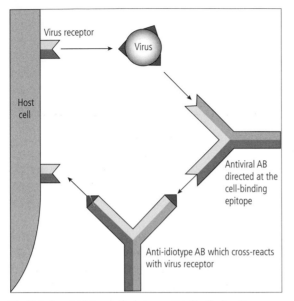

Fig. 11.3 An anti-idiotype antibody, to an antiviral antibody, acting as an autoantibody. In this instance there is 'molecular mimicry' between the idiotype and the autoantigen.

However, considerable advances have been made in recent years in understanding how these auto-immune reactions may arise.

Family studies and HLA gene associations have been useful in identifying those individuals who are at risk of developing disease. The innovation of molecular biology techniques should enable further characterization of these disease susceptibility genes as well as looking for associations elsewhere in the genome. Much emphasis is being placed on the role of the environment in disease induction, particularly with viral infection and by using highly specific molecular analysis it is possible to identify traces of viral DNA that may provide important clues.

The ultimate goal in immunotherapy is to arrest disease and return the individual to a state of tolerance. Considerable research efforts are being focused on the mechanisms of tolerance and how these mechanisms are bypassed or deficient for certain autoantigens. Manipulation of the cytokine network using monoclonal antibodies should be useful in increasing our understanding of auto-immune diseases and for the therapy of those diseases where the target autoantigen is not yet known.

Key points

1 A critical feature of the immune system is its ability to discriminate between foreign and self-antigens (i.e. exercise self-tolerance). Autoimmunity occurs when mechanisms of tolerance break down.

2 Autoimmune diseases are classified as organ-specific (autoantigen located in one tissue) or systemic (autoantigen is widespread). Animal models have been useful in understanding autoimmune diseases.

3 Autoimmunity develops at the cellular and humoral levels. Autoreactive T cells and the cytokines they secrete are important in the induction of autoimmunity. Autoreactive B cells produce autoantibodies to self-components. These autoantibodies may or may not be directly pathogenic.

4 A number of factors influence the susceptibility of an individual to autoimmune disease. These include genetic, hormonal and environmental (infectious agents and drugs) factors.

5 Mechanisms which lead to autoimmunity include mimicry between foreign and self-antigens, failure of suppressive mechanisms and release of self-antigens not normally exposed to the immune system.

6 Improvements in our understanding of autoimmune pathogenesis are leading to the application of new forms of therapy (e.g. re-establishment of tolerance, or inhibition of the activity of T cells or cytokines).

Further reading

Janeway C.A., Travers P., Walport M. & Capra J.D. (1999) Autoimmunity: responses to self antigens. In: *Immunobiology: The Immune System in Health and Disease* (4th edn), pp. 490–509. Churchill Livingstone/Garland.

Roitt I., Brostoff J. & Male D. (1998) Autoimmunity and autoimmune disease. In: *Immunology* (5th edn), pp. 367–379. Mosby, London.

Steinman L. (1993) Autoimmune disease. *Scientific American* **269**: 74–83.

Immunodeficiency

The immune system is composed of cells (B and T lymphocytes, monocytes and neutrophils) and their secretory products (antibodies, cytokines and serum complement). These function in an integrated manner for host defence against foreign microorganisms and the generation of inflammatory responses. Although no single component functions without the participation of others, four conceptually different systems for host defence can be identified —*humoral immunity, cell-mediated immunity, phagocytosis* and *complement*. Deficiencies of each of the functional systems occur, some on the basis of genetically determined traits, others due to the effects of the environment such as exposure to drugs (e.g. corticosteroids or cyclosporin A) or viral infections (e.g. the human immunodeficiency virus (HIV), measles virus or Epstein–Barr virus).

Understanding the physiological basis of immune deficiency has contributed to an understanding of how the immune system serves to protect the normal host from infection. In fact, the biological significance of many host defence functions has been defined by recognition of the specific problems that occur in patients with inborn errors of individual components of host defence.

This chapter will briefly illustrate how abnormalities of individual components lead to increased susceptibility to infection and other illnesses. Specific examples of immunodeficiency states are selected to illustrate principles. The following sections should therefore be regarded as illustrative rather than comprehensive.

Drug- or virus-induced immunodeficiency is not discussed as these topics are considered elsewhere (see Chapter 9 and case study 4). It is worth noting that some immunodeficiency states are also associated with an increased incidence of certain forms of cancer. This subject is dealt with more fully in Chapters 21–23.

Deficiency of humoral (antibody-mediated) immunity

X-linked agammaglobulinaemia

X-linked agammaglobulinaemia (XLA) is the prototypic disorder of humoral immunity. XLA results from a deficiency of the enzyme Bruton's tyrosine kinase (Btk) and B-lymphocyte development is arrested at the stage of pre-B cells. Males with this disease do not have mature immunoglobulin-bearing B lymphocytes in peripheral blood, do not have plasma cells or secondary lymphoid follicle formation in lymphoid tissues, and have severe hypogammaglobulinaemia (reduced levels of immunoglobulin in blood). No other compartment of immune function is affected by lack of Btk. In particular, T-cell function and cell-mediated immunity are completely intact. Therefore, individuals with XLA serve as a model for discerning the role of antibody in host defence.

The *Btk* gene has been mapped to the X chromosome, and XLA is therefore not the result of abnormal structural genes on the somatic chromosomes that

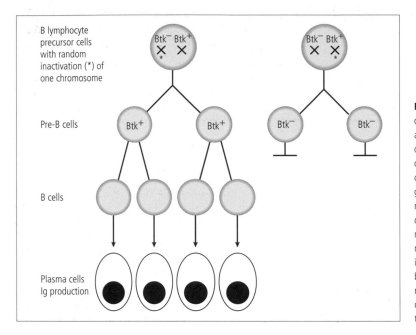

B lymphocyte precursor cells with random inactivation (*) of one chromosome

Pre-B cells

B cells

Plasma cells Ig production

Fig. 12.1 B lymphocyte growth and differentiation in a female carrier of X-linked agammaglobulinaemia. Early in embryological development, inactivation of one of the X chromosomes occurs in each cell. If the chromosome carrying the abnormal *Btk* gene (*Btk⁻*) is inactivated (*), *Btk* function is normal and subsequent B-cell growth and differentiation of the daughter cells occur normally. If the chromosome carrying the normal gene (*Btk⁺*) is inactivated, *Btk* function is abnormal and B-cell differentiation is blocked. Carrier females are immunologically normal because the surviving B cells can diversify and grow sufficiently for those cells that never develop.

encode the immunoglobulins themselves. An interesting demonstration of the X chromosome effect on B-lymphocyte differentiation is observed in the female carriers of XLA, all of whom are immunologically normal. In normal females, one of the two X chromosomes in each cell is randomly inactivated. This is also observed in all of the cells of XLA carrier women, except among their B lymphocytes. The latter cells all inactivate a single X chromosome, the one with the defective *Btk* gene. Lack of expression of the normal gene blocks B-cell differentiation, and therefore only the B cells with the normal X chromosome active are able to differentiate fully (Fig. 12.1). Analysis of X chromosome activation patterns of peripheral blood was used to determine carrier status, even before abnormalities in the *Btk* gene were identified as the cause of XLA.

The differential diagnosis of hypogammaglobulinaemia in infancy includes transient hypogammaglobulinaemia of infancy, immunoglobulin deficiency with increased immunoglobulin M (IgM), severe combined immunodeficiency disease (SCID) and rare cases of HIV infection. Quantitation of B and T lymphocytes in peripheral blood is helpful in distinguishing among these possibilities. Boys with XLA have no detectable B lymphocytes but have

normal numbers of T lymphocytes. In contrast, infants with transient hypogammaglobulinaemia generally have normal numbers of B and T lymphocytes; children with SCID have decreased numbers of T lymphocytes with normal, decreased or increased numbers of B cells; and children with HIV infection have decreased numbers of CD4+ T lymphocytes.

Boys with XLA are usually protected from infection by transplacentally acquired maternal IgG for their first 3–4 months of life (Fig. 12.2). Thereafter, chronic or recurrent bacterial and viral infections are the predominant clinical manifestation of XLA. Otitis media, pneumonia (Fig. 12.3), diarrhoea and sinusitis occur most often, usually in combination with each other. Infections with heavily encapsulated bacteria such as *Streptococcus pneumoniae* and *Haemophilus influenzae* are common because the host defence against these organisms relies upon the ability of antibody to bind to the polysaccharide capsule with subsequent complement activation and phagocytosis (opsonization). Infections may begin on mucosal surfaces, but are not limited to them because there is absence of serum immunoglobulin. As a result, localized bacterial infections may be spread through the blood stream to

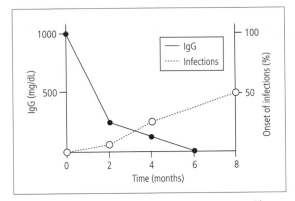

Fig. 12.2 Boys with X-linked agammaglobulinaemia are protected from infection during the first few months of life by transplacentally acquired maternal IgG. As the maternal IgG levels fall (half-life of IgG is approximately 23 days), there is an increasing incidence of infections.

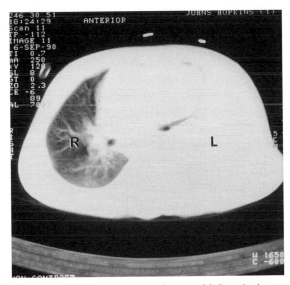

Fig. 12.3 CT scan of a child with X-linked agammaglobulinaemia who presented with pneumococcal pneumonia and empyema predominantly affecting the left lung. The pneumonia in the left lung (L) is represented as a pale area on the CT scan and may be compared with the relatively normal appearance of the right lung (R).

other tissues such as the meninges, joints and bones.

Patients with XLA generally recover uneventfully from viral infections, but not without exception. Enteroviruses (such as coxsackie virus, echovirus and poliovirus), which usually cause a self-limiting mild gastroenteritis in normal children, are prone

to cause chronic disseminated infections in XLA patients. Chronic hepatitis, meningoencephalitis (inflammation of the meninges and brain) and dermatomyositis (coexistent inflammation of skin and muscle) can result from enterovirus infections. These are often fatal, although therapy with γ-globulin containing virus-specific antibodies may be helpful.

Selective IgA deficiency

This provides an important contrast to XLA. In this disorder, individuals have a complete or almost complete lack of serum and mucosal IgA, but have normal levels of all other immunoglobulin classes and have normal cell-mediated immune function. Many of the clinical features of this disease can be explained by the unique biological properties of IgA. It is the predominant immunoglobulin class on mucosal surfaces, although IgA comprises only 15% of immunoglobulin in serum. IgA is secreted onto mucosal surfaces as a macromolecular complex consisting of two IgA molecules joined to a J chain and a secretory component. The majority of patients with IgA deficiency lack both serum and secretory IgA, but there are rare cases in which there is a deficiency of secretory but not serum IgA.

Unlike the major serum immunoglobulin classes, IgG and IgM, IgA is largely silent as a mediator of inflammatory responses. It does not activate complement or promote opsonization, but functions in antimicrobial defence by inhibiting microbial adherence and by neutralizing viruses and toxins. IgA also has an important role in antigen clearance, preventing soluble antigens from penetrating the mucosa and entering the systemic circulation.

Some patients with selective IgA deficiency have an increased susceptibility to infection, although there is disagreement about the relative risk of infection that IgA deficiency imposes upon the host. Because IgA is the predominant immunoglobulin on mucosal surfaces and only a minor component of serum immunoglobulin, most infections in IgA-deficient patients are confined to the mucosal surfaces of the respiratory tract (e.g. otitis media, sinusitis, bronchitis and pneumonia) and gastrointestinal tract (e.g. viral gastroenteritis), and systemic infections such as meningitis and bacterial sepsis are no more common than among the general population.

It is interesting that IgA-deficient patients also appear to have an increased susceptibility to atopic and autoimmune diseases (see Chapters 10 and 11). Atopic disorders such as allergic rhinitis, asthma, urticaria, eczema and food allergy, occur in 20–30% of individuals with IgA deficiency. It has been postulated that lack of secretory IgA allows inhaled and ingested antigens to penetrate the mucosal epithelium and to elicit allergic antibody (IgE) responses in the bronchial and gastrointestinal lymphoid tissues. A particularly hazardous allergic reaction in IgA-deficient patients is the development of anaphylactic reactions following the infusion of plasma or γ-globulin. The IgA in these products is recognized as a foreign protein in individuals who have no detectable IgA.

A variety of autoimmune diseases have also been associated with selective IgA deficiency. These include juvenile rheumatoid arthritis, systemic lupus erythematosus, autoimmune thyroiditis and pernicious anaemia. The precise mechanisms leading to these clinical manifestations of IgA deficiency cannot be fully explained by the absence of IgA antibodies. It has been hypothesized that disordered immune regulation underlies both IgA deficiency and susceptibility to autoimmune disease. The structural genes for IgA are intact in virtually all IgA-deficient patients, while abnormalities of helper T lymphocytes and cytokine production have been demonstrated. These observations suggest that factors other than the serum IgA level are important in determining the clinical expression of this disease.

Deficiency of cell-mediated (T-cell) immunity

DiGeorge syndrome

DiGeorge syndrome is a genetically determined abnormality that results from abnormal neural crest migration into the third and fourth pharyngeal pouches during early fetal development. The majority of cases are caused by a deletion of the chromosomal region 22q11.2, but the specific causative gene or genes in that region have not yet been identified.

This deletion causes a number of congenital anomalies, including abnormal development of the thymus gland. Patients may have thymic hypoplasia (underdevelopment) or aplasia (thymus gland fails to develop). Since the thymus is the gland within which T lymphocytes develop, thymic hypoplasia leads to T-lymphocyte deficiency. All T-cell subpopulations are affected equally, so that there is deficiency of both CD4 helper cells and CD8 cytotoxic cells. Affected infants have low levels of lymphocytes in the blood circulation (the majority of peripheral blood lymphocytes are T cells) and are depleted of lymphocytes in the paracortical areas of lymph nodes and spleen. The deficiency of cell-mediated immunity results in increased susceptibility to infections with fungi, the protozoan *Pneumocystis carinii*, and *Mycobacterium* spp., because these organisms are intracellular pathogens. That is, they are ingested by monocytes and other phagocytic cells, but are not easily killed without the participation of T lymphocytes. DiGeorge syndrome patients are also highly susceptible to viral infection because they lack cytotoxic T cells which kill virus-infected host cells (Chapter 9). As a result, relatively common viruses such as varicella-zoster virus (chickenpox) and rotavirus (gastroenteritis) may cause fatal infections in affected children. Most patients with DiGeorge syndrome have sufficient residual T cells to allow normal or near normal growth and differentiation of B lymphocytes.

Severe combined immunodeficiency

SCID describes a group of disorders, which are characterized by severe functional abnormalities of both B and T lymphocytes. Individuals with this disorder lack virtually all humoral and cell-mediated immune function. They are susceptible to the widest possible array of bacterial, viral, fungal and protozoan pathogens. If untreated, most die of infections within the first year of life.

A number of underlying defects have been identified, each of which is able to produce the SCID phenotype. A congenital absence of lymphoid stem cells leads to complete deficiency of lymphocytes and thus to SCID. However, it is interesting that many of the known causes of SCID are the result of

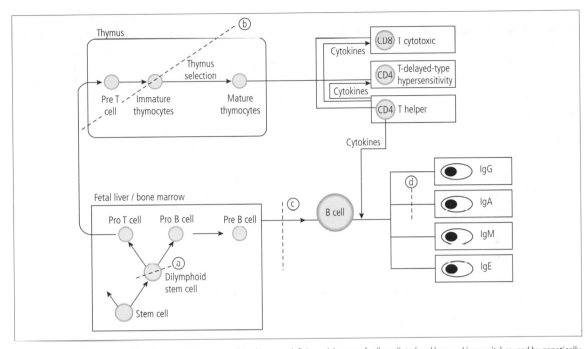

Fig. 12.4 Primary deficiencies of lymphocytes. (a) Severe combined immunodeficiency (absence of cell-mediated and humoral immunity) caused by genetically determined absence of lymphoid stem cells; (b) DiGeorge syndrome (decreased numbers or absence of T lymphocytes) caused by thymic aplasia or hypoplasia. Because T helper lymphocytes produce cytokines that are necessary for B-cell development, there may be associated defects in humoral immunity; (c) X-linked agammaglobulinaemia (absence of humoral immunity) caused by deficiency of *Btk* with block in B-lymphocyte differentiation; (d) selective IgA deficiency, aetiology unknown in most cases.

defects in T lymphocytes with secondary abnormalities of the B lymphocytes. For example, a defect in the gene encoding the cytokine receptor γ_c chain (cytokines or interleukins are growth and differentiation factors largely produced by T lymphocytes, and the γ_c chain is common to receptors for interleukins 2, 4, 7, 9 and 15) leads to SCID. In these cases, the near total arrest of T-lymphocyte development prevents helper T lymphocyte production of cytokines that are essential for B-lymphocyte growth and differentiation. Such patients can be treated by transplanting T lymphocytes from a normal individual. As the donor T lymphocytes mature, they secrete cytokines and allow the recipient's own B cells to develop. The relationship between T and B lymphocyte deficiences is outlined in Fig. 12.4.

Deficiency of phagocytic cell function

Neutrophils together with monocytes and macro-

phages are the most important of the body's cells that possess the ability to phagocytose foreign antigens and microorganisms. Many phagocytic cells are mobile and can move from the blood stream through tissues to the site of microbial invasion or inflammation, while other phagocytic cells are fixed in the spleen and lymph nodes where they clear microorganisms and other particulate matter from the blood and lymphatic circulation, respectively.

Monocytes also have the ability to serve as antigen-presenting cells and to secrete a variety of pro-inflammatory substances including cytokines and complement components. In order to function properly, phagocytic cells must attach to a substrate (*adherence*), move through tissues toward the site of microbial invasion (*chemotaxis*), attach to opsonized microbes and ingest them (*phagocytosis*), and kill the microbes (*intracellular killing*). Abnormalities of any of these steps will lead to deficiency in host defence.

Table 12.1 Leucocyte adhesion deficiency.

α-chain	β-chain	Function
CD11a(α_L)	CD18(β_2)	LFA-1 mediates cellular adhesion for interactions of immune cells
CD11b(α_M)	CD18(β_2)	CR3 mediates phagocytosis of C3bi-coated targets
CD11c(α_X)	CD18(β_2)	p150, 95 mediates adhesion of phagocytes to substrate and to C3bi

Leucocyte adhesion deficiency results from a defect in a gene on chromosome 21 encoding the β-chain (CD18). The gene cluster for α-chains is on chromosome 16.

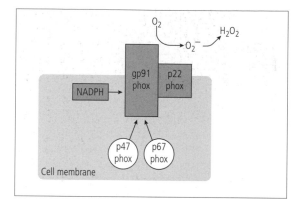

Fig. 12.5 NADPH oxidase system. Chronic granulomatous disease results from mutation in either the *gp91-phox* (encoded by the X chromosome), *p22-phox* (chromosome 16), *p47-phox* (chromosome 7) or *p67-phox* (chromosome 1) subunits of the NADPH oxidase assembly. Cytochrome b$_{558}$ is the membrane-bound heterodimeric complex of *gp91-phox* and *p22-phox*; *p47-phox* and *p67-phox* are cytosolic components. When the NADPH oxidase system functions normally, molecular oxygen is reduced to superoxide anion (O_2^-) which leads to the formation of H_2O_2.

Leucocyte adherence deficiency

This is an autosomal recessive trait that results from the lack of expression of the CD11/CD18 family of leucocyte-associated *integrin* molecules [CD11a/CD18 (LFA-1), CD11b/CD18 (Mac-1 or complement receptor 3) and CD11c/CD18 (p150,95)] necessary for phagocyte adherence (Table 12.1). The disease results from a defect in the gene encoding the β-chain common to each of these glycoproteins. The inability to adhere to tissue substrate impairs leucocyte mobility. Affected individuals have an increase in the number of circulating blood leucocytes because the cells cannot adhere to vascular endothelium (see Chapter 5). They also have difficulty mobilizing those leucocytes to the sites of infection and are unusually susceptible to bacterial infections, especially those that begin along body surfaces such as the skin, gingivae, perirectal area and the lungs.

Chronic granulomatous disease

Chronic granulomatous disease results from a different abnormality of phagocyte function, the inability to kill ingested microorganisms. In the normal individual, ingestion of a microorganism by the phagocytic cell results in activation of the myeloperoxidase–H$_2$O$_2$–halide system by which molecular oxygen is reduced to superoxide through a series of reactions involving reduced nicotinamide adenine dinucleotide phosphate (NADPH) oxidase.

The superoxide in turn undergoes further reactions leading to the generation of reduced oxygen derivatives such as hydrogen peroxide and hydroxyl radicals. Myeloperoxidase catalyses the reaction of hydrogen peroxide with chloride to create hypochlorite ions. The net effect of these toxic derivatives of reduced molecular oxygen is to kill microorganisms within the phagocytic vacuole. Individuals with chronic granulomatous disease lack one of the components of the NADPH oxidase system (Fig. 12.5), and are therefore unable to kill most ingested microorganisms. Their phagocytic cells have normal mobility and normal phagocytosis, and microorganisms are effectively trapped within phagocytic cells. However, because the microorganisms cannot be killed, granulomas (see Chapters 5 and 10) and abscesses form within various tissues including the skin, lymph nodes, spleen and liver (Figs 12.6 and 12.7).

The complement system

The complement system is composed of a large number of serum proteins that act in a cascade to mediate defensive and inflammatory reactions (see Chapter 5). The majority of the biologically

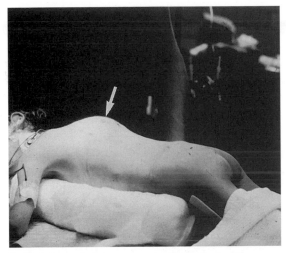

Fig. 12.6 Paravertebral abscess represented by an area of swelling (arrowed) in a boy with chronic granulomatous disease. The abscess in this case was the result of infection with the fungal organism *Aspergillus fumigatus*.

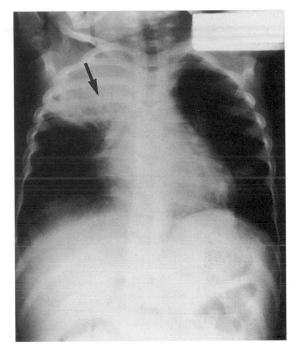

Fig. 12.7 Chest radiograph from a child with chronic granulomatous disease. The patient had previously been immunized with bacillus Calmette–Guérin (BCG). This is a live attenuated strain of the organism *Mycobacterium bovis* which has been used for the vaccination of children against tuberculosis. The patient developed pneumonia, shown on the radiograph as an area of opacity in the right upper lobe (arrowed). Later, the pneumonia was shown to be the result of infection with the BCG organism. In the normal host BCG is non-pathogenic; however, in patients with chronic granulomatous disease it may produce severe, potentially life-threatening, infections.

significant effects of the complement system are mediated by the third component (C3) and the terminal components (C5–C9). However, in order to perform their biological functions, C3 and C5–C9 must first be activated by other complement components via either the classical or alternate pathway. The classical pathway is activated by antigen–antibody complexes; the alternate pathway can be activated by molecules with repeating chemical structures such as bacterial polysaccharides or lipopolysaccharides and does not require specific antibody. Once activated, C3 can be covalently bound to the surface of an invading microorganism, thereby making it more susceptible to phagocytosis (opsonization). C5 can initiate formation of a membrane attack complex, a multimolecular assembly of C5b, C6, C7, C8 and C9, that inserts into cell membranes and thereby lyses the target cell.

Patients with a genetically determined deficiency of a complement component generally have an increased susceptibility to bacterial infection. The kind of bacteria that most often cause these infections depends upon the role of the specific complement component that is missing. For example, deficiencies of the early components (C1, C4, C2 and C3) interfere with the opsonic action of complement,

and affected individuals have increased susceptibility to infection from heavily encapsulated bacteria (e.g. *S. pneumoniae*, *H. influenzae*) for which opsonization is the primary host defence (Fig. 12.8). Individuals with deficiencies of the terminal components (C5–9) have an increased susceptibility to microorganisms against which the bacteriolytic actions of complement are most important. These include Gram-negative bacteria, particularly *Neisseria* species. Some individuals with complement deficiency also have a propensity to develop autoimmune disease, including systemic lupus erythematosus (see Chapter 11), and immune complex-mediated disease (see Chapter 10) such as immune complex glomerulonephritis.

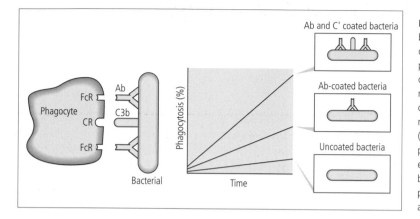

Fig. 12.8 Host defence against encapsulated bacteria involves the coordinated interaction of antibody (Ab), complement (C') and phagocytes. Ab binds to the extracellular capsule, leaving the Fc portion of the Ab molecule available to bind to Fc receptors (FcR) on phagocytes (opsonization). C' is activated most efficiently via the classical pathway (by bound Ab), but also via the alternate pathway (by bacterial polysaccharides). In either case, C3b is covalently bound to the bacterial surface. Ingestion of bacteria by phagocytes is enhanced by binding to FcR and complement receptors (CR).

Key points

1 Immunodeficiency can be genetically determined or acquired by drug treatment or viral infection (e.g. HIV).

2 Genetically determined deficiencies of each of the four main components of the immune system (T lymphocytes, B lymphocytes, phagocytes and complement) can be identified.

3 Immunodeficiency results in varying degrees of susceptibility to infection and other illnesses. The precise nature of this susceptibility depends upon the nature of the immune defect.

4 Because of the integrated nature of the immune system, a deficiency in one component can affect the function of another.

Summary

This chapter has described deficiencies of individual components of the immune system. More than 50 genetically determined defects have been identified, affecting virtually all individual components of the immune system. However, it is important to recognize that each of these discrete deficiencies of cells or their products will have multiple effects on immune function because of the interactive nature of the components. For example, deficiency of antibody interferes with activation of the complement cascade via the classical pathway. The secondary deficiency of complement activation, as well as the primary deficiency of antibody, impair opsonization and thereby interfere with the function of phagocytic cells. Study of the primary immunodeficiency diseases has helped our understanding of the complex nature of host immune defence, and its role in the pathophysiology of disease.

Further reading

Fischer A., Cavazzana-Calvo M., De Saint Basile G. *et al.* (1997) Naturally occurring primary deficiencies of the immune system. *Annual Review of Immunology* **15**: 93–124.

Ochs H.D., Smith C.I.E. & Puck J.M. (1999) *Immunodeficiency Diseases. A Molecular and Genetic Approach.* Oxford University Press, New York.

Puck J.M. (1997) Primary immunodeficiency diseases. *Journal of the American Medical Association* **278**: 1835–1841.

WHO Scientific Group (1997) Primary immunodeficiency diseases. *Clinical Experimental Immunology* **109** (suppl.): 1–28.

Transplantation Immunology

Transplantation is the relocation of cells, tissues or organs. An autologous transplant or *autograft* involves relocation within the same individual (e.g. the use of skin tissue from one part of the body to repair damage in another; the removal, modification and restoration of bone marrow to the same individual). In an *isograft* relocation is from a donor to a genetically identical (*syngeneic*) recipient. Unfortunately few individuals have identical twins and therefore in clinical practice, the vast majority of transplants are *allografts* between genetically different (*allogeneic*) donors and recipients. To the recipient (or host) the graft is 'foreign' and the immune system of the host is stimulated to attack and destroy the graft (graft rejection). The most significant problem in improving the success rate of transplantation is that of minimizing and controlling graft rejection. Unfortunately, many transplants that are clinically indicated are not possible because of the shortage of suitable donor organs. This has stimulated research into transplantation between animals of different species (*xenografts*), particularly grafts from pigs to humans. The genetic (*xenogeneic*), immunological and more general physiological differences between donor and recipient are complex and need to be more clearly understood before the significant problems of xenograft rejection can be resolved (Fig. 13.1).

Types of rejection

Allograft rejection most commonly occurs several days to weeks after transplantation. This is referred to as *acute allograft rejection*.

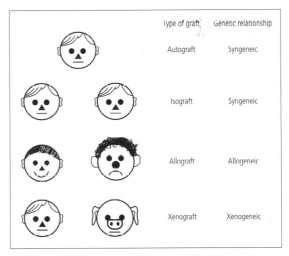

Fig. 13.1 There are several types of graft which differ in the genetic relationship between donor and recipient.

A much more rapid immune response is sometimes encountered. This *hyperacute rejection* can take place within 24 h of transplantation and results from the presence in the host of preformed antigraft antibodies. These antibodies on encountering graft antigens, activate complement and stimulate an acute inflammatory response (see Chapter 5) against the graft. The presence of preformed antibodies implies the presence of memory B cells, formed by a previous exposure to antigens present on the graft. There are three ways in which the host might have been previously exposed to antigens from another individual.

• Through repeated blood transfusions leading to exposure to surface antigens on donor white blood cells which are common to graft antigens.

• In females, through exposure during pregnancy to fetal antigens, encoded by paternally inherited genes, which are common to antigens on the graft.

• Through a previous graft displaying antigens which are common to the newly transplanted organ.

Fortunately hyperacute rejection is normally avoided through blood grouping and monitoring for the presence of antigraft antibodies in the potential host prior to transplantation.

Chronic rejection takes place over a much longer time scale (months or years). The mechanisms of this process are still not fully understood, but may include more general, long-term physiological damage to the graft in addition to specific immunological rejection.

Characteristics of acute allograft rejection

Early studies of acute allograft rejection in the 1940s revealed key aspects of the mechanism of rejection. Studies of skin grafts in mice showed that grafts between mice of the same strain (syngeneic) were successful, whereas grafts between different strains resulted in rejection within 10–14 days. If a second graft from the same donor strain was made to the same recipient mouse, rejection occurred within 5–6 days. This demonstrated a 'memory' component to the acute rejection response. The initial 'first set' response was shown to result from the activation of naïve T lymphocytes in response to graft antigens. On secondary exposure to the same graft antigens, memory T cells formed in the primary response are activated in the more rapid 'second set' or *accelerated rejection* (Fig. 13.2).

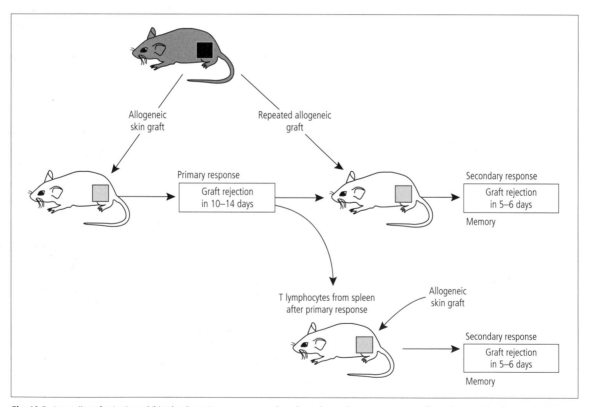

Fig. 13.2 Acute allograft rejection exhibits the slow primary response and accelerated secondary response on regrafting, characteristic of immunological memory. These responses are dependent on the activation of antigraft T cells.

Other studies focused on determining the genetic basis of allograft rejection. These studies used congenic strains of mice that were of the same genetic background but with particular genes or sets of genes differing from this common background in each of the different strains. The results of skin grafts between different donor and recipient strains allowed the identification of the genes involved in encoding antigenic differences that were important in stimulating tissue rejection. These are described as histocompatibility (tissue compatibility) antigens. The most significant of these are the *major histocompatibility antigens* encoded by the *major histocompatibility complex* (MHC) of genes.

The major histocompatibility complex

Function of MHC

The major histocompatibility molecules are proteins that are synthesized in the endoplasmic reticulum, modified to form glycoproteins in the Golgi body and then transported to the cell surface (Fig. 13.3). Their transport to the cell surface is dependent on the binding of peptides that may be derived from processed antigens. The presentation of these antigenic peptides by MHC on the surface of cells triggers the clonal expansion and differentiation to effector function of T cells with an appropriate receptor specificity. (Chapter 6 gives a more detailed description of the events of antigen processing and presentation.)

Genetic organization of MHC

The genes of the MHC exhibit some interesting characteristics. There are two classes of MHC gene and three principal genes within each class. The MHC encodes the production of MHC proteins that in humans are referred to as *human leucocyte antigens* (HLA). The MHC class I genes encode HLA-A, -B and -C, and the MHC class II genes encode HLA-DP, -DQ and -DR (Fig. 13.3 shows the arrangement of these genes on the chromosome). Each individual may have two different alleles for each gene. These alleles are coexpressed. That is each of the alleles can encode a different MHC protein molecule that will be expressed at the cell surface. Within the

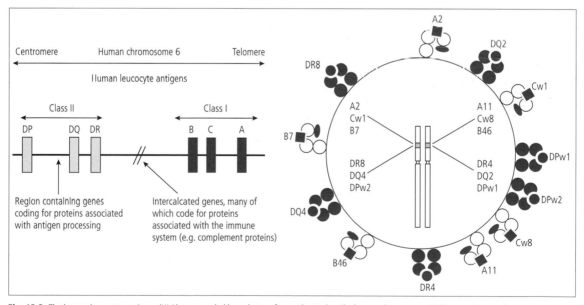

Fig. 13.3 The human leucocyte antigens (HLA) are encoded by a cluster of genes located on the human chromosome 6. They are the most important genes in determining tissue (in)compatibility—the major histocompatibility complex. Although the genes have many different forms (polymorphic) within the population, each individual inherits only two alleles for each gene. The alleles are codominantly expressed.

population there are a large number of different alleles, which are translated into many different proteins (a high degree of *polymorphism*). The polymorphic differences are located in the amino acid sequence that determines the structure of the binding site. Different MHC molecules have different binding site structures, different specificities and therefore bind different sets of peptides. It is important to note that each individual will inherit only two alleles (one from each parent) for each of the three class I genes, and two for each of the three class II genes. The high degree of polymorphism is in the population, not within the individual.

Polymorphism of MHC

This high level of polymorphism confers a significant evolutionary advantage in protecting the population against infection. Unfortunately the immune system did not evolve to facilitate transplantation. Clearly the higher the level of polymorphism, the more difficult it is to find genetically matched donor and recipient pairs to reduce or eliminate the problems of transplant rejection.

There is evidence that the better the match between the MHC of donor and recipient (the greater the number of common alleles), the less the problems with rejection leading to enhanced transplant survival rates. It is important to note that the MHC genes are not equally polymorphic. HLA-B is the most polymorphic class I gene (currently 286 different alleles identified in the population) followed by HLA-A (144 alleles). HLA-DR (226 alleles) is the most polymorphic of the class II genes. Similarly HLA genes are not all equally expressed at the cell surface. Tissue typing of donor and recipient focuses on matching HLA-A, -B and -DR as closely as possible.

Initially tissue typing employed serological methods, differentiating between different forms of HLA proteins. These methods have been supplemented by the application of molecular genetics, initially restriction fragment length polymorphism (RFLP) and more recently the use of polymerase chain reaction (PCR) based techniques. These methods identify differences in the DNA of different allelotypes. It is evident that genotyping is far more precise, enabling the detection of small differences in the

nucleotide sequences which form the code for the polymorphic amino acids that characterize the peptide binding site specificities of the HLA molecules. The serotype HLA-A2, for example, can be resolved into about 30 different genotypes.

Inheritance of MHC genes

The HLA genes are 'tightly linked', that is they are located close together (in a complex) on the same chromosome—the short arm of chromosome 6. During meiosis there is only a very low chance of a cross-over occurring between genes and they are therefore usually inherited as a block. There is a 1 in 4 chance that siblings will have the same HLA alleles.

The presentation of graft antigens

For a T-cell response to be activated, graft antigens must be processed to form peptides. These are then presented at the cell surface by MHC molecules, activating the clonal expansion of those T cells that are able to recognize the MHC–peptide complexes.

MHC class II positive antigen-presenting cells of the host could process graft antigens by the exogenous pathway in a similar way to which they process other foreign antigens such as bacteria. This is referred to as *indirect presentation* of graft antigens. It is a conventional 'self restricted' response in which T cell and presenting cell are of the same MHC type—they are both host cells.

However, it has been observed that the T-cell response to allogeneic graft antigens is especially vigorous. It seems that host T cells are activated directly by peptides presented by MHC molecules expressed on the surface of graft cells. By definition, in an allograft, this is an allo-response to allo-MHC and is not 'self restricted'.

At first this might seem to be contrary to the concept of 'self restriction'. It should be remembered, however, that developing T cells are 'tested' in the thymus for their ability to recognize 'self' MHC. Those that are able to do so are positively selected and go on to form mature peripheral T cells. This does not preclude the possibility that they will also recognize other types of MHC (allo-MHC). They are simply not tested against other types. Transplanta-

Fig. 13.4 Graft antigens may be processed and presented by host cells in a similar way to other foreign antigens. This is indirect presentation. The graft peptides are presented by host major histocompatibility complex (MHC) to host T cells of the same MHC type. This is the conventional 'self restricted' response. The T cell and presenting cell are of the same MHC type. Acute allograft rejection involves a very vigorous T-cell response in which graft peptides are presented by graft cells to host T cells. In an allograft the graft and host cells are by definition of different MHC type. This direct presentation involves an allo-response. MHC class II positive cells in the graft may be passenger cells (e.g. dendritic cells) carried within the graft. They migrate in the host to lymph nodes where they stimulate the proliferation of helper T (Th) cells. The Th cells return to the graft and 'help' cytotoxic T cells that recognize and lyse graft cells.

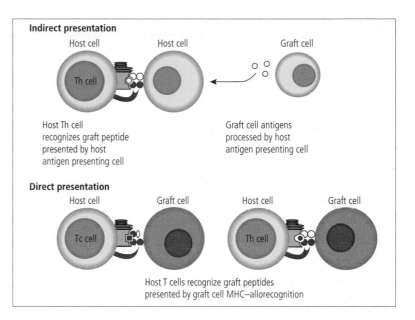

tion is one of the few occasions when T cells are challenged by allo-MHC molecules.

In transplant rejection then, there is a vigorous T-cell response. CD4+ T cells from the host respond to peptide presented by allo-MHC class II molecules on graft cells or on class II positive passenger cells, such as dendritic cells, contained in the graft. It is thought that passenger cells pass to the host secondary lymphoid organs where they activate the clonal expansion of T cells, which then return to the graft to carry out their effector function. It is worth remembering that only a few cell types express MHC class II. The T-cell response induced by a graft will be partly determined by its content of class II positive cells. CD8+ T cells from the host are able to recognize peptides presented by allo-MHC class I molecules on the surface of graft cells resulting in their lysis. These responses result from *direct presentation* of graft antigens by MHC on the surface of graft cells to host T lymphocytes (Fig. 13.4).

Allo-responses result therefore from cross-reaction by host T cells that have been positively selected in the thymus to recognize foreign antigen presented on 'self MHC'. Allo-responses are far more vigorous than self restricted responses as many more T-cell clones are activated. This may partly be due to minor variations in the structure of proteins in dif-

ferent individuals (minor polymorphisms) but is principally a result of the role of MHC in selecting peptides for presentation to T cells. The graft (allo-) MHC molecules will have peptide binding sites with different structures and therefore different specificities. They therefore present a completely different set of peptides even when the peptides are derived from identical proteins. It is this presentation of such a diverse range of different peptides by graft MHC that results in the activation of such a large number of host T-cell clones.

T-cell effector functions

Although the magnitude of T-cell responses to graft antigens is greater than that to foreign infectious agents, the range of effector functions invoked is similar (see Chapter 6 and Fig. 13.5).

Lymphokines produced by activated helper T cells enhance the inflammatory response against the graft.

They 'help' the proliferation of cytotoxic T lymphocytes in direct response to graft antigens. These cytotoxic T cells are able to lyse graft cells.

Lymphokines also 'help' the activation and differentiation of B cells leading to the production of anti-graft antibodies by plasma cells. These antibodies

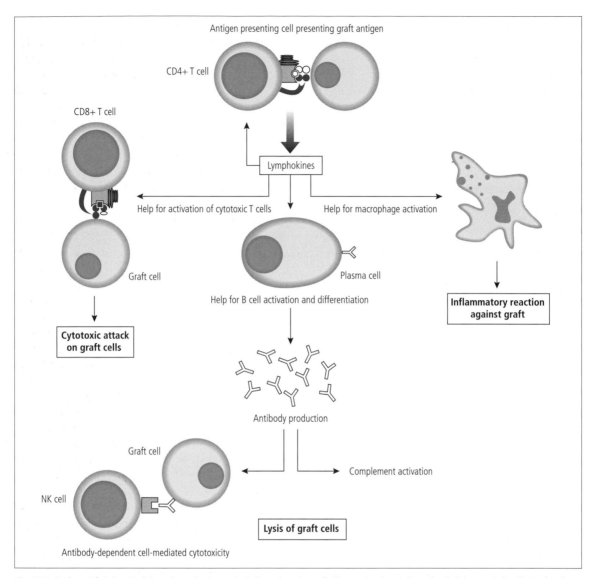

Antigen presenting cell presenting graft antigen

CD4+ T cell

CD8+ T cell

Lymphokines

Help for activation of cytotoxic T cells

Help for macrophage activation

Graft cell

Plasma cell

Help for B cell activation and differentiation

Cytotoxic attack on graft cells

Inflammatory reaction against graft

Antibody production

Graft cell

Complement activation

NK cell

Lysis of graft cells

Antibody-dependent cell-mediated cytotoxicity

Fig. 13.5 Graft-specific helper T cells coordinate the immunological attack on the graft. They produce lymphokines that 'help' cytotoxic T-cell lysis of graft cells, the production of antigraft antibodies and the initiation of an inflammatory reaction against the graft.

stimulate the complement-mediated lysis of graft cells and antibody-dependent cell-mediated cytotoxic attack on graft cells, mediated by natural killer cells.

The control of rejection

Allograft survival depends on the effective control of immunological rejection. As syngeneic grafts are not rejected, there are clearly advantages in trying to ensure a close match of HLA alleles between donor and recipient. However, whilst the majority of studies show a positive relationship between graft survival and the number of matched HLA alleles the situation is complex to analyse as:

• Minor histocompatibility antigens (potentially any other proteins that show polymorphism within the population) also contribute to tissue incompatibilities and consequently rejection.

- In many cases tissue matching has been carried out serologically which for unrelated donor/recipient pairs lacks the precision of genotyping.
- In virtually all cases, allograft survival is assessed in the context of one of a variety of immunosuppressive regimens.
- The emphasis, in most studies, is on the number of HLA mismatches where specific qualitative allelic mismatches for different genes may be of greater relevance.

Organ differences in transplantation

In a brief consideration of the immunological basis of graft rejection there is a danger of over generalization. Different organs and tissues, composed of different cell types, will express MHC class II antigens to differing degrees. Additionally they will differ in their content of MHC class II positive passenger cells. This will have a significant impact on their immunogenicity in the context of their induction of direct allo-responses by host T cells.

Organs and tissues will also differ in the extent to which they are subjected *in situ* to immune surveillance. There are also clear differences between organs that influence donor availability, pre- and post-transplant procedures and survival rates. Some of these differences for commonly transplanted organs are considered below.

Renal transplantation

Kidney transplantation is the treatment of choice for the majority of patients with end-stage renal failure. Recipients can be maintained in a stable condition by dialysis allowing adequate time for extensive HLA matching. There is potential availability of related living donors in addition to unrelated cadaver donors (there are interesting ethical dimensions in the increasing market for organs from unrelated living donors). The most extensive studies of the importance of HLA matching in graft survival have been carried out for renal transplantation. Although there is evidence that HLA matching of donor and recipient (particularly HLA-A and HLA-DR) improves graft survival rates, it is equally clear that effective immunosuppression can largely overcome the immunological consequences of using a mismatched graft.

Cardiac transplantation

In contrast in cardiac transplantation, in which recipients are almost always terminally ill and rely on the availability of a heart from a patient on 'life support', there is often insufficient time for full HLA matching. Improved graft survival rates are largely attributable to effective immunosuppression together with early detection of rejection by histological examination of endomyocardial biopsy samples and the timely use of appropriate 'rescue therapy' to counteract the rejection process (see below).

Bone marrow transplantation

Bone marrow or blood stem cell transplants are routinely used for the treatment of patients with haematological malignancies and solid tumours. *Autologous* transplants use bone marrow or blood stem cells collected form the patient, purified, and returned by infusion after the patient has received high dose chemotherapy or myeloablative therapy which destroys cancer cells as well as many normal cells including those of the bone marrow. Advanced breast cancer and lymphoma are now the most common indications for autologous transplants, although several other malignant diseases such as ovarian cancer, germ cell cancer, neuroblastoma and sarcoma are now treated in this way. *Allogeneic* bone marrow/stem cell transplants (using bone marrow or blood stem cells collected from HLA-matched donors) after myeloablative therapy are used in the treatment of acute and chronic leukaemias. Other applications of bone marrow transplants include the treatment of inherited blood disorders such as sickle cell anaemia and thalassaemia as well as immune-related diseases such as rheumatoid arthritis and multiple sclerosis. Allogeneic bone marrow transplantation requires careful HLA matching of donor and recipient, and extensive registers of potential bone marrow donors are now kept to increase the chances of finding well-matched donors.

One of the major complications of allogeneic bone marrow transplantation is the development of acute or chronic graft versus host disease (GvHD). GvHD occurs when immunologically competent T lymphocytes derived from the donor (graft) make an immune response against antigens expressed on recipient (host) tissues. This response may be additional to the more usual host versus graft rejection response. The symptoms of GvHD are arbitrarily classified as those that are present within the first 100 days after transplantation. They are of four clinical grades of severity reflecting the extent of the damage caused by the immunological attack by graft-derived lymphocytes on cells of the skin, gastrointestinal tract or liver. Chronic GvHD can be either limited (involving skin damage and/or liver dysfunction), or extensive (with more severe damage to both the liver and other target organs). After bone marrow transplantation, humoral and cellular immunity in the recipient is reconstituted from the transplanted stem cells. This immune reconstitution is delayed or prevented by GvHD and the treatment of GvHD, which utilizes immunosuppressive drugs.

Stem cell purification technology has developed to allow the removal of residual cancer cells from bone marrow or mobilized blood stem cells, and/ or the separation and purification of stem cells to reduce transplant-related complications. The depletion of T lymphocytes from bone marrow decreases the incidence of GvHD, but can also be associated with an increased recurrence of leukaemia. Emerging technologies now allow the generation of therapeutic quantities of haematopoietic stem/ progenitor cells from small volumes of bone marrow. There is also the potential for *ex vivo*, cell-based, gene therapy designed to increase the utility of stem cell transplants for the treatment of a range of defects.

Liver transplantation

The early graft survival rates for liver transplantation were low, largely as a result of the complexity of the surgical procedures involved. Irreversible damage to the liver as a consequence of congenital abnormalities, viral disease or damage by toxic chemicals, including alcohol, require transplantation. The liver is a large organ and can often be divided between more than one recipient. In some cases auxiliary transplants are made where the graft is inserted alongside the bulk of the recipient's liver. As with heart transplants there is often little scope for HLA matching. The liver has low immunogenicity reducing the problems of graft rejection. This seems particularly to be the case with hyperacute rejection, which is rarely encountered in liver transplantation.

Corneal transplantation

Thousands of corneal transplants are performed each year, saving or restoring the vision of the newborn, industrial workers, athletes, contact lens wearers, the elderly and a variety of others with corneal diseases. Corneal disease is characterized by blurred vision or blindness stemming from damage to the cornea. Causes vary from congenital abnormalities to trauma in industrial workers and sports participants, eye infections in contact lens wearers and complications resulting from cataract surgery.

Corneal transplantation is often required because the corneal endothelium cannot replace or repair itself. Recently, human corneal endothelial cells have been successfully grown and induced to divide repeatedly. Unlike native corneal endothelium, cultured corneal endothelium can be frozen for later use.

One common feature of all allografts is that the effective control of rejection depends on pharmacological intervention or the use of procedures such as total lymphoid irradiation to suppress the activities of the immune system.

Immunosuppression

The fundamental immunological response in transplant rejection is the clonal expansion of T cells that are specific for graft antigens. The helper T cells orchestrate a variety of effector responses (see above). The goal of immunosuppressive therapy is to specifically inhibit proliferation and/or effector function of these graft-specific T cells. This 'gold standard' has not yet been achieved.

Two of the earliest drugs used in immunosuppression were azathioprine and corticosteroids such as prednisolone. These illustrate different mechanisms of immunosuppression. *Azathioprine* is a base analogue that interferes with DNA replication and hence blocks cell division including lymphocyte proliferation. *Corticosteroids* in contrast reduce the number of circulating lymphocytes and have an anti-inflammatory action. They reduce MHC expression and antigen presentation which are involved in the sensitization phase of the T-cell response, and also inhibit effector functions such as the activation of macrophages.

The most widely used immunosuppressive drug, which has significantly improved graft survival, with the consequent expansion of transplant programmes, is the fungal macrolide cyclosporin. *Cyclosporin* selectively inhibits the production of interleukin 2 (IL-2) by T cells. The more recently introduced *FK-506* has a similar mode of action, whilst the related compound *rapamycin* blocks signal transduction from the IL-2 receptor. Binding of IL-2 to IL-2 receptors is essential to the activation and proliferation of T lymphocytes.

Whilst these compounds have a more specific effect than azathioprine, they share the same disadvantages in that they fail to control chronic rejection, enhance the risk of opportunistic infections, lead to an increased incidence of spontaneous neoplasms and induce direct or indirect toxic side-effects.

In clinical practice using the drugs in combination, dual or triple therapy regimens reduces these side-effects. These therapies are commenced shortly before transplantation and continue as long as the graft functions.

Monoclonal antibodies, or preferentially humanized forms of monoclonal antibodies, are used in *'rescue therapy'* to control and reverse rejection episodes particularly in cardiac transplantation. They are most commonly used against T-cell surface antigens such as CD3, CD4 and CD25 (IL-2R) to interfere with the function of cells that are co-ordinating the immunological attack on the graft.

Summary

The vast majority of organ and tissue transplants are allografts between genetically different hosts and recipients. The immune system mounts an attack on the 'foreign' graft. The response of host T lymphocytes to antigen presented by allo-MHC on graft cells is the key component of this vigorous response.

Although MHC matching can improve graft survival this is ultimately dependent on the control of rejection through effective immunosuppression.

Key points

1 Grafts are of different types, classified on the basis of the genetic differences between donor and recipient. Allografts, between genetically different donor/recipient pairs, are clinically the most important.

2 The immune system recognizes allografts as 'foreign' and responds by attacking and destroying graft cells. The nature and timing of the immune response is dependent on previous exposure of the recipient to graft antigens.

3 The activation and proliferation of T cells that coordinate the immune response against graft antigens is the key event in acute allograft rejection.

4 The highly polymorphic antigens encoded by the MHC present graft antigens to host T cells to generate a direct allo-response, which is more vigorous than the normal self restricted response to foreign antigens derived from infectious agents.

5 Different transplanted organs or tissues show distinct physiological and immunological properties which determine pre- and post-transplant procedures and influence graft survival.

6 Graft survival can be improved by HLA matching, and for some organs this effective matching seems essential. In all cases, allograft survival depends on effective pharmacological interventions to suppress immune activity and control rejection.

Further reading

Brostoff J., Scadding G.K., Male D. & Roitt I.M. (1991) *Clinical Immunology.* Gower Medical.

Goldsby R.A., Kindt T.J. & Osborne B. (2000) *Kuby Immunology* (4th edn). W.H. Freeman, New York.

Gould D.S. & Auchinloss H. Jr. (1999) Direct and indirect recognition: the role of MHC antigens in graft rejection. *Immunology Today* **20**: 77–82.

Rich R.R., Strober W., Fleischer T.A., Schwartz B.D. & Shearer W.T. (1995) *Clinical Immunology Principles and Practice.* Mosby, St. Louis.

CHAPTER 14

Anaemia

Anaemia is defined as a reduction in blood haemoglobin concentration. This is reflected in a reduction in circulating red cell mass and in the oxygen-carrying capacity of the blood. Anaemia is a consequence of one of a number of disorders underlying defective erythrocyte (red blood cell) production or excessive loss of erythrocytes from the circulation. Therefore, whenever a patient is found to be anaemic it is essential to investigate further to identify the underlying cause. This chapter considers the fundamental causes of different types of anaemia and concludes with an overview of the basic laboratory investigations used to classify anaemia.

Blood formation

Red cell formation

Haemopoiesis (blood cell production) takes place in bone marrow. All blood cells (erythrocytes, leucocytes and platelets) are derived from a single clone of primitive cells—the *pluripotent stem cell*. Stem cells have the ability to divide and differentiate under the influence of specific cytokines (growth factors), released by *stromal* cells in the bone marrow, including macrophages and fibroblasts. Initially the differentiated stem cells form *myeloid* and *lymphoid* stem cells (Fig. 14.1). Myeloid stem cells give rise to the progenitors of three principal cell lines:
• The myeloid–monocyte series (producing granulocytes and monocytes).
• The megakaryocyte series (producing platelets).

• Erythroid progenitor cells (producing erythrocytes—the red blood cells).

Erythropoiesis is the aspect of haemopoiesis which produces mature red blood cells. Erythropoiesis takes place in several stages as erythroid precursor cells develop from relatively undifferentiated pronormoblasts to late normoblasts. The normoblasts lose their nucleus before being released into the circulation as *reticulocytes* (young erythrocytes). Normal erythropoiesis is dependent on the availability of nutrients including folate and vitamin B_{12}.

Haemoglobin synthesis

Haemoglobin is the oxygen-carrying component of erythrocytes. A typical red blood cell contains over 600 million haemoglobin molecules, each of which is a tetramer of four *haem* groups (Fig. 14.2) and four globin chains.

The assembly of haem takes place in the mitochondria of erythrocyte precursor cells in red bone marrow. Four haem molecules each combine in the cell cytoplasm with α- or β-globin chains synthesized in ribosomes to form haemoglobin (Fig. 14.3). Normal adult haemoglobin contains two types of globin chain—two α-chains (each 141 amino acids) and two β-chains (each 146 amino acids).

Several factors can interfere with the synthesis of haemoglobin including lack of essential nutrients (as in iron deficiency), inherited structural abnormalities, usually in the globin chains, or defects in the efficient assembly of haemoglobin molecules.

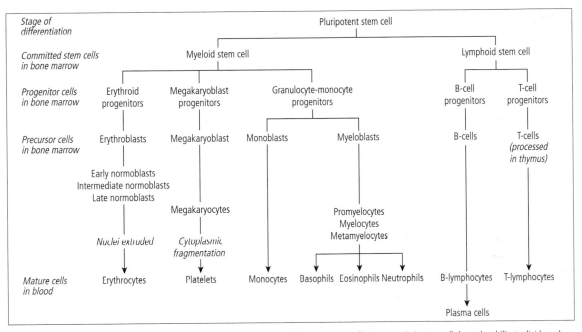

Fig. 14.1 An outline of haemopoiesis. All mature blood cells are derived from pluripotent stem cells. Haemopoietic stem cells have the ability to divide and differentiate under the influence of specific growth factors. Lymphoid stem cells give rise to B- and T-cell lines. B lymphocytes undergo further differentiation into plasma cells for antibody production. T-lymphocyte precursors are processed in the thymus to produce T cells—T-helper, T-suppressor and cytotoxic T cells. Myeloid stem cells give rise to three types of progenitor cell which produce erythrocytes, platelets or cells of the monocyte and granulocyte series.

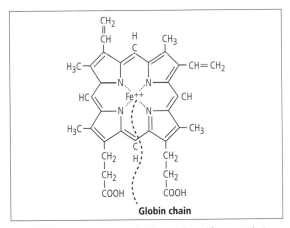

Fig. 14.2 The structure of haem. Each haem is formed from a porphyrin ring into which is inserted ferrous iron. An α- or β-globin chain attaches to each haem, four of which combine to form each haemoglobin molecule.

Causes of anaemia

A preliminary diagnosis of anaemia is based on establishing a reduction in total blood haemoglobin concentration, though this gives no indication of the cause. The reference range for haemoglobin concentration differs for males and females—it is usual for adult females to have rather lower haemoglobin levels than their male counterparts. Furthermore, a low haemoglobin concentration does not always signify anaemia: an increase in plasma volume causes an apparent anaemia (pseudoanaemia) though the total body haemoglobin content is normal. This is seen, for example, in pregnancy (during which a mild reduction in blood haemoglobin concentration is a frequent finding) and can be difficult to differentiate from genuine anaemia in pregnancy. The basic causes of anaemia are summarized in Table 14.1.

Anaemia is characterized by a reduction in the concentration of haemoglobin in the blood or in

125

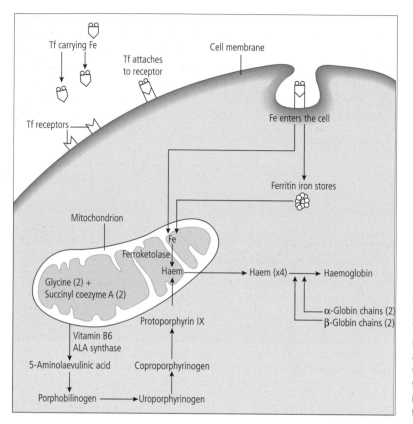

Fig. 14.3 Haemoglobin synthesis in developing erythroblasts. The essential components for the synthesis of haem are pyrrole rings and iron, together with the enzymes which assemble these into iron-containing porphyrin rings. Iron is transported to developing red blood cells in the bone marrow by the carrier protein transferrin (Tf). Tf attaches to specific receptors on the cell membrane and the whole complex (iron, Tf and receptor) is taken into the cell. The iron then either enters cellular iron stores (as ferritin) or passes to mitochondria where it combines with protoporphyrin IX to form haem.

Table 14.1 Principal causes of anaemia.

Defective haemoglobin synthesis
Diminished erythrocyte production
Excessive erythrocyte destruction
Blood loss

numbers of circulating erythrocytes. Usually if one of these is reduced then the other is reduced also, because haemoglobin is contained within erythrocytes. However, there are circumstances in which total blood haemoglobin concentration may be mildly reduced, but with a normal red blood cell count. This occurs in the early stages of *iron deficiency* anaemia and some *thalassaemia syndromes*. In such cases, despite the normal red cell numbers, individual erythrocytes are reduced in size and contain a lowered amount of haemoglobin. As the condition progresses and anaemia becomes more severe, the red cell count falls. Most other types of anaemia are characterized by reduction in both total haemoglobin concentration and red cell count, with erythrocytes of normal or increased cell size.

Defective haemoglobin synthesis

Defective haemoglobin synthesis falls into two groups—defects of haem synthesis and defects of globin synthesis. Defects in haem synthesis can be due to lack of available iron at the site of synthesis or to failure of the enzyme mediated assembly of porphyrin rings. Defective globin chain synthesis may be *qualitative* (resulting in structurally abnormal haemoglobins) or *quantitative* (resulting in delayed synthesis of one or other globin chain). Defects in haemoglobin synthesis generally result in red blood cells which are smaller than normal and contain reduced amounts of haemoglobin (*microcytic* and *hypochromic* cells—see later).

Iron deficiency

Iron deficiency, the cause of the commonest nutritional anaemia, results in diminished haem synthesis, and hence reduced haemoglobin within erythrocytes. Iron deficiency anaemia also occurs when the rate of erythropoiesis increases to compensate for blood loss or the demands of pregnancy. This is because dietary sources of iron may be adequate to support a normal rate of erythropoiesis but are insufficient to maintain a higher rate.

Chronic blood loss is an important cause of iron deficiency anaemia. During haemorrhage, iron is irretrievably lost from the body and dietary sources of iron are insufficient to compensate for the loss. Malabsorption of iron (as in coeliac disease, case study 18) is another possible cause of iron deficiency. Iron deficiency is characterized by low serum iron, low serum ferritin (reflecting depleted iron stores) and a raised concentration of serum transferrin which indicates an increase in iron transport capacity.

Causes of apparent iron deficiency (blood count results which mimic those of iron deficiency with low serum iron) include defects in plasma iron transport in chronic inflammatory diseases such as rheumatoid arthritis. Laboratory results differ from those in iron deficiency in that serum ferritin concentrations are often normal or high and serum transferrin is usually low. This type of anaemia is normally unresponsive to iron therapy.

Porphyrias

Defects in the assembly of porphyrin rings are known as porphyrias. Porphyrias are a rare group of inherited disorders characterized by deficiencies of enzymes controlling haem synthesis. The rate-limiting step in haem synthesis, the condensation of glycine and succinate to form 5-aminolaevulinic acid (ALA), is catalysed by ALA synthase (Fig. 14.3). Product inhibition normally controls ALA synthase activity, so faulty haem synthesis results in overproduction of porphyrins or their precursors. Clinical effects of the porphyrias include photosensitivity, dermatitis and neurological disorders resulting from accumulation of porphyrins in the tissues. King George III (*The Madness of King George*) is reputed to have suffered from a form of congenital porphyria.

A rare type of anaemia characterized by abnormal accumulation of iron in erythrocyte precursors (sideroblastic anaemia), which can be congenital or acquired, may be due to a similar defect in haem synthesis. Prolonged exposure to high concentrations of lead (see also Chapter 18), which inhibits several stages of porphyrin synthesis, may be accompanied by a similar form of mild anaemia.

Inherited defects in globin chain synthesis

Thalassaemia syndromes

Alpha- and beta-globin chains are required in sufficient quantity to enable the synthesis of haemoglobin molecules with two of each type of chain. The *thalassaemias* are quantitative globin chain defects associated with an imbalance in the rate of synthesis of α- and β-globin chains, usually due to depression of synthesis of one or other chain. The effects are variable, depending on the degree to which globin chain synthesis is suppressed, but can be life threatening.

Two closely linked genes on the short arm of chromosome 16 code for α-globins, so synthesis of these chains is controlled by four genes in each cell. *Alpha-thalassaemia* is characterized by deletion or alteration of one or more of these genes, the severity of the clinical outcome varying with the number of genes deleted. Severe forms of α-thalassaemia, with deletion of all four genes, are incompatible with life, and pregnancy with an affected fetus frequently fails to reach full term. Less severe forms of α-thalassaemia (deletion of three of the four genes) are associated with variable survival and quality of life. Typically there is moderate anaemia and the formation of unstable β-chain tetramers (haemoglobin H) may be a feature. Alpha-thalassaemia traits (deletion of one or two genes) are of little clinical significance to affected individuals, but genetic counselling is essential for affected partners in a child-bearing relationship.

Beta-globin chains are coded for on the short arm of chromosome 11. Severe *β-thalassaemia* is associated with profound anaemia from the first year of life and dependence on regular transfusions. Iron overload due to these transfusions becomes a problem, and may contribute to morbidity, though the risk of this can be reduced by the active use of iron chelating agents. Beta-thalassaemia minor is much less severe, with a blood picture superficially similar to that of iron deficiency.

Haemoglobinopathies

The correct sequence of amino acids in the four globin chains is essential to the efficient function of the haemoglobin molecule. Structural globin chain defects (haemoglobinopathies) are usually due to base substitutions (point mutations) in the DNA which codes for the polypeptide globin chains, resulting in single amino acid substitutions. Such changes have variable outcomes, depending on the nature and site of the amino acid substitution, ranging from no clinical effect to severe consequences such as altered oxygen affinity, or destabilization of the haemoglobin molecule resulting in reduced erythrocyte lifespan.

One of the most important of the single amino acid substitution defects is the replacement of glutamic acid by valine at position 6 in the β-chain of haemoglobin A to produce *sickle haemoglobin*. When inherited as the homozygous condition (known as sickle cell disease), under conditions of low oxygen tension haemoglobin S precipitates as long filaments, distorting the shape of the erythrocytes. The resulting sickle cells lodge in small blood vessels causing painful *infarctions* (death of surrounding areas of tissue following sudden deprivation of blood supply) and reduction in red cell lifespan (see also case study 21). Another of the haemoglobinopathies, haemoglobin C disease, is also characterized by reduced red cell lifespan, and is due to the replacement of glutamic acid by lysine at the same β-chain locus as haemoglobin S. When either condition is inherited as the heterozygous 'trait' (one gene coding for normal haemoglobin and the other coding for haemoglobin S or C) some normal adult haemoglobin is produced alongside the defective haemoglobin and subjects are symptom-free. In each case the heterozygous condition confers some protection against malaria due to the protozoon parasite *Plasmodium falciparum*, which helps to explain their natural geographical distribution (see case study 5).

The precise cause of anaemia in the different haemoglobinopathies and thalassaemia syndromes is often complex. Increased rates of *haemolysis*, leading to reduction in erythrocyte lifespan and ineffective erythropoiesis (see later) both contribute. Combinations of inherited structural haemoglobin defects and thalassaemia minor can produce complex and very severe forms of anaemia.

Diminished erythrocyte production

In this group of anaemias, haemoglobin synthesis is normal, but erythropoiesis is reduced. Defects in erythropoiesis may be due to nutrient lack, bone marrow *hypoplasia* (underactivity), infiltration of bone marrow with malignant cells or to various chronic disease states.

Nutrient lack

Certain vitamins and other nutrients are essential for normal blood formation. Of particular importance in erythropoiesis are the B group vitamins, vitamin B_{12} and folate, which are essential for DNA synthesis. Lack of either of these vitamins is associated with disordered maturation of erythrocyte precursors in the bone marrow. In prolonged vitamin B_{12} or folate deficiency erythrocyte precursor cells display a characteristic morphological alteration in which nuclear maturation lags behind that of the cytoplasm (*megaloblastic change*). These abnormal cells are known as *megaloblasts*, to distinguish them from their normal counterparts (*normoblasts*). The mature erythrocytes resulting from megaloblastic erythropoiesis are much larger than their normal counterparts and are known as macrocytes, though they are significantly reduced in number. An additional complication in severe, prolonged vitamin B_{12} deficiency is subacute combined degeneration of the spinal cord, which results in characteristic neurological changes. Deficiencies of vitamin B_{12} and folate have three potential causes—dietary insufficiency, malabsorption and metabolic interference as discussed below.

Vitamin B_{12}

• Dietary deficiency of vitamin B_{12} is rare, but since the vitamin is present only in foods of animal origin strict vegetarians are susceptible.

- Absorption of vitamin B_{12} from the intestinal tract requires the presence of a glycoprotein, *intrinsic factor* (IF), secreted by parietal cells in the fundus and body of the stomach. IF binds to vitamin B_{12} and the complex is absorbed in the distal ileum, so lack of IF results in vitamin B_{12} malabsorption. The most common disorder associated with vitamin B_{12} malabsorption is *pernicious anaemia*, an autoimmune condition characterized by the presence of autoantibodies to parietal cells and/or intrinsic factor.
- Disturbance of vitamin B_{12} metabolism is rare but prolonged exposure to nitrous oxide anaesthesia has been shown to cause megaloblastic change.

Folate
- Folate deficiency can arise due to dietary lack, particularly in times of increased requirements, such as in pregnancy, or in disorders associated with rapid cell turnover (psoriasis, neoplastic and haemolytic disorders).
- Malabsorption is a feature of some digestive tract disorders: for example in coeliac disease (see case study 18), serum and red cell folate assays may be used to monitor progress.
- The drug methotrexate, mainly used in the treatment of leukaemia, competes with folate for the enzyme *folic acid reductase*, thus reducing purine synthesis and causing megaloblastic change in the bone marrow.

Bone marrow hypoplasia
Reduced erythropoiesis can also be due to bone marrow damage, leading to *hypoplastic* or *aplastic* anaemia (anaemia due to reduced haemopoietic activity). There are several potential causes, though many cases are of unknown aetiology. Some are *iatrogenic* (physician induced), caused by exposure to cytotoxic drugs, chemicals or radiotherapy. Thyroid, liver or renal disease, or viral infection may also result in bone marrow hypoplasia.

Ineffective erythropoiesis
Ineffective erythropoiesis (IE) is a failure of erythrocyte precursor cells to reach maturity, resulting in their destruction in the bone marrow. Some degree of IE occurs in normal haemopoiesis affecting up to one in eight erythrocyte precursors.

An increase in IE contributes to many forms of anaemia, including those seen in the thalassaemia syndromes, megaloblastic anaemia and some leukaemias.

Chronic disease states
Inflammatory or neoplastic disease may cause diminished red cell production, though in certain chronic inflammatory disorders (e.g. rheumatoid arthritis) anaemia may be due to a defect in iron utilization. Chronic renal failure is associated with impaired erythropoiesis because the kidney is a major source of the hormone *erythropoietin*, which stimulates the later stages of red cell production.

Malignant blood disorders
Leukaemias and other malignant blood diseases are an important cause of anaemia due to reduced erythropoiesis. Leukaemias are categorized as *acute* or *chronic* depending on the degree of maturation of the predominant cells, and are further subdivided according to the particular haemopoietic cell line involved (see case studies 29 and 30). Characteristically, the bone marrow contains large numbers of immature leukaemic cells which displace normal haemopoietic cells, and there may also be some megaloblastic changes in erythropoiesis. Most leukaemias are characterized by anaemia (often severe in the acute forms of leukaemia), *thrombocytopenia* (reduction in blood platelet count) and *neutropenia* (reduction in circulating neutrophils). These cause patients to be highly susceptible to spontaneous bleeding and to severe bacterial infection.

Excessive erythrocyte destruction (haemolytic disorders)

The normal red cell has a mean lifespan in the circulation of 110–120 days. Reduced erythrocyte lifespan may result in anaemia, though this is not always the case because the bone marrow is usually able to increase production of erythrocytes to compensate for the premature loss. Despite this, if red cell lifespan is very short or the defect is permanent, premature cell death may not always be fully compensated by an increase in the rate of erythropoiesis and anaemia results.

There are two major groups of haemolytic disorder—those due to *intrinsic* and those due to *extrinsic* erythrocyte defects.

Intrinsic erythrocyte defects

Intrinsic erythrocyte defects leading to haemolytic disorders are usually congenital and can be subdivided into three categories. These are defects of: (a) haemoglobin; (b) intracellular enzymes; (c) the erythrocyte membrane.

• Alterations in haemoglobin structure can cause reduction in erythrocyte lifespan due to instability of the haemoglobin molecule itself or its defective interaction with other cell structures.

• Deficiencies or structural defects of intracellular enzymes, such as *pyruvate kinase* (PK) or *glucose-6-phosphate dehydrogenase* (G6PD), affect the ability of erythrocytes to metabolize nutrients and provide for their energy needs. The cells do not survive for their normal duration in the circulation, particularly, in the case of G6PD deficiency, if exposed to oxidative stress.

• Erythrocyte membrane defects, usually associated with abnormalities of the cytoskeleton, become clinically significant if they alter the biconcave disc shape and reduce erythrocyte deformability. This reduces the ability of the cells to enter and pass through small blood vessels. The affected cells become trapped in the splenic sinusoids and are removed from the circulation prematurely.

Hereditary spherocytosis

One example of this group of disorders is *hereditary spherocytosis*, in which an inherited defect in the spectrin group of cytoskeletal proteins results in spherical erythrocytes which have a reduced lifespan. The rate of erythropoiesis increases to compensate for this, but if the rate of production fails to keep pace with the rate of destruction then anaemia results. There is normally a substantial reserve capacity in the bone marrow which can compensate for reduced red blood cell lifespan, though periodically the bone marrow may fail to compensate fully, particularly if the patient has an infection or health is compromised in some other way. Thus, patients experience occasional periods of anaemia ('*haemolytic crisis*') interspersed with months or years of good health.

Extrinsic erythrocyte defects

Extrinsic defects are usually acquired and affect erythrocytes which are not intrinsically abnormal in any way. Examples include infection with malarial parasites (case study 5), other systemic infections, severe trauma or burns, or heart valve defects. The acquisition of autoantibodies to antigens on the red cell surface (such as those of the rhesus system) is a cause of *autoimmune haemolytic anaemia*, which can be triggered by exposure to some drugs. Immune-mediated haemolytic transfusion reactions, though rare, also cause significant reduction in erythrocyte lifespan.

Nutritional aspects of haemolytic disorders

In most haemolytic disorders haemoglobin is broken down extravascularly, usually in the spleen, and the iron and globin chains are recycled for further use within the body. For this reason, there is not usually any iron deficiency in most haemolytic disorders. However, the increased rate of erythropoiesis which is necessary to compensate for increased red cell destruction can deplete folate and cause megaloblastic changes. For this reason folic acid is often administered in chronic haemolytic disorders to avoid any megaloblastic changes which could arise due to folate depletion.

Blood loss

Haemorrhage (blood loss) results in erythrocytes leaving the circulation prematurely. The effects on erythropoiesis vary depending on whether the blood loss is *acute* or *chronic*. Acute haemorrhage (i.e. sudden and of short duration) of more than 1 L leads to a fall in total blood haemoglobin over the first 24 h. Normally, the bone marrow makes up the deficit in red cell numbers within a few weeks, as long as bleeding does not continue. If anaemia results from acute blood loss it is temporary, is not associated with any obvious morphological changes to the erythrocytes, other than reduction in total red cell count and is described as *normochromic* and *normocytic* (see below).

In the early stages of prolonged (or chronic) blood loss similar compensatory mechanisms are initiated. However, a continuous supply of iron is needed for the synthesis of haemoglobin and there is often insufficient iron available from dietary sources to compensate for that which continues to be lost. Thus, in chronic blood loss of a degree sufficient to cause anaemia the eventual outcome is invariably iron deficiency. Lack of iron leads to impaired haemoglobin synthesis and this, added to the requirement for increased erythropoiesis to replace lost red blood cells, results in *microcytic hypochromic anaemia* (see below). Chronic blood loss, including that due to menstruation, is an important cause of iron deficiency anaemia. However, as mentioned earlier, iron deficiency may also be due to malabsorption or to poor diet.

Classification of anaemia

When a patient is first recognized to be anaemic the underlying cause is not always immediately apparent, so laboratory data are used as a basis for further investigations. Anaemia is initially classified on the basis of erythrocyte size and morphology. The average size of the erythrocytes, measured as *mean cell*

Table 14.2 Laboratory classification of anaemia.

	Hb	RBC	MCV	MCH
Microcytic hypochromic	Low	Normal/low	Low	Low
Normocytic normochromic	Low	Low	Normal	Normal
Macrocytic normochromic	Low	Low	High	Normal/high

Hb, haemoglobin concentration; MCH, mean red cell haemoglobin content; MCV, mean red cell volume; RBC, red cell count.

volume (MCV) is most useful in defining the type of anaemia, which is provisionally classified as *normocytic* (normal MCV), *microcytic* (reduced MCV) or *macrocytic* (high MCV). *Mean cell haemoglobin* (the amount of haemoglobin in the average erythrocyte) and the microscopic morphology (appearance) of erythrocytes on stained blood films are both important. If staining intensity is reduced the red cells are described as *hypochromic*, which usually correlates with reduced mean cell haemoglobin (MCH). Measurement of total haemoglobin concentration, erythrocyte count (RBC), MCV and MCH enable

Table 14.3 Classification of anaemia on the basis of cell size.

	May be	Examples
Microcytic anaemia Reduced mean cell volume (MCV < 80 fl approx.)	Microcytic and hypochromic or microcytic without hypochromic red blood cells	Iron deficiency anaemia Anaemia of chronic inflammatory disease (e.g. rheumatoid arthritis) Thalassaemia
Macrocytic anaemia Increased mean cell volume (MCV > 95 fl approx.)	Two types: megaloblastic or non-megaloblastic (i) Megaloblastic (macrocytosis due to megaloblastic erythropoiesis)	Vitamin B_{12} or folate deficiency or acute leukaemia with megaloblastic changes in the bone marrow
	(ii) Non-megaloblastic (macrocytosis without megaloblastic change)	Some cases of liver disease Alcoholism (but note that folate deficiency may have a role) Some haemolytic anaemias
Normocytic anaemia Normal mean cell volume	Usually normochromic, normocytic anaemia	Acute blood loss Some haemolytic anaemias Some anaemias of chronic disorder (e.g. chronic renal failure) Hypoplastic or aplastic anaemias, malignancy, pregnancy

Key points

1 The four basic causes of anaemia are defective haemoglobin synthesis, diminished erythrocyte production, excessive erythrocyte destruction and blood loss.

2 Iron deficiency anaemia can arise from poor diet or malabsorption; chronic blood loss is also an important cause.

3 The haemoglobinopathies and thalassaemia syndromes are inherited conditions affecting haemoglobin synthesis and structure.

4 Vitamin B_{12} and folate deficiencies cause megaloblastic changes to erythropoiesis.

5 Erythropoiesis is also reduced in aplastic anaemia and in infiltration of bone marrow by leukaemic or other malignant cells.

6 Haemolytic disorders may be inherited or acquired. Some inherited haemolytic disorders have a defined geographical distribution and a high incidence in certain population groups.

7 Anaemia may be provisionally classified on the basis of cell size and morphology.

different types of anaemia to be described as *microcytic hypochromic*, *macrocytic normochromic* and *normocytic normochromic* (Table 14.2).

Classification of anaemia on the basis of cell size gives little information on the specific *aetiology* (underlying cause) in individual cases. However, it does indicate some possible causes and helps to exclude others, so that further investigations to identify the precise cause(s) of the anaemia can be initiated. As with other disorders the aetiology of anaemia can be multifactoral: Table 14.3 shows some possible causes of microcytic, normocytic and macrocytic anaemias.

Summary

The aim of this chapter has been to review the major causes of anaemia. In this volume, it is possible only to give an overview, and readers wishing to consider the subject in greater depth are advised to refer to the texts below.

Further reading

Bain B.J. (1996) *A Beginners Guide to Blood Cells*. Blackwell Science Ltd., Oxford.

Hoffbrand A.V., Pettit J.E. & Moss P. (2000) *Essential Haematology* (4th edn). Blackwell Science Ltd., Oxford.

Hughes Jones N.C. & Wickramasinghe S.N. (1996) *Lecture Notes on Haematology* (6th edn). Blackwell Science Ltd., Oxford.

Mehta A.B. & Hoffbrand A.V. (2000) *Haematology at a Glance*. Blackwell Science Ltd., Oxford.

Schiffman F.J. (1998) *Hematologic Pathophysiology*. Lippincott–Raven, Philadelphia.

Nutritional Disorders

Diseases resulting from inappropriate intake of nutrients are numerous, ranging from micronutrient deficiencies through starvation ('protein-energy malnutrition') to obesity and related diseases. Deficiency diseases resulting from malnutrition are now relatively rare in the UK and the rest of the developed world. A far more significant group of disorders which form a substantial and growing health and economic burden in both developed and many developing countries are the so-called 'diseases of affluence', in particular obesity. The incidence of obesity has reached epidemic proportions in these countries with an average of some 40% of the adult population being overweight or obese. Associated with obesity are a number of severe diseases including type II diabetes and vascular disease.

This chapter briefly considers some of the more common deficiency diseases and discusses the possible genetic and environmental factors contributing to the increasing incidence of obesity, diabetes and vascular disease. Other 'eating disorders' such as anorexia nervosa will also be considered.

Protein-energy malnutrition

Malnutrition is now relatively uncommon in the developed world, except in instances of eating disorders such as anorexia nervosa (see above). In some developing countries it can be a major problem, however, especially during food shortages brought about by natural disasters such as drought or by military conflicts.

Such malnutrition, resulting from inadequate food intake, is generally referred to as *protein-energy malnutrition* as it is now recognized that it is not due to lack of protein in the diet, but to a general lack of food-energy intake. Although there is a nutritional requirement for certain amino acids ('essential' amino acids) which the body is unable to synthesize in sufficient quantities for itself, undernutrition does not usually result in a deficiency of essential amino acids and protein content of the diet may indeed be relatively high. Unfortunately, if there is a deficiency in total food intake, the protein may be used as a fuel rather than for use in growth or to replace tissue protein. In individuals with low stores of fat, an inadequate intake of metabolic energy results in weight loss which over prolonged periods will result in breakdown and utilization of the body's tissue proteins in order to supply energy requirements. As well as its use in defining obesity, the body mass index (BMI)* is a useful measure of the degree of protein-energy malnutrition in adults (Table 15.1).

Table 15.1 Definitions of 'underweight' and 'malnutrition' using the BMI.

Category	BMI*
'Desireable'	20–25
Underweight	18.5–19.9
Moderate protein-energy malnutrition	17–18.4
Moderately severe protein-energy malnutrition	16–17
Severe protein-energy malnutrition	< 17

* For method of calculation of BMI see p. 136.

Marasmus and kwashiorkor

These are extreme forms of protein-energy malnutrition. *Marasmus* is an inevitable consequence of a long-term shortage of food often exacerbated by acute famine, or may result from such famines alone. Sufferers exhibit extreme emaciation with no adipose reserves, muscle wastage and eventually loss of protein from critical organs such as liver, heart and kidneys (although these are preserved as long as possible). The catabolism of protein is associated with reduced synthesis of protein in general and hence immune responses are impaired with consequential increase in infections. Intestinal mucosal cell regeneration is drastically reduced with a resulting impairment of absorption (the intestinal mucosa becomes more secretory than absorptive under these conditions). Diarrhoea is a major problem in marasmus sufferers and thus worsens the malnutrition; furthermore, it presents severe problems when re-feeding is attempted.

Kwashiorkor is only observed in children. Children suffering from severe protein-energy malnutrition exhibit the same characteristic features as in marasmus, i.e. muscle wasting, impaired immunity and malabsorptive intestinal mucosa, but in addition they suffer from oedema and liver enlargement. These latter effects produce the misleading abdominal enlargement and limb puffiness which from a distance give an illusion of plumpness. Hair and skin colour and texture are affected also. At one time it was believed that the additional severity of kwashiorkor resulted from a lack of protein in the diet, even if total energy intake was adequate. This is now known not to be the case, and it is still far from clear what additional factors result in kwashiorkor rather than simply marasmus, although it is likely that general food deficiency coupled to reduced ingestion of antioxidants (such as vitamins C and E, see below) is implicated.

Micronutrient deficiencies

Whilst protein-energy malnutrition is a major issue in developing countries, deficiency of individual nutrients, especially of micronutrient *vitamins* and *minerals*, where overall energy intake is adequate is also a considerable problem. The most common micronutrient deficiencies are discussed below.

Vitamin A deficiency

This is the most important cause of blindness in children worldwide, with some 14 million children under school age having a clinically apparent deficiency. Vitamin A, or *retinoic acid/retinol* is a vital component of the visual pigment rhodopsin and its deficiency leads to impaired vision (and in the longer term to xerophthalmia, keratinization and ulceration of the cornea, and hence blindness). Retinoic acid, acting via nuclear receptors, has important functions in the regulation of cell differentiation and turnover. Excess vitamin A is toxic. *Carotenoids*, found in many coloured vegetable foods, act as *provitamin A* being broken down in the intestinal mucosa to vitamin A. Beta-carotene has very low toxicity (unlike vitamin A itself) and has potent antioxidant properties which may be beneficial in the prevention of cancer, vascular disease and diabetic complications.

Vitamins B_1 and B_2 deficiencies

Deficiency of these vitamins is a considerable problem in Africa and much of Asia. B_1, *thiamin*, is required as a coenzyme in carbohydrate metabolism. Many tissues are affected by thiamin deficiency, the most common result of long-term deficiency (coupled with relatively high carbohydrate intake) being beriberi which features peripheral nervous damage and muscle weakness. Central nervous system damage (Wernicke–Korsakoff syndrome) can also result from thiamin deficiency, especially that seen in alcoholics.

B_2, *riboflavin*, is involved in redox reactions in fuel metabolism and deficiency results in various skin lesions.

Vitamin D deficiency

Vitamin D is derived primarily from the action of sunlight on 7-dehydrocholesterol in the skin. This results in the production of *cholecalciferol*, vitamin D_3, which acts as a precursor for a steroid-like (secosteroid) hormone *calcitriol* (1,25-dihydroxy-vitamin D), synthesized in the kidney. A synthetic vitamin D, derived from ultraviolet (UV) irradiation of the plant sterol, *ergosterol*, and known as vitamin D_2 is sometimes used as a dietary supplement and can be used identically for calcitriol synthesis.

Calcitriol stimulates expression of a calcium-binding protein in intestinal mucosa and in bone which is vital for the normal uptake of calcium and its use in bone formation. Deficiency of vitamin D, most usually due to inadequate exposure to sunshine (and when dietary supplementation is absent), results in *rickets* in children (undermineralization of the bones) or its equivalent in adults—*osteomalacia*.

Vitamin D deficiency is now relatively rare in the UK, except in some ethnic groups, and the toxicity of high intakes of vitamin D has resulted in reduced supplementation of foods with the vitamin.

Other vitamin deficiencies

Rarer deficiencies include those of vitamin B_6, B_{12} (pernicious anaemia), folic acid (megaloblastic anaemia; in addition folate supplementation in pregnancy may reduce the risk of spina bifida and other neural tube defects in the infant) and vitamin C (scurvy; larger doses of this vitamin, ascorbic acid, may have antioxidant benefits).

Iodine deficiency

Iodine is necessary for synthesis of thyroid hormones T_3 and T_4. In areas of the world far from the sea (seawater is rich in iodine), especially in upland limestone areas where iodine is readily leached from the soil and thus not taken up by food plants, *goitre* is prevalent. Goitre involves enlargement of the thyroid glands in the neck and the deficiency results in low metabolic rate and mental impairment.

Iron deficiency

Iron deficiency results in *anaemia*, a reduced synthesis of haemoglobin, because of the absolute need for iron in the *haem* moiety of the protein and related ones such as myoglobin and the cytochromes. Anaemia is particularly common in women because of

loss of iron in menstrual blood. In some developing countries intestinal parasites cause loss of blood in the faeces and can result in anaemia in both sexes (see also Chapter 14).

Appetite disorders

Disorders associated with the regulation of appetite and energy expenditure have been increasing worldwide. In technologically advanced countries where food is plentiful and relatively inexpensive the incidence of obesity has been steadily rising making it the most common chronic disease in the developed world (Fig. 15.1). For example, in 1998 it was estimated that 25% of the population of the UK were obese; in the USA the problem is more severe, some 35% of women and 31% of males being classed as obese. However, in such societies where obesity is prevalent there has also been a marked increase in other diseases associated with defective control of appetite such as anorexia nervosa and bulimia. Perhaps the cultural preoccupation with body image and weight gain is exacerbated by the obesity problem so that any fat is conceived to be 'bad'. Treatment for disorders associated with appetite is often difficult and relapse is frequent; however, recent advances in the understanding of the genetics of obesity and in appetite regulation at the molecular level may hold the key to developing future therapies.

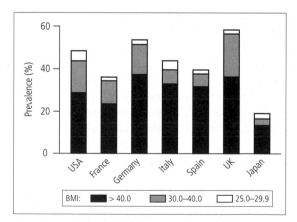

Fig. 15.1 Obesity is becoming a very common problem in affluent countries.

Table 15.2 Definitions of 'overweight' and 'obese' using BMI.

Category	BMI
Underweight	< 20
'Desireable'	20–25
Acceptable	25–27
Overweight	25–30
Obese	30–40
Severely obese	> 40

Obesity

It is obvious that obesity cannot be defined by body weight alone since the latter will clearly vary with height. Ideally it should be assessed in terms of excess adiposity and its relationship to morbidity and mortality, but this is impractical in routine measurement since quantification of body fat content needs elaborate laboratory measurements. An index derived from the relationship between body surface area and weight is the *BMI* which is calculated as the weight (kg) divided by the square of the height (m²) and is thus given in units of kg/m^2. Calculations of the associated risks of disease and premature mortality have led to definitions of bands of BMI being defined as normal, overweight, obese and so on (Table 15.2).

A BMI of below 20 is associated with undernutrition and is considered underweight. Very low BMI in women (e.g. anorexic or athletes) is often associated with lack of ovulation, suggesting that some body fat is required for female fertility. This suggestion is supported by the fact that the 'normal' body fat content of women is ~30% compared with ~16% for men. A 'desirable' BMI of 20–25 is associated with the lowest morbidity whereas health risks are increased in the overweight and especially in the obese and severely obese categories. The health problems associated with obesity include hypertension, cardiovascular disease, increased risk of stroke, type 2 (non-insulin dependent) diabetes and the development of some cancers. It has, however, been recognized for some time that the risks of adverse health consequences from obesity are affected by the anatomical distribution of adipose tissue. Epidemiological studies have shown that upper body or *'android'* obesity, in which adipose tissue accumulates around the abdominal region (giving an 'apple' shape to the body), is closely associated with metabolic disorders such as cardiovascular disease and diabetes. By contrast in the case of peripheral *'gynoid'* obesity, where there is accumulation of subcutaneous fat particularly in the gluteal and thigh region (sometimes referred to as a 'pear' body shape), there is little association with metabolic disease. Android obesity is common in men and postmenopausal women but is rarer in younger women who predominantly exhibit gynoid obesity.

By the laws of thermodynamics it can be demonstrated that obesity must result 'simply' from an imbalance between energy intake and energy expenditure, thus the first approach to treatment will usually entail a controlled energy intake (diet) coupled with an exercise programme. Either, or both, of these approaches is designed to achieve an energy intake that is lower than energy expenditure, with the result that the *negative energy balance* is compensated for by the loss of adipose tissue. Less desirably loss of muscle tissue can occur if the balance is too negative, as in the case of 'very low calorie diets' which can amount to 'starvation'. It is also recognized, however, that the body has homoeostatic mechanisms by which it can compensate for changes in energy intake and expenditure in order to maintain a 'set-point' body weight.

Research into the genetics of obesity and in the regulation of appetite has made significant advances in recent years following the discovery of the sequence of the *ob* (obesity) gene. This gene was first identified in mice with a recessively inherited genetic obesity (*ob/ob* mice, Fig. 15.2); its cloning using 'positional cloning' methodology was reported by Jeffrey Friedman *et al.* in the journal *Nature* in December 1994 (Zhang *et al.* 1994). Because of the potential significance of the gene and its product there has since been an explosion of published research on it (in excess of 2000 papers by late 1999). Friedman *et al.* predicted that the sequence of the normal (wild-type) gene encoded a secreted protein which, in view of the finding that its expression was primarily in adipose tissue, was able to signal the size of the adipose depot back to the areas of the

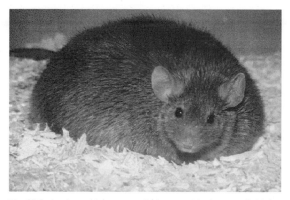

Fig. 15.2 An obese *ob/ob* mouse weighing some 90 g (compared with the average weight of a lean littermate of 25 g).

brain which control appetite and energy expenditure (in particular parts of the *hypothalamus*). The normal gene product, which is a 167 amino acid protein, is called *leptin* from the Greek word *leptos* (λεπτοο) meaning thin. Leptin behaves as a hormone and interacts with leptin receptors in the hypothalamus and elsewhere (Fig. 15.3a). Obese mice have a mutation in the leptin (*lep*) gene, formerly referred to as the *ob* gene and more recently as the *lep^ob* gene which results in an absolute deficiency in leptin production (Fig. 15.3b).

The importance of leptin in the control of appetite, and of leptin deficiency in obesity, was evident from the characteristics of the genetically obese mouse which is hyperphagic, hyperinsulinaemic and has a thermogenic defect resulting in an inability to maintain body temperature at low environmental temperatures. Treatment of *ob/ob* mice by injection with leptin produced by recombinant technology completely normalizes their eating behaviour, body weight and metabolism. Another genetically obese mouse, the 'diabetic' (*db/db*) mouse, has a mutation in the leptin receptor gene and exhibits an identical phenotype to that of the *ob/ob* mouse. Unlike the *ob/ob* mouse, but as predicted, it has very high levels of circulating leptin and it is unresponsive to both the endogenous and injected hormone.

Leptin has been shown to affect neuronal circuits in the brain that regulate feeding and metabolism. By acting on its receptors in several hypothalamic centres it modulates a number of neuropeptides which are involved in control of feeding. It downregulates *neuropeptide Y*, an extremely potent peptide which is known to increase food intake (an effect which can be demonstrated even when it is injected into the brain of fully fed animals). Other neuropeptides which may be modulated by leptin include melanocyte concentrating hormone (MCH) (stimulates feeding), cholecystokinin (CCK) and glucagon-like peptide-1 (7–36) amide (GLP-1) (inhibits feeding). Leptin inhibits insulin secretion via neural pathways and also by acting directly on insulin-producing cells. Conversely, insulin stimulates leptin production by adipocytes, implying that a classical feedback loop exists between insulin and leptin.

Leptin and human obesity

As yet it is not clear to what extent defects in the leptin signalling system play a part in human obesity. Initial studies of both lean and obese subjects showed a clear positive correlation between body weight/adiposity and plasma leptin levels. Thus the circulating leptin concentration is a clear reflection of the human adipose tissue mass in most humans. There was, however, no evidence of leptin deficiency in these groups although it was proposed that a 'leptin-receptor deficiency' could be present. Since there was also no evidence of abnormalities in the leptin receptors in these groups it was suggested that 'leptin resistance' might be occurring. Such resistance would account for the continuing tendency of obese people to 'overeat' in the face of high leptin levels. It is, however, far from clear whether such resistance results from a simple 'receptor downregulation' (as observed with other hormones) or from the influence of higher brain centres in humans. It may be argued that humans, being self-aware, can override lower circuits of feeding behaviour regulation; thus the pleasurable sensations of eating 'tasty' food may be stronger than the leptin inhibition of feeding at the hypothalamic level.

Recent research, however, has demonstrated that leptin-signalling deficiencies can and do occur in humans with the predicted result of overeating and extreme obesity. Professor Steven O'Rahilly and his group at Cambridge reasoned that genetic defects in leptin signalling analogous to those in rodents

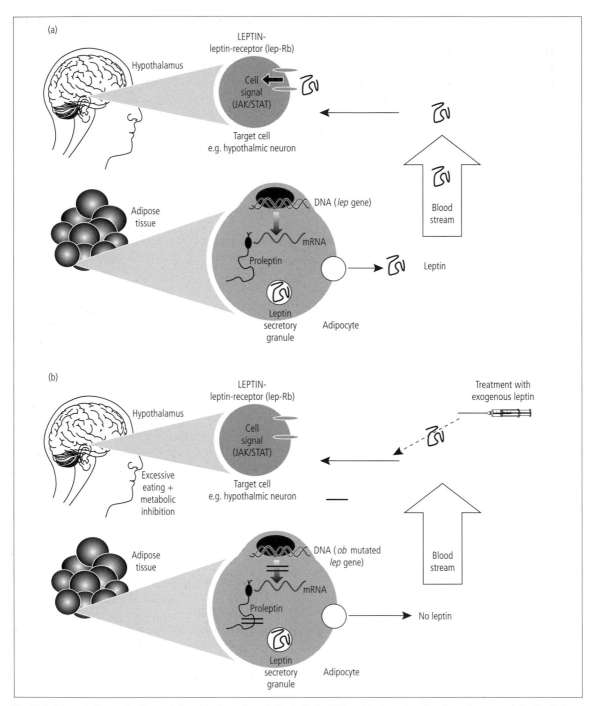

Fig. 15.3 Schematic diagram showing regulation of feeding and metabolism by leptin. (a) Normal leptin produced by adipose tissue controls food intake by binding to leptin receptors in the hypothalamus. (b) Mutation in leptin genes leads to deficiency of leptin and hence no activation of saitiety pathways in the brain. This can be corrected by treatment with recombinant leptin.

should be evident from a very early age as they are in mice. In 1997 they reported that a survey of obese children had revealed two very obese individuals from the same family with no detectable circulating leptin (Montague *et al.* 1997). Genetic analysis confirmed that the cousins have a mutation in the leptin gene similar to that of the *ob/ob* mouse. These children have been treated with recombinant leptin and have responded emphatically with reduced appetite and weight. Other mutations in leptin and leptin receptor genes, resulting in extreme obesity, have since been identified in Turkey and France, respectively. Whilst these mutations are rare, they do demonstrate the need for an intact leptin system for normal weight homoeostasis.

Other possible physiological roles of leptin

Leptin also provides a mechanism to explain *amenorrhoea* (the lack of ovulation) in very thin females since it has been demonstrated to modulate normal reproductive function in both animals and humans (*ob/ob* female mice and leptin-deficient women are infertile) and to interact with the hypothalamopituitary–gonadal axis. Interestingly, placenta expresses leptin almost as highly as adipose tissue.

Anorexia nervosa and leptin

Another eating disorder in which leptin has been proposed to have a role is that of anorexia nervosa. Anorexic individuals appear to lose normal feeding instincts. This would predictably happen if leptin levels were inappropriately high. There is no evidence that this is the case, and studies have shown low levels of leptin consistent with the low adipose tissue mass.

Relationship of obesity to other metabolic diseases: 'insulin resistance syndrome'

As mentioned above, the incidence of cardiovascular disease, type II diabetes and other disorders is much higher in clinically obese subjects, to the extent that it has been proposed that these diseases are linked in a common syndrome which was described by Gerald Reaven in 1988 and is known as *'insulin resistance syndrome'* (or 'syndrome X' or 'metabolic syndrome'). Obesity is characterized

by hyperinsulinaemia in both animal models and in humans. Insulin resistance (reduced sensitivity of insulin-sensitive tissues such as skeletal muscle and adipose tissue) is necessarily present as well, although there is some debate as to whether the insulin resistance occurs in order to compensate for the hyperinsulinaemia (which otherwise would result in severe hypoglycaemia and possibly death!) or whether hyperinsulinaemia is compensatory for the insulin resistance. It is possible to argue both cases although opinion generally favours the second explanation. Insulin resistance and hyperinsulinaemia are also strong factors in the pathogenesis of vascular diseases and the former is the major feature of type II diabetes.

The highest incidence of these associated diseases occurs in a number of populations around the world who have recently moved from a traditional 'hunter–gatherer' lifestyle to an affluent Western style of life. It has been suggested that such groups have been under strong selection pressures to enable them to survive in their traditional environment, which involves brief periods of plenty (e.g. when rains come and wild food and game animals are plenty) interspersed with longer periods of scarcity (e.g. during dry season droughts). This selected *'thrifty genotype'* would result in a propensity to 'hypersecrete' insulin, which combined with selective muscle insulin resistance would favour accumulation of adipose tissue triacylglycerol (Fig. 15.4). Such stores of tissue fat then provide energy during the periods of scarcity. The thrifty genotype hypothesis then predicts that the same people confronted with a continuing, overabundant supply of the high-fat, high-energy affluent diet would continually oversecrete insulin, developing insulin resistance, obesity, vascular disease and diabetes. Indirect support for the hypothesis comes from epidemiological studies of groups such as the Pima Indians of Arizona or Australian Aborigines where the incidence of obesity in adults approaches 100% and that of diabetes nearly 50%. More direct support is available, including studies on a group of Australian Aborigines with diabetes who returned to their traditional lifestyle for 7 weeks and who exhibited a dramatic improvement in their diabetes and other metabolic abnormalities (Table 15.3).

Parameter	Before	After 7 weeks	Significance
Body weight (kg)	81.9 ± 3.4	73.8 ± 2.8	$P < 0.001$
BMI (kg/m^2)	27.2 ± 1.1	24.5 ± 0.8	$P < 0.001$
Fasting glucose (mmol/L)	11.6 ± 1.2	6.6 ± 0.5	$P < 0.001$
Glucose 2 h after OGTT (75 g)	18.5 ± 1.3	11.9 ± 0.9	$P < 0.001$
Fasting insulin (µm/L)	23 ± 3	12 ± 1	$P < 0.001$
Insulin 2 h after OGTT (75 g)	49 ± 9	59 ± 11	n.a.
Fasting triglycerides (mmol/L)	4.02 ± 0.46	1.15 ± 0.10	$P < 0.001$
Fasting cholesterol (mmol/L)	5.65 ± 0.23	4.98 ± 0.34	n.s.
Blood pressure: systolic (mmHg)	121 ± 5	114 ± 5	$P < 0.08$
Blood pressure: diastolic (mmHg)	80 ± 2	72 ± 2	$P < 0.02$
Bleeding time (min)	4.1 ± 0.4	5.9 ± 0.4	$P < 0.01$

Table 15.3 Thrifty genes: effect of changes in lifestyle in Australian Aborigines. The table shows a major change in metabolic abnormalities of diabetes and other risk factors for cardiovascular disease in a group of diabetic Aborigines response to 7 weeks reversion to a traditional hunter–gatherer lifestyle (mean $\pm$ SE, $n = 10$). Adapted from O'Dea (1984).

n.a., Not applicable; n.s., not significant.

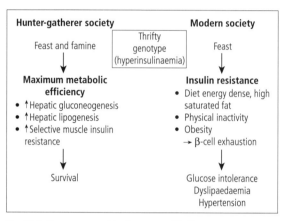

Fig. 15.4 Diagram summarizing the proposed 'thrifty genotype hypothesis'.

Summary

Nutritional disorders range widely from deficiencies including undernourishment which are of significance mainly in developing countries to so-called 'diseases of affluence' which are a major health problem in Western countries. This chapter has surveyed the most common disorders with particular attention paid to the obesity and related diseases, which are of particular significance in the UK, and has discussed recent genetic advances which have identified an important system of weight and metabolic control involving the hormone leptin.

Key points

1 Obesity is the commonest, and most rapidly increasing, nutritional disorder and a major health problem in 'developed' countries.

2 Protein-energy malnutrition and micronutrient deficiency are still common, primarily in underdeveloped countries.

3 Obesity has genetic and environmental components and is linked, especially in the case of 'abdominal' upper-body obesity, with diabetes and cardiovascular disease as well as with other metabolic disorders.

4 Metabolic disorders including obesity, diabetes and vascular diseases are associated with insulin resistance ('insulin-resistance syndrome').

5 The 'thrifty-gene hypothesis' suggests that insulin resistance and hyperinsulinaemia may be survival advantages in a hunter–gatherer society, and have thus been selected for during human evolution, but become pathogenic, causing metabolic disorders, in developed societies.

6 The appetite-regulating hormone *leptin* is produced by adipose tissue, and defects in the leptin signalling system may have a role in the pathogenesis of eating and metabolic disorders.

Further reading

Bender D.A. (1997) *Introduction to Nutrition and Metabolism* (2nd edn). Taylor & Francis, London.

Friedman J.M. & Halaas J.L. (1998) Leptin and the regulation of body weight in mammals. *Nature* **395**: 763–770.

References

Montague C.T. *et al.* (1997) Congenital leptin deficiency is associated with severe early-onset obesity in humans. *Nature* **387**: 903–908.

O'Dea K. (1984) Marked improvement in carbohydrate and lipid metabolism in diabetic Australian aborigines after temporary reversion to traditional lifestyle. *Diabetes* **33**: 596–603.

Reaven G.M. (1988) Role of insulin resistance in human disease. *Diabetes* **37**: 1595–1607.

Ur E. (ed.) (2000) Neuroendocrinology of leptin. In: Grossman A.B. (ed.) *Frontiers of Hormone Research* **26**. Karger, Basel.

Zhang Y. *et al.* (1994) Positional cloning of the mouse *obese* gene and its human homologue. *Nature* **372**: 425–432.

Disorders of Haemostasis

The normal haemostatic (or 'blood coagulation')
system helps to ensure that blood is confined to,
and flows freely within, the circulatory system. The
process involves platelets, vascular endothelium,
the blood coagulation cascade and several substances which promote or inhibit clot formation.
Haemostatic mechanisms thus contribute to the
maintenance of efficient blood flow, and to the
arrest of bleeding from injured blood vessels. This
chapter considers basic haemostatic processes and
some disorders which result from defects in
haemostasis.

Overview of haemostasis

Complex processes have evolved to prevent excessive blood loss after injury and to maintain circulatory integrity. These haemostatic processes depend
upon the interaction of the following:
• The blood vessel wall, in which damage to the
endothelium initiates clotting processes.
• Circulating blood platelets, which are activated
by vessel wall injury or other tissue damage.
• The blood coagulation and fibrinolytic mechanisms, and their respective inhibitors.

Depending on its nature, disturbance of haemostasis can lead to either bleeding or *thrombosis*
(formation of a clot within the vascular system).
Expressed very simply, most bleeding disorders are
due to underactive haemostasis, and some thrombotic disorders are due, at least in part, to overactive
haemostatic mechanisms.

Arrest of bleeding

The physiological process underlying the arrest of
bleeding following damage to a blood vessel is
twofold, each of which helps prevent further blood
loss. These are *vasoconstriction* (narrowing of blood
vessels) and the formation, at the site of injury, of a
haemostatic plug (or 'clot'). The haemostatic plug is
derived initially from platelets and incorporates
fibrin strands, into which erythrocytes and leucocytes also become trapped. The fibrin strands are
formed from activation of the blood coagulation
cascade culminating in the conversion of fibrinogen
to fibrin (Fig. 16.1).

Because the 'clotting' process is so potent, control
mechanisms are required to prevent extension of a
clot once it has formed. The control mechanisms
include the following.
• Blood flow (which washes away activated coagulation factors).
• The production, by vascular endothelium, of
prostacyclin (PGI_2) (which inhibits platelet activity).
• Activation of *fibrinolysis* (which dissolves clots).
• The presence of inhibitors of plasma coagulation
factors.

Under normal circumstances haemostasis is held
in check by its naturally occurring inhibitors, thus
preventing the formation of 'unwanted' blood clots.

Platelet structure and physiology

Platelets have a fundamental role in haemostasis.

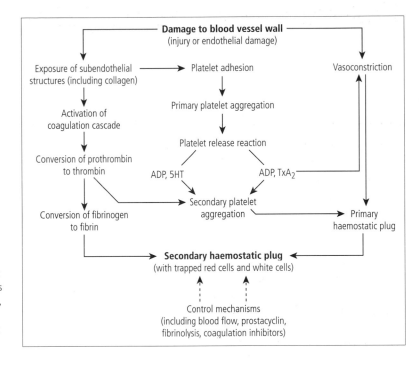

Fig. 16.1 Fundamentals of haemostasis showing involvement of blood vessels, platelets, the blood coagulation cascade and control mechanisms. Vascular injury and exposure of the subendothelium cause vasoconstriction and activation of platelets and the blood coagulation cascade. Complex interactions between these three mechanisms result in the conversion of fibrinogen to fibrin, and the formation of primary and secondary haemostatic plugs. Control mechanisms limit any unnecessary extension of the clot.

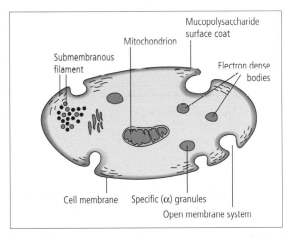

Fig. 16.2 Platelet ultrastructure. A diagrammatic representation of a blood platelet in section. The outer zone consists of a mucopolysaccharide surface coat, submembranous filaments and open and closed membrane systems which provide phospholipid for participation in the coagulation cascade. Within the cytosol are further membrane systems, microfilaments and microtubules. Electron-dense bodies contain adenosine diphosphate (ADP), serotonin and calcium, all of which participate in the platelet release reaction. Specific (α) granules contain growth factors, fibrinogen and other procoagulant substances. Platelets are rich in mitochondria which satisfy their high demand for energy.

They are cytoplasmic fragments derived from mega-karyocytes and are able to survive in the circulation for up to 10 days. Electron microscopy of platelets reveals three zones (Fig. 16.2) as listed below.

The *outer zone*, which is membrane associated. This has a role in platelet adhesion and aggregation and interacts with the blood coagulation cascade. Platelet membrane phospholipid participates in blood coagulation and several plasma coagulation factors, including fibrinogen, are present on the platelet surface.

The *sol gel zone* (*cytosol*) which contains contractile proteins, microfilaments and microtubules. The cytosol contents contribute to platelet shape change, adhesion, aggregation and the 'release reaction' (see below).

Platelet organelles (dense bodies, α-granules and lysosomes), containing a variety of haemostatically active compounds which are released during platelet activation.

Once activated, usually as a result of tissue damage, normal platelets adhere to the damaged vessel wall and aggregate to one another. They then release

143

their granule contents, which include adenosine diphosphate (ADP), 5-hydroxytryptamine (5-HT), adrenaline and thromboxane A_2 (TXA_2). The release of these compounds further potentiates platelet aggregation. This phase culminates in the formation of a *primary haemostatic plug* of platelets at the site of injury. Simultaneous activation of the coagulation cascade, initiated in part by platelet activation, results in the incorporation of fibrin into the clot, which is now called a *secondary haemostatic plug*.

Blood coagulation cascade and its control

The *blood coagulation cascade* results in the production of fibrin, which is incorporated into the haemostatic plug. Once activated, a sequence is initiated in which a series of enzymes (usually serine proteases) act on substrates which are cleaved by the enzyme, and which themselves then have enzymic activity (Fig. 16.3).

The blood coagulation cascade exhibits the typical

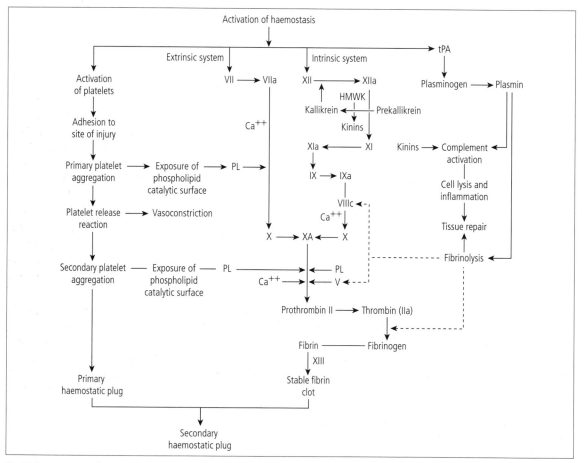

Fig. 16.3 An overview of haemostasis showing integration of the blood coagulation cascade with other haemostatic mechanisms. Vascular injury activates the coagulation cascade, platelets and fibrinolysis. Activation of coagulation factor XII causes generation of kallikrein and kinins, which initiate complement activation and inflammation. The conversion of plasminogen to plasmin causes both complement activation and fibrinolysis. Platelet activation results in release of a range of procoagulant substances, particularly platelet phospholipid, which provides a catalytic surface for the coagulation cascade. The 'extrinsic' and 'intrinsic' systems of the coagulation cascade are shown as distinct entities, but there is thought to be interaction between the two *in vivo*. Coagulation factors: XIII, XII, XI, IX, X, VII, II (proenzymes); XIIa, XIa, IXa, Xa, VIIa, IIa (activated serine proteases); VIIIC, V (cofactors); FGN, fibrinogen; PL, platelet phospholipid; tPA tissue plasminogen activator.

features of other biological cascades, i.e. amplification, specificity and control. This potent mechanism is balanced by several naturally occurring inhibitors which help prevent fibrin clot formation (notably the *serine protease inhibitors* or SERPINS) and the fibrinolytic system which digests clots once they are formed.

When shown diagrammatically (as in Fig. 16.3) it is convenient to depict two separate, quite distinct mechanisms with a common final pathway. These represent early observations that clotting in blood removed from the body and exposed only to a glass or similar surface (intrinsic coagulation) was a different process to that stimulated by tissue extracts (extrinsic coagulation). This led to the development of *in vitro* laboratory procedures which test separately for components of intrinsic and extrinsic systems, enabling differentiation of a range of coagulation factor defects. However, there is evidence that, *in vivo*, there is close integration of the extrinsic and intrinsic coagulation cascades, interaction with platelets (via membrane phospholipid) and also a relationship to inflammatory events (via the complement and kinin systems, see Chapters 5 and 6). In addition, there are several examples of feedback within the coagulation cascade, and a simultaneous activation of the fibrinolytic system (Fig. 16.3).

Prostaglandin metabolism in platelets and blood vessels

We have seen that *platelet aggregation* is stimulated by exposure to a range of substances including *collagen* and *thrombin*, the latter being formed in the coagulation cascade. Thrombin binds to receptors on the vascular endothelium and on platelet membranes. This causes release of arachidonic acid which is metabolized by cyclooxygenase to prostaglandin G_2 (PGG_2). PGG_2 is further metabolized to TXA_2 in platelets, and to PGI_2 (prostacyclin) in the vascular endothelium.

TXA_2 and PGI_2 have opposing effects on platelet adenylate cyclase: PGI_2 stimulates activity of this enzyme causing an increase in cyclic adenosine monophosphate (cAMP), thus lowering free calcium ion concentrations and reducing platelet adhesion and aggregation. In addition to its inhibitory effect on platelets, PGI_2 is a vasodilator, whereas TXA_2 has the opposite effect, acting as a vasoconstrictor and a potent inducer of platelet aggregation (Fig. 16.4).

Regular ingestion of low dose aspirin (acetylsalicylic acid) is recommended to susceptible patients to protect against the development of arterial thrombosis. Aspirin inhibits the activity of platelet cyclooxygenase, thereby reducing TXA_2 production for the life of those platelets in circulation at the time. The inhibition of endothelial cyclooxygenase is transient, so the overall effect is an excess of PGI_2 over TXA_2, thus reducing platelet activity.

Role of the vascular endothelium in haemostasis

In the presence of small amounts of thrombin, healthy vascular endothelium opposes coagulation by producing PGI_2, which inhibits platelet aggregation. Other substances opposing clot formation include tissue plasminogen activator (tPA) which stimulates fibrinolysis, and the coagulation inhibitors antithrombin III and thrombomodulin.

Conversely, endothelial cells synthesize von Willebrand factor, a procoagulant protein which promotes platelet adhesion and aggregation, and acts as a carrier for the factor VIII coagulation factor. Thus, healthy vascular endothelium contributes to both promotion and inhibition of blood coagulation.

Damage to vascular endothelium activates platelets and blood coagulation mechanisms. This may be desirable (to arrest bleeding) or undesirable— for example, when damage to the intima of the blood vessel promotes the formation of a *thrombus* (an unwanted clot which forms within a blood vessel).

Factors contributing to bleeding and thrombosis

Activation of haemostasis may result from the following damage.
• Trauma or other physical damage requiring activation of haemostatic mechanisms to prevent blood loss.

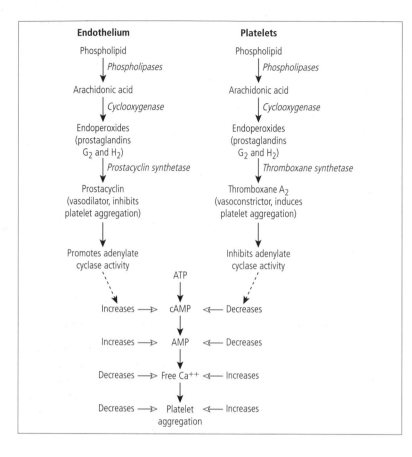

Fig. 16.4 The synthesis of prostaglandins in vascular endothelial cells and in platelets. Arachidonic acid metabolism follows different paths in vascular endothelial cells and platelets. In endothelial cells PGI_2 synthetase catalyses the conversion of endoperoxides to PGI_2, whereas in platelets the equivalent reaction is catalysed by thromboxane synthetase to form TXA_2. PGI_2 and TXA_2 have opposing actions on blood platelets.

• Endothelial damage, often associated with atherosclerosis, causing abnormal haemostatic activation which can result in formation of a thrombus, possibly leading to vessel occlusion.

A reduction in platelet numbers or in the concentration of blood coagulation factors limits the ability to form effective haemostatic plugs and results in a bleeding tendency. Conversely, an increase in haemostatic activity may predispose to thrombosis.

Clinical conditions arising from disturbed haemostasis

Haemostatic disorders can thus be divided into two types.
• Disorders of underactivity: bleeding disorders such as *haemophilia A*, *Christmas disease* or *thrombocytopenic purpura*.

• Disorders of overactivity (Table 16.1): thrombotic disorders such as *thrombotic stroke*, *coronary heart disease* and *deep vein thrombosis*.

However, it should be emphasized that in many thrombotic disorders, additional factors contribute to the pathogenesis of the disorder, including lipid imbalances associated with atherosclerosis (see Chapter 17).

Haemostatic involvement in thrombotic and bleeding disorders

Bleeding disorders

Abnormal bleeding may arise from deficiencies in platelet numbers or function, blood coagulation factor disorders (either congenital or acquired) or defects in the vascular wall. Of these, platelet defects are the most common, followed by coagula-

Table 16.1 Haemostatic involvement in bleeding and thrombotic disorders.

	Haemostatic activity	
	Reduced	Increased
Possible clinical consequence	Bleeding	Thrombosis
Contributory haemostatic factors		
Abnormalities of the vessel wall	Cut or rupture of blood vessel	Atheroma
		Exposure of subendothelium
Platelets	Reduced numbers	Increased numbers
	Reduced platelet function	Increased reactivity
Blood coagulation factors	Reduced concentration	Increased concentration
	Abnormal structure	
Blood coagulation inhibitors	Increased concentration of inhibitors	Reduced concentration of inhibitors (e.g. protein S, C or antithrombin III)
Fibrinolysis	Increased fibrinolytic activity	Decreased fibrinolytic activity
Other causes		Reduced blood flow
		Increased blood viscosity
		Hyperlipidaemia

tion factor disorders. Bleeding due primarily to vascular disorders is rare. Increased fibrinolytic activity or raised coagulation inhibitors may also be implicated in excessive bleeding.

Platelet disorders

Platelet disorders are usually acquired. *Thrombocytopenia* (reduction in platelet numbers) usually presents with superficial bleeding (*petechiae* or bruising) and may be due to failure of platelet production or shortened platelet survival. Most cases of *idiopathic thrombocytopenic purpura* (ITP) are now understood to be autoimmune in origin, and in such cases circulating immunoglobulin G (IgG) antibodies to platelets can often be identified. Drugs can also induce an autoimmune response to platelets, resulting in thrombocytopenia, though some drugs also depress megakaryocyte production. Other conditions linked with thrombocytopenia include bone marrow disorders such as aplastic anaemia (see Chapter 14) and leukaemia (case studies 29 and 30).

Defects in platelet function rarely cause major spontaneous bleeding, though they may cause blood loss after dental extraction or surgery. Ingestion of aspirin or other non-steroidal anti-inflammatory agents blocks the activity of platelet cyclooxygenase, causing a characteristic transient defect in platelet function. However, this is rarely sufficient to cause bleeding alone, but may exacerbate bleeding from other lesions, e.g. ulceration or malignancy in the gastrointestinal tract.

Congenital coagulation disorders

The best known of the congenital bleeding disorders are *haemophilia A* and *haemophilia B* (Christmas disease) due to deficiencies of factor VIIIC and factor IX, respectively. Both conditions are uncommon, the incidence of Christmas disease being approximately one-fifth that of haemophilia A. The inheritance of both disorders is X-linked and both are characterized by painful spontaneous bleeding into joints and muscles, depending on the severity of the deficiency. The concentration of the deficient coagulation factor is typically in the region of 0–5% of normal, corresponding to a range of clinical severity from severe to mild haemophilia. Treatment of active bleeding is by administration of the deficient coagulation factor (factor VIII or factor IX) in the form of a concentrate, while some patients with severe deficiency utilize coagulation factor replacement on a prophylactic basis.

Von Willebrand's disease (vWD) is an inherited autosomal bleeding disorder due to deficiency of von Willebrand factor, resulting in reduced factor VIII coagulant activity and abnormal platelet function. Again severity varies, and in most cases is mild, with patients experiencing episodic bleeding particularly after a haemostatic challenge such as minor surgery or dental extraction. In contrast to haemophilia bleeding in vWD tends to be superficial, typically from mucous membranes, rather than deep as in muscles and joints. However, a small number of patients with vWD experience spontaneous bleeding similar to that in haemophilia A, requiring treatment with factor VIII, either in the form of a concentrate or as cryoprecipitate (see case study 17).

Acquired bleeding disorders

Examples of acquired coagulation factor disorders are seen in liver disease and *disseminated intravascular coagulation* (DIC). The liver synthesizes most coagulation factors resulting in their deficiency in liver disease. In addition, because of the malabsorption associated with *cholestatic* ('obstructive') liver disease there is often a reduction in several blood coagulation factors, particularly factors II, VII, IX and X which depend on vitamin K for their synthesis. DIC is characterized by widespread deposition of *microthrombi* with a consequent depletion in platelets and coagulation factors, and a high risk of spontaneous bleeding. This is often exacerbated by a dramatic increase in fibrinolytic activity which digests the flimsy clots which are able to form. DIC is often associated with leukaemias, other malignant blood disorders and complications in pregnancy and childbirth.

Thrombotic disorders

Thrombosis

During the nineteenth century Virchow described three factors contributing to the onset of thrombosis, which later became known as *Virchow's triad*.
- Damage to the inner surface of the vessel wall.
- Disturbed blood flow.
- Altered 'blood mechanisms'.

Virchow's 'blood mechanisms' are now known to be haemostatic systems involving complex interactions between the vascular endothelium, platelets and the blood coagulation cascade. One or more of Virchow's triad contribute to most arterial and venous thromboembolic disorders. However, it appears that different parts of the haemostatic system may predominate in venous and arterial thrombosis. In general, venous thromboembolism is often triggered by changes in blood coagulation factors or their inhibitors together with reduced blood flow, while arterial thrombosis is usually associated with damage to the vascular endothelium and increased platelet activity. However, these are not mutually exclusive: for example, increased blood fibrinogen concentration has been linked to increased risk of coronary artery occlusion, and platelets are certainly implicated in venous thrombosis.

Venous thromboembolism

An embolus is defined as a clot (or other form of solid material, such as fat, or an air bubble) carried in the circulatory system. *Thromboembolism* is the occlusion of a blood vessel by a clot which originated in a larger vessel and which has been carried in the circulatory system from its original site. Typically, venous thrombi form initially in the deep veins of the leg(s) after surgical operations which are followed by prolonged bed rest. This is associated with reduced blood flow and the postoperative hypercoagulable state, which is characterized by raised concentrations of most blood coagulation factors. The fibrinolytic system is activated and gradually dissolves any clots, but fragments may break off to form emboli. These pass through the vena cava and the right chambers of the heart, but lodge in the pulmonary circulation resulting in *pulmonary embolism* (PE). PE results in reduced perfusion of the lungs, varying in severity depending on the site and size of the occluded vessel. Acute chest pain and *haemoptysis* (coughing up of blood-stained sputum) are among the typical clinical features, but these vary: small pulmonary emboli may produce few signs and symptoms and large emboli can result in sudden death.

The causes of most venous thrombosis, e.g. that following surgery, can be readily explained. However, in a small proportion of patients other factors are thought to be responsible. For example, unexplained or recurrent venous thrombosis is sometimes associated with oestrogen therapy, pregnancy or malignant diseases. The rare inherited deficiencies of coagulation inhibitors, particularly of *protein C*, its cofactor *protein S* and *antithrombin III*, are recognized as causes of *thrombophilia* (increased tendency to venous thrombosis). The presence of the paradoxically named *'lupus anticoagulant'*, an autoantibody to phospholipid which prolongs clotting times *in vitro*, is also associated with an increased risk of thrombosis. However, at the time of writing, the commonest known cause of inherited thrombophilia in Western countries is *factor V Leiden*. This is due to an abnormal gene for coagulation factor V which is present in approximately 5% of the population. Its effect is to reduce the inhibitory effect of protein C on factor V, thereby increasing the potency of the coagulation cascade.

Patients at risk of recurrent venous thrombosis, including those who have recently experienced a deep vein thrombosis or PE, may be treated with an anticoagulant drug such as *heparin* or *warfarin*. Heparin, which must be administered subcutaneously or intravenously enhances the activity of antithrombin III, thus inhibiting a number of coagulation factors. Warfarin, given orally, often after initial treatment with heparin, reduces plasma concentrations of the vitamin K dependent coagulation factors (factors II, VII, IX and X) thereby reducing the risk of further clot formation.

Arterial thrombosis

The presence of *atheroma* (see Chapter 17) predisposes to arterial thrombosis. Interaction between blood platelets and atheromatous deposits appears to be fundamental to the development of thrombotic arterial occlusion. These events may be briefly summarized as follows.

• Atheromatous damage to the arterial intima or exposure of components of the subendothelial vessel wall (including collagen) triggers platelet activation.

• This is followed by adhesion of platelets to the site of injury, platelet shape change and primary aggregation, the platelet release reaction and further aggregation.

• Platelets secrete a range of compounds, including *platelet-derived growth factor* (PDGF) during the release reaction. PDGF causes mitotic division of intimal smooth muscle cells, and migration of medial smooth muscle cells to the arterial intima. Thus, localized activation of platelets exacerbates damage to the intima of the blood vessel.

• Simultaneous activation of the blood coagulation cascade also occurs, enhanced by the platelet release reactions, and fibrin becomes associated with the platelet aggregates, trapping red cells. The resulting thrombus may extend, partially or fully occluding the vessel, although fibrinolytic mechanisms are also activated to limit this spread.

The precise aetiology of arterial atheromatous change has not yet been clearly elucidated. Fatty streaks are common in young people and may be reversible, though they may progress to form *atheromatous plaques*, which are less easy to reverse and are associated with intimal damage. The cause of the initial endothelial damage is unclear, though it is postulated that atheroma may form as a reaction to free radical damage (see Chapter 17).

The clinically important result of haemostatic activation in atherosclerosis is vessel occlusion. This denies an area of tissue of its blood supply (causing *ischaemia*). If this occurs in the coronary arteries which supply the heart muscle (*myocardium*), reduced blood flow results in myocardial ischaemia, and this in turn can lead to chest pain on exertion (*angina pectoris*). Complete coronary artery occlusion results in death of an affected area of heart muscle, a condition known as *myocardial infarction* (MI). Among predisposing factors for MI are raised blood lipid concentrations, the presence of atherosclerosis, increased platelet activity, raised blood coagulation factors, high blood pressure (*hypertension*) and vasoconstriction or arterial spasm.

Summary

Effective haemostasis depends on a complex interaction of compounds released from vascular endothelium, the activity of platelets, the blood coagulation cascade and all their integrating,

Key points

1 Activation of haemostatic mechanisms involving blood platelets and the coagulation cascade follows damage to the vascular endothelium.

2 Following physical or traumatic damage, haemostatic mechanisms are triggered to prevent excessive blood loss.

3 Disorders of haemostasis cause a number of bleeding disorders, both congenital and acquired.

4 Haemostatic imbalance is also associated with certain arterial and venous thromboembolic disorders.

5 Reduced blood flow and venous stasis, together with raised coagulation factor concentrations (particularly postoperatively), or reduced coagulation inhibitors, predispose to venous thromboembolism.

6 In arteries, where endothelial injury is associated with atheromatous deposits, haemostatic activation appears to exacerbate the damage, often resulting in thrombus formation.

7 Therapeutic measures to reduce platelet reactivity reduce the risk of arterial thrombosis. Oral anticoagulant drugs reduce plasma concentrations of vitamin K dependent coagulation factors thereby reducing the likelihood of further clot formation, particularly after deep vein thrombosis or PE.

promoting and inhibitory factors. This chapter has briefly reviewed the haemostatic imbalances which contribute to bleeding and thrombosis.

Our current concepts of the detailed contribution of haemostatic mechanisms to the aetiology and pathogenesis of bleeding and thrombotic disorders are constantly being refined, with important developments in understanding currently taking place. Some oversimplification has been necessary in the presentation of these complex systems, and readers are referred to more specialist texts for more detail.

Further reading

Hoffbrand A.V., Pettit J.E. & Moss P. (2000) *Essential Haematology* (4th edn). Blackwell Science Ltd., Oxford.

Hughes Jones N.C. & Wickramasinghe S.N. (1996) *Lecture Notes on Haematology* (6th edn). Blackwell Science Ltd., Oxford.

Mehta A.B. & Hoffbrand A.V. (2000) *Haematology at a Glance*. Blackwell Science Ltd., Oxford.

Schiffman F.J. (1998) *Hematologic Pathophysiology*. Lippincott–Raven, Philadelphia.

CHAPTER 17

Atherosclerosis

Atherosclerosis is an inflammatory disease, one clinical manifestation of which is coronary heart disease (CHD), a major cause of disability and death in the Western World. Although the causes of CHD are known to be multifactorial, much attention has been paid to the effects of raised blood cholesterol concentration as a risk factor for atherosclerosis. However, the damage associated with atherosclerosis is due to a number of cellular and molecular responses which promote an inflammatory response.

Overview

The pathogenesis of atherosclerosis is complex and is not yet completely understood. Atherosclerosis is characterized by a progressive accumulation within the arterial wall of cholesterol-containing particles, cell fragments and support matrix materials. These lesions occur principally in the large and medium sized elastic and muscular arteries and so can lead to a reduction in the blood supply to the heart, brain or extremities, resulting in the development of *ischaemia* (reduced oxygen supply) in the tissues supplied by the affected arteries. Clinical examples of the effects of ischaemia are *angina pectoris* (chest pain on exertion due to oxygen lack to the heart muscle) or *intermittent claudication* (pains in the calves and legs when walking). Furthermore, rupture of the atherosclerotic lesion may occur and if this develops in the coronary arteries that supply the myocardium the resulting ischaemia may cause death of an area of myocardial tissue (*myocardial infarction*) producing the clinical effects of a 'heart attack'. There are many factors which induce

inflammation and atherosclerosis, and typical risk factors which can promote and accelerate the atherosclerotic lesion include smoking, hypertension and diabetes.

Aetiology and pathogenesis

The normal human artery is composed of several layers (Fig. 17.1).
• The tunica intima, an inner smooth uninterrupted monolayer of endothelial cells overlying a thin layer of connective tissue matrix scattered within which are a small number of smooth muscle cells, together with collagen and glucose aminoglycans (GAG). The intima is bounded by elastic tissue (the internal elastic lamina).

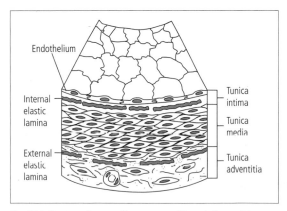

Fig. 17.1 Structure of a normal human artery. The main layers of the arterial wall are the intima, media and adventitia, with the internal and external elastic lamina separating these layers.

- The tunica media, a thick layer of smooth muscle cells separated by small amounts of elastin, collagen and GAG.
- The tunica adventitia, an external layer of connective tissue separated from the media by external elastic lamina. The adventitia consists of collagen, fibroblast and GAG.

Atheromatous plaques usually arise in the arterial intima, typically causing narrowing of the lumen. This may lead to complete occlusion of the vessel lumen, particularly if there is also activation of haemostasis, resulting in thrombus formation. Alternatively rupture of the atherosclerotic plaque may occur with release into the artery of its contents. This can lead to haemostatic activation and cause sudden and catastrophic thrombus formation within the artery, typified by myocardial infarction. There are many factors which contribute to the development of atherosclerosis and these will be discussed in some detail.

Many studies in animals and humans have lead to the characterization of the events that lead to atherosclerotic plaque formation. The most recent of the resulting hypotheses emphasize endothelial dysfunction as the most potent cause of the atherosclerotic event. Release of cytokines from, and expression of adhesion molecules by, endothelial cells is important in the recruitment of monocytes into the subendothelial space. Lipid-laden monocytes and macrophages deposit lipid in the artery wall to form fatty streaks, which are the earliest histological lesions identified as atherosclerosis becomes established. The resulting endothelial cell disruption leads to release of a variety of cellular constituents which activate the blood coagulation cascade and other haemostatic mechanisms (see Chapter 16), resulting in the generation of thrombin and fibrin, the activation of platelets and the secretion of local growth factors from endothelial cells. The possible causes of endothelial dysfunction include those noted in Table 17.1, each of which is considered later.

Progression of atherosclerosis

Over time, a simple fatty streak, the earliest lesion seen in atherosclerosis, can progress to form a 'complicated' plaque which may potentially either

Table 17.1 Possible causes of endothelial dysfunction.

Hypercholesterolaemia, modified lipids and lipoproteins
Homocysteine
Hypertension
Infection

occlude a vessel or rupture. In more detail three phases may ensue as follows.
- The necrotic centre can stabilize and produce an ever-widening and protruding fibrous plaque. With gradual evolution the plaque can slowly occlude the arterial lumen.
- A more catastrophic endpoint is the rupture of the necrotic centre through the middle of the fibrous plaque into the arterial lumen. Matrix metalloproteases released from macrophages appear to be involved in plaque destabilization by digesting collagen fibres. The 'shoulder' of the plaque is most prone to rupture. The release of contents from the necrotic centre can activate coagulation causing thrombus formation and leaving a blockage within that part of the lumen.
- Alternatively, the arterial flow may take the contents and/or any thrombus to an arteriole distal to the rupture where occlusion could occur, an event known as embolism.

Lipid transport

Lipids (fats) are transported in the blood stream in a variety of particles containing greater or lesser amounts of cholesterol and triglyceride. The major particles which transport lipids are chylomicrons (triglyceride-rich), very low density lipoproteins (VLDL, triglyceride-rich), low density lipoproteins (LDL, cholesterol-rich) and high density lipoproteins (HDL, cholesterol-rich). A schematic diagram of plasma lipoprotein metabolism is shown in Fig. 17.2.

Not all of these lipids transported in the blood are implicated in the development of atherosclerosis. For example, HDL confers some protection against CHD, in contrast to LDL, the major particle carrying cholesterol in the blood, which is highly atherogenic. LDL can be derived from the metabolism

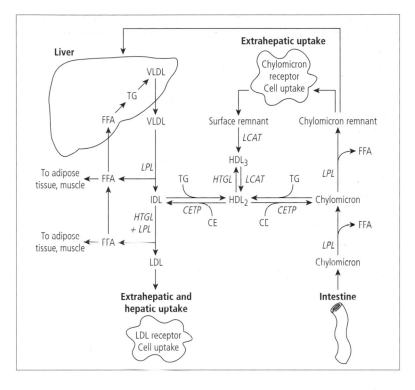

Fig. 17.2 An overview of lipoprotein metabolism. Dietary fats and cholesterol are absorbed from the gut and assembled as triglyceride-rich chylomicrons. Lipoprotein lipase (LPL), in the capillary walls of muscle or adipose tissue, releases free fatty acids (FFA) and monoglycerides. As the fats are removed, the chylomicrons reduce in size, their density increases and the remaining cholesterol is carried as high density lipoprotein (HDL). HDL circulates in the blood and is taken up by liver cells where some is metabolized to very low density lipoprotein (VLDL). Circulating VLDL is a substrate for LPL and is converted via intermediate density lipoprotein (IDL) to HDL or LDL. Specific cell receptors allow the capture of LDL for cell membrane synthesis and energy requirements. Excess LDL in the blood predisposes to atheroma formation. Lipid subfraction: CE, cholesterol; TG, triglycerides. Enzymes: CETP, cholesterol esterase transfer proteins; HTGL, hepatic triglyceride lipase; LCAT, lecithin cholesterol acyl transferase.

of VLDL, through an intermediary lipoprotein called intermediate density lipoprotein (IDL), or directly from secretion of LDL by the liver. LDL is normally cleared by peripheral cells and the liver by uptake on specific receptors (apolipoprotein B_{100}). However, if LDL particles become trapped in an artery they can be internalized by macrophages leading to the formation of lipid peroxides.

The accumulation of these lipid peroxides and cholesterol esters within arterial cells leads to subtle changes and they ultimately form foam cells. As more and more foam cells are formed the atherosclerotic plaque enlarges in size and becomes progressively more unstable. Modified oxidized LDL particles will promote a greater inflammatory response releasing mediators of inflammation such as tumour necrosis factor α, interleukin 1 and macrophage colony-stimulating factor. The presence of these inflammatory molecules leads to more uptake of LDL from the circulation into the artery thus promoting an increasing inflammatory response.

Antioxidants

Antioxidants have been shown in animal models to prevent the tissue lesions caused by the oxidation of LDL. In contrast to the clinical trials which have demonstrated a reduction in clinical events after cholesterol concentrations are decreased by drugs, or by other means, no well-designed clinical trials have shown any direct antioxidant protective effect in humans. In particular antioxidants such as β-carotene have been shown to have no benefit, and indeed may have clinically negative effects.

Homocysteine

Rare homozygous metabolic defects in the enzymes necessary for homocysteine metabolism have been shown to be associated with advanced atherosclerosis in children who inherit this syndrome. In children with enzyme defects such as cystathione β-synthase or methylene tetrahydrafolate reductase, severe atherosclerosis can develop and a first myocardial infarction can occur by the age of 20 years. Homocysteine is toxic to endothelium, is prothrombotic, increases collagen production and decreases availability of nitric oxide. Studies have demonstrated that plasma homocysteine concentrations are elevated in many patients who have no enzymatic defect and these individuals have an increased risk of symptomatic atherosclerosis of the coronary, peripheral, and cerebral arteries. Trials using folic acid as a supplement to reduce the increased homocysteine concentrations are underway, but as yet there are no definitive conclusions.

Hypertension

In patients with hypertension, concentrations of angiotensin-II (the principal product of the renin–angiotensin system) are often increased. Angiotensin-II is a potent vasoconstrictor and can also stimulate the growth of intimal smooth muscle cells, which is a feature of atherogenesis. Hypertension is associated with a number of additional proinflammatory activities which increase the concentrations of hydrogen peroxide and free radicals, reduce the formation of nitric oxide and in turn increase peripheral resistance to arterial blood flow. It is of note therefore that free radicals are implicated in hypertension, hyperlipidaemia and atherosclerosis.

Infection

An interesting hypothesis has been the incidence of atherosclerosis in the presence of infectious agents, notably herpesvirus and *Chlamydia pneumoniae*, both of which have been identified in coronary arteries at postmortem examination. Furthermore, increased concentrations of antibodies with specificity to these organisms have been demonstrated. However, there are no direct data to support the hypothesis that these infectious agents can directly cause atherosclerotic lesions.

Other factors in atherosclerosis

Smoking
Smoking causes a variety of changes within arteries.

These include vasoconstriction (as a direct result of the action of nicotine), reduced metabolism of VLDL and an increase in the production of IDL particles, which are important in the development of atherosclerosis since they are not taken up by the classical apolipoprotein B_{100} receptor-mediated pathway. IDL particles may also directly contribute to the inflammatory response in atherosclerosis. Smoking has been shown to reduce antioxidant protection in plasma, which may also exacerbate the process of oxidation of lipoproteins. Another of the changes associated with smoking is an increase in plasma fibrinogen concentration. This increases the likelihood of fibrin clot formation, thus promoting platelet aggregation and further initiating activation of the coagulation cascade in areas already affected by vascular damage.

Diabetes mellitus
Diabetes mellitus causes a variety of tissue changes which are the result of high concentrations of plasma glucose (see case study 14) and disturbance in lipid metabolism caused by insulin deficiency and/or insulin resistance (the inability of some tissues to respond properly to insulin). Changes in endothelial function and increased glycation and oxidation of LDL occur as a result of high glucose concentrations. The net effect, particularly in type II diabetes mellitus, is that VLDL particles decrease in density. With their density altered transfer of triglyceride and cholesterol ester between VLDL and LDL occurs resulting in LDL particles that become smaller and more dense. Smaller, denser LDL particles are more prone to uptake in atherosclerotic lesions and additionally more prone to oxidation. This helps to explain the increased problem of CHD in diabetic patients which is at least twice as common as in non-diabetic subjects.

Summary

Atherosclerosis develops over a period of years and can cause gradual arterial occlusion which, when this affects the myocardial blood supply, often presents as *angina pectoris*. Alternatively, it may present with the more sudden and catastrophic event of myocardial infarction. Endothelial injury, hyperlipidaemia, activation of the blood coagulation cascade and activation of platelets all contribute to its pathogenesis. The most effective strategy to reduce the incidence of CHD is to prevent atherosclerosis. Risk factors for atherosclerosis should be identified in individual patients and treatment plans tailored to reduce risk factors, principally by modification of lifestyle. Lifestyle changes should therefore focus on the following.

• Cessation of smoking.

• Identification and treatment of individuals with hypertension.

• Reduction of the saturated fat content in the diet.

• Identification and treatment of diabetes mellitus.

• Modification of haemostatic mechanisms in patients with a high risk of thrombosis.

Further reading

Ross R. (1999) Atherosclerosis—an inflammatory disease. *New England Journal of Medicine* **340**: 115–126.

Smith A.F., Beckett G.J., Walker S.W. & Rae P.W.H. (1998) Disorders of plasma lipids and lipoproteins. In: *Lecture Notes on Clinical Biochemistry* (6th edn). Blackwell Science Ltd., Oxford.

Ounpuu S., Anand S. & Yusuf S. *The Global Burden of Cardiovascular Disease.* http://www.medscape.com/medscape/cardiology/2000/v04.n02/mc0428.ounp/mc0428.ounp.html.

Lipoproteins and Atherosclerosis: The Role of HDL Cholesterol, Lp(a), and LDL Particle Size. Speakers: Alan Fogelman, UCLA School of Medicine, Los Angeles, CA; H. Robert Superko, Cholesterol, Genetics, & Heart Disease Institute and Berkeley Heart Lab, San Mateo; Calif Reporter: Carlos S. Ince, MD. Reviewer: Michael J. Czarnecki, DO, FACP. http://www.medscape.com/medscape/CNO/1999/ACC/eng/03.07/0107.carl/0107.carl.html.

Toxicology and Poisoning

Toxicology is routinely described as the *science of poisons*, which invites the question—what is a poison? A familiar answer lies in the famous quotation *'Alle ding sind gifft . . . allein die dosis macht das ein ding kein gifft ist'* ('Everything is a poison . . . it is only the dose that makes it not a poison'; Paracelsus, 1493–1541). More specifically, a poison is any chemical with the potential to cause harm, even death, to an organism. Such a compound, by interacting with the organism, from molecular to tissue level may alter that organism's homoeostasis to the extent that normal function is compromised. Poisons may be conveniently classified as drugs, food additives, environmental pollutants, industrial chemicals, natural toxins and household poisons. However, a number of other terms may be used to classify toxic agents without any particular systematic basis, such as its target organ (e.g. liver), usage (e.g. pesticide), source (e.g. animal toxin), effect (e.g. carcinogen) or biochemical mode of action (e.g. sulphydryl group inhibitor).

Toxicology may embrace a number of areas such as descriptive toxicology, which concerns toxicity testing to provide information by which the evaluation of risk to humans can be evaluated. In turn this relates to regulatory toxicology which uses this descriptive information to make policy decisions on the use of different chemicals. Mechanistic toxicology attempts to describe the mode of action by which chemicals exert their effect on organisms. There are three specialized areas of toxicology, forensic toxicology, a hybrid of analytical chemistry and fundamental toxicology, concerned primarily with the harmful effects of chemicals in humans and establishing the cause of death. Clinical toxicology which involves investigating diseases caused by, or associated with, toxic substances and specializing in emergency medicine and poisoned patient management. Environmental toxicology, including ecotoxicology evaluates the impact of chemical pollutants on the environment and population dynamics within ecosystems.

Exposure

Before any substance can inflict its toxic effect, it must gain entry to the body. Exposure can occur under a number of circumstances, intentional ingestion, occupational and environmental exposure and accidental or intentional poisoning. With some exceptions, the most likely routes of entry are via the skin, lungs or gastrointestinal tract. For a given toxin, exposure can be defined by the means of entry, how many exposures take place, the concentration of the toxin and the time scale of repeated exposures. The ease of entry and subsequent distribution depends very much on the physicochemical properties of the toxin, in particular the degree of water and lipid solubility. Generally speaking lipid-soluble substances will move through cell membranes with greater ease than more ionic forms which may make use of carrier systems present for

Table 18.1 Instances and examples of toxic effects.

Instances of toxic effect	Example
Interference with excitable membranes	Tetrodotoxin blocks sodium channels particularly along the nerve axon—the inward action potential is inhibited Both sensory and motor nerves are affected and death may occur as a result of skeletal paralysis
Interference with ATP production	Inhibition of the tricarboxylic acid cycle (e.g. fluoroacetate) or the alteration of electron transport chain function (e.g. cyanide inhibits, or 2,4-dinitrophenol uncouples the electron transport chain) results in diminished (ATP) energy production
Binding to biomolecules	Carbon monoxide by binding to iron atom of the haem molecule by competing with oxygen. Haemoglobin binds more readily with carbon monoxide than oxygen, tissues become deprived of oxygen resulting in ischaemia. Aerobic energy production declines, anaerobic respiration is increased which results in an acidosis from lactic acid accumulation
Binding to intracellular thiols	Oxidation, cross-linking, formation of mixed disulphides of SH groups can inhibit key enzyme activities particularly those involved in mitochondrial function and membrane permeability. Lead and other heavy metals are capable of binding to –SH groups
Interference with calcium homoeostasis	Reaction with sulphydryl groups will inhibit Ca^{2+} ATPases (lead and other heavy metals) Direct damage to plasma membrane results in increased influx of calcium, e.g. carbon tetrachloride Depletion of ATP gives a rise in intracellular calcium, e.g. uncoupling agents 2,4-dinitrophenol
Interference with nucleic acid synthesis and function	Cytosine arabinoside inhibits DNA polymerase Actinomycin D intercalates with DNA by binding to guanine and blocking the movement of RNA polymerase. This prevents transcription and ultimately protein synthesis Cycloheximide prevents RNA transfer
Interference with lipids	Carbon tetrachloride causes necrosis by the formation of a reactive electrophilic intermediate—trichloromethyl peroxy radical that covalently binds to microsomal lipid and directly reacts with membrane phospholipid
Carcinogenicity	A toxic effect that causes the uncontrolled proliferation of tissues (see Chapter 21), examples of carcinogenic agents are legion but include polycyclic aromatic hydrocarbons, aflatoxins and vinyl chloride
Mutagenicity	A toxic effect that results in specific damage to the genetic material of the cell, hence the effect is heritable (see Chapter 21), examples would be the nitrogen mustard derivatives and nitrosoureas
Teratogenicity	A toxic effect on the development of the embryo or fetus whilst it is still in the uterus. Usually teratogenicity is the effect of toxic substances on the somatic cells rather than germ cells. Developing tissue is often especially vulnerable to toxic insult. Examples comprise ionizing and non-ionizing radiation, environmental and industrial pollutants, dietary deficiency and drugs such as thalidomide, diethyl stilboesterol and alcohol
Immunotoxicity	Toxic insult to primary and secondary lymphoid tissue can inhibit or reduce immune function, e.g. organophosphorus compounds, dibenzodioxins Conversely, stimulation of the immune system may occur as in hypersensitivity reactions such as anaphylaxis (tartrazine), cytolytic (e.g. aminopyrine), Arthus reactions (hydralazine) and delayed hypersensitivity (halothane)

endogenous substrates. Distribution will also be influenced by the extent of binding to endogenous macromolecules.

Concentration of a toxin will be influenced by metabolism. Any xenobiotics (foreign compounds) are likely to be metabolized in a number of sites in the body but predominantly the smooth endoplasmic reticulum of the liver. This process occurs initially by hydrolysis, reduction or oxidation reactions, generally referred to as phase I, they are usually catalysed by mixed function oxygenase enzymes. Of these enzymes cytochrome P-450, a haem protein, is the most important. Phase I is often, though not necessarily invariably, followed by phase II reactions which result in formation of conjugates via groups such as glucuronyl, sulphate or methyl. As a consequence the xenobiotic is rendered less toxic and is often more water soluble and thereby readily excreted in the urine. Metabolism and subsequent excretion will contribute to the time of residence in the body. The general rule is that if the rate of excretion does not exceed the rate of entry then accumulation will occur, which increases the toxic potential of a given toxin. Degree of toxicity does appear to demonstrate dose dependency.

Acute exposure to a substance refers to a single application of that substance to an organism resulting in a toxic effect which occurs within minutes or hours of exposure. Chronic exposure is the repeated delivery over a period of time such that the substance accumulates in the body resulting in a toxic effect. Once the toxin has entered the body there are a number of effects which can lead to a pathological consequence which may be comprised of direct physiological disturbance of tissues/organs, mutagenesis, carcinogenesis (see Chapter 21) or teratogenesis. These effects may include those shown in Table 18.1.

The following relatively familiar examples illustrate ways in which various chemicals may elicit some of the toxic effects listed above.

Tartrazine

An example of a potential toxic substance, which also illustrates the somewhat equivocal nature of some aspects of toxicology, is the orange dye tartrazine. This dye has often been used as a food additive particularly in orange juice to intensify the orange colour. Two toxic effects have been reported for tartrazine, it is claimed that it induces hyperkinetic behaviour in children and causes uriticaria and skin rashes. The induction of hyperkinetic behaviour has been the subject of a number of studies which have focused on comparison of selected groups of individuals who have been administered diets free from food additives. Conclusions drawn from these studies have been uncertain. Some reports indicate a clear effect whilst others indicate that there was no effect of the additive on behaviour. Hyperkinetic behaviour is difficult to quantify and may not necessarily result from a single cause; other factors in a child's environment may well contribute to its behaviour.

However, the appearance in some subjects of urticaria is a definite adverse reaction to the ingestion of tartrazine. In such subjects there is an itching sensation and the appearance of red weals on the skin surface. These effects may be due to the release of the autacoid histamine, which dilates blood vessels by an action on histamine H_1-receptors. The general 'reddening' is because of dilatation of small arterioles precapillary sphincters and the weal as a result of increased permeability of the postcapillary venules. The itching is likely to be due to stimulation of sensory nerve endings. The mechanism whereby tartrazine effects histamine release is unknown, though it does not appear to involve production of antibodies or interfere with prostaglandin synthesis. It is interesting to note that there may be subjects who are predisposed to an allergic reaction, not only to tartrazine but also to other colouring additives and some cross-reactivity has been noted. Asthma has also been reported as a symptom of response in a limited number of subjects.

Bleach and other household substances

Bleach, dishwasher powder, kettle descalers and drain cleaners are all examples of household products with toxic properties. The effects recorded are a consequence of the corrosive nature of their constituents. A number of cases involve accidental poisoning of young children but more serious effects are seen in instances where the poisoning is intentional. Drinking of household bleach will cause severe burning of the mouth and oesophagus leading to considerable oedema in the pharynx and larynx. On entering the stomach, reaction with the hydrochloric acid present will release hypochlorous acid—an irritant and chlorine gas, which if inhaled is toxic to the lungs. In an individual who had drunk kettle descaler, containing formic acid, the postmortem revealed almost entire corrosion of the stomach and severe ulceration of mouth and throat.

Paracetamol

Paracetamol, a non-steroidal anti-inflammatory drug (NSAID), readily purchased as an over-the-counter drug, is commonly used as an analgesic and antipyretic drug. At therapeutic doses of 325 to 1000 mg the drug is relatively safe. However, overdose (10–25 g paracetamol), particularly in episodes of attempted suicide, results in potentially serious intoxication. The first symptoms of paracetamol poisoning include nausea, vomiting, anorexia and abdominal pain. Within 2–4 days plasma aminotransferase and bilirubin levels are increased and prothrombin clotting time is lengthened. These indications of hepatic damage may be confirmed at biopsy by slight steatosis—the accumulation of triglycerides in hepatocytes and inflammation may also be present. Centrilobular necrosis is also apparent. This region of the liver is particularly sensitive to damage from toxic compounds, the phenomenon is partly explained by the high levels of cytochrome P-450 and reduced nicotinamide adenine dinucleotide phosphate (NADPH) cytochrome P-450 reductase present. Paracetamol has been shown to bind more in the centrilobular region than any other site. In some cases, acute renal damage also occurs. The biological half-life of paracetamol is also increased. In cases of serious poisoning hepatic coma followed by death will occur.

An explanation lies in the hepatic metabolism of paracetamol. The majority of the drug is metabolized by conjugation to paracetamol glucuronide or paracetamol sulphate (Fig. 18.1). However, some 5% is metabolized to mercapturic acid via glutathione. None of these metabolites is toxic but the conversion of paracetamol to mercapturic acid, occurs via a reactive intermediate N-acetyl-p-benzoquinone imine (NAPQI). When overdose occurs, the usual detoxification of this intermediate by glutathione is saturated and NAPQI will accumulate.

NAPQI will bind covalently to cysteine residues in hepatic protein and although the developmental mechanism is unclear, this process contributes to hepatic necrosis. By an alternate pathway, NAPQI can also conjugate with glutathione, oxidize glutathione and be itself reduced back to paracetamol. As a result of the depletion of glutathione, protein sulphydryl groups may become oxidized. The significance of this action is that proteins involved in cellular transport systems are affected, in particular calcium-transporting proteins thus altering calcium homoeostasis and also Na^+-K^+-dependent adenosine triphosphatase (ATPase). Similar reactions may occur in the kidney; renal cortical necrosis has been reported, including loss of brush border membranes, loss of cells into the tubule, breakdown of the basement membrane and alteration to mitochondria.

As a consequence of glutathione depletion and also necrosis of liver cells, the ability to metabolize paracetamol will become increasingly compromised and the half-life of paracetamol will be lengthened. Quite clearly this exacerbates toxicity and will continue unless some intervention occurs. In cases of serious intoxication, intensive support therapy allied to administration of sulphydryl agents, particularly N-acetyl-cysteine is essential. However, it should be noted that treatment needs to be instituted no later than 15–20 h after overdose.

Lead

Lead is an element that has been used for centuries and the toxicology of which is reflected by its many uses. In Roman times it was used in pipes to carry water and to 'improve' wine when added as 'sweet sugar of lead' or lead acetate. In the Middle Ages lead chromate was added to cakes to give them a richer yellow colour. The Industrial Revolution had many uses for lead because of its physical and chemical properties whilst the motor car in the twentieth century used lead acid batteries and

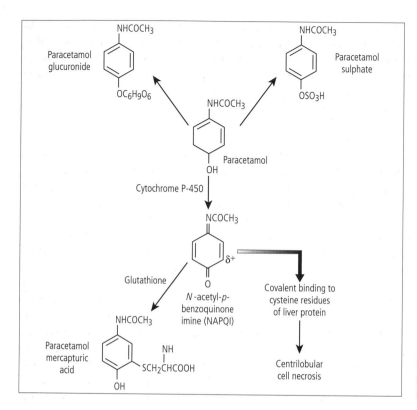
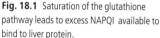

Fig. 18.1 Saturation of the glutathione pathway leads to excess NAPQI available to bind to liver protein.

added lead to petrol for over half a century as an 'antiknocking' agent. Poisoning by lead has been well documented, particularly by occupational clinicians. Exposure may be a consequence of occupation or environment.

Signs and symptoms of a non-specific nature are comprised of a metallic taste, appetite loss, constipation, pale appearance, weakness, insomnia, irritability, headache, muscle and joint pains, fine tremors and colic. Most of these effects are related to the impact of lead poisoning on the nervous system, the renal system and the haematological profile. Less well understood effects involve the reproductive system, where sterility, abortion and neonatal morbidity and mortality were common features in the population occupationally exposed to lead.

In the central nervous system, symptoms include ataxia, stupor, coma and convulsions. Lead encephalopathy will present with cerebral and cerebellar oedema with endothelial swelling and proliferation. Extravasation of periodic acid–Schiff (PAS) positive protein material has been observed; other vascular changes include capillary endothelial necrosis, hyalinization and thrombus formation. Axonal degeneration and necrosis with some demyelination is also a feature of this symptom of lead poisoning. Whilst these effects are apparent in severe lead intoxication, even low levels of lead may contribute to hyperactivity, decreased attention span and decrease in IQ, particularly in young children. Neurotransmission can also be impaired; this includes cholinergic transmission, dopamine uptake mechanisms and γ-aminobutyric acid function. Indeed the impairment in cholinergic function, along with the demyelination-related fall in nerve conduction velocity may have been the cause of two of the classical symptoms of peripheral neuropathy (wrist drop and foot drop) noted in workers occupationally exposed to lead.

Lead has a number of haematological effects. In lead poisoning a microcytic, hypochromic anaemia with increased reticulocytes and basophilic stippling of red blood cells has been reported. The stippling is thought to be the consequence of inhibition of pyrimidine-5-nucleotidase. Lead also affects certain steps in haem synthesis, particularly the enzymes aminolaevulinate synthetase, aminolaevulinate dehydrase, ferrochetolase, haem oxidase and coproporphyrinogen oxidase (see Chapter 14). This means that there will be more protoporphyrinogen available but because ferrochetolase is inhibited, protoporphyrinogen becomes part of the globin moiety rather than haem and the iron is replaced by zinc. Insufficient haem results in negative feedback control on aminolaevulinate synthetase which in turn results in increased synthesis of aminolaevulinate. In consequence there is a decrease in haemoglobin synthesis and anaemia results. Lead also increases the fragility of the red blood cell membrane which tends to shorten its life in the blood. The basis for this effect is unknown but there is a concomitant inhibition of Na^+–K^+-dependent ATPase.

In the renal system, acute lead poisoning can cause reversible tubular dysfunction which is most pronounced in the proximal tubular cells. With prolonged exposure an irreversible interstitial pathology is observed with vascular sclerosis, tubular cell atrophy and interstitial fibrosis. A characteristic feature is the presence of inclusion bodies which under light microscopy appear as dense, homogeneous, eosinophilic bodies. These are lead–protein complexes and much of the lead in the cell may be associated in this form. In early exposure to lead these may be seen to confer a protective effect by sequestering the lead. However, cells containing these inclusion bodies are swollen and have altered mitochondria. Direct effects of lead on the renal system are manifested in disturbances in the transport properties of tubular cells, amino acid, glucose and electrolyte reabsorption is particularly affected.

The impact of lead insult can be related to events at the cellular level. Lead will react readily with carboxyl groups of glutamate and aspartate residues, the sulphydryl group of cysteine and the phenoxy group of tyrosine. Lead is also capable of displacing calcium ions at a number of binding sites with the consequence of altered calcium homoeostasis. Lead has a strong affinity for mitochondrial membranes and induces an increase in membrane permeability.

In addition, mitochondrial respiration and oxidative phosphorylation are impaired. It is a possibility that the mitochondrion is a key site for lead intoxication, which may explain a number of the clinical symptoms observed.

Thalidomide

Metabolically active and developing tissue is often at high risk from potentially toxic substances. During organogenesis the embryo is at greatest risk from toxic agents. The impact of a toxin may result in structural and/or functional abnormality of the fetus and, unless death or abortion intervene, the neonate. The classical example of teratogenicity is the impact of the drug thalidomide. In the mid to late 1950s, thalidomide, a sedative drug, was prescribed in the UK as a treatment for morning sickness in pregnancy. The drug had a low maternal toxicity and was successful in treating the condition. However, between 1958 and 1962 the number of congenital malformations per thousand births rose from 0.2 to 3.2; epidemiological studies revealed that this rise could be linked to use of thalidomide. The physical manifestations of thalidomide toxicity were phocomelia (foreshortened limbs) and malformation of facial features and internal organs. As Table 18.2 shows, teratology occurred if thalidomide was taken between days 34 and 50 of pregnancy and the degree of malformation appeared to be related to the period when the drug was used.

Needless to say thalidomide use in pregnancy ceased immediately.

Despite considerable research, the mechanism of teratogenic action has yet to be fully elucidated. Toxicity testing has shown that chirality is important in that the $S(-)$ enantiomer of thalidomide

Table 18.2 Teratological effects of thalidomide in early pregnancy.

Days into pregnancy	Malformation
34–39	Ears and cranial nerves
39–42	Reductions in arm length
43–46	Reductions in lower extremity length
47–50	Digital malformation

rather than the $R(+)$ enantiomer is far more toxic. In addition, it appears that the effect is the consequence of a metabolite rather than the drug itself. A minor form of the enzyme cytochrome P-450 is responsible for generating a reactive metabolite, the identity of which is unknown but believed to be an epoxide. Of major significance to toxicology, thalidomide was a xenobiotic with low adult/maternal toxicity reported following testing. In consequence of the thalidomide disaster, investigations in pregnant animals became a more extensive and established practice in xenobiotic testing.

Asbestos

Asbestos is a term used for a variety of compounds which are fibrous mineral silicates. From an industrial point of view, their important properties lie in their ability to withstand heat and provide insulation. There are several forms of asbestos, preeminent amongst these are chrysolite (or white asbestos) which is thought to be biologically inert and crocidolite (or blue asbestos) which is far more dangerous biologically. Crocidolite has been indicated as the causative agent for mesothelia, bronchial carcinoma, gastrointestinal tumours and malignant haematological disease. Individuals are most likely to have been exposed to asbestos in factories manufacturing asbestos products, with inhalation as the predominant route of entry. In addition, demolition workers are at considerable risk in situations where asbestos is a part of the fabric of a structure undergoing demolition. Some water filters may have contained asbestos, beverages may have been a route of entry in the past. A particular problem may arise where white asbestos is contaminated with the blue variety and unwitting exposure occurs.

A curious feature of asbestos is that it is chemically inert yet the fibres are quite cytotoxic and can even haemolyse red blood cells. It is the physical shape and dimensions of asbestos fibres that are associated with the toxicity of asbestos and its ability to act as a carcinogen. Toxicity is dose related and depends on exposure for a considerable period of time. The major pathological conditions associated with asbestos are interstitial fibrosis of the

lung (asbestosis), benign pleural disease, bronchial carcinoma and malignant mesothelioma. In asbestosis, fibres are found in fibrotic areas of the lung and sputum. The air spaces are often virtually obliterated by collagen. At the same time, the asbestos fibres can become covered with iron-containing protein. Hardly surprisingly, the sufferer will be extremely breathless.

Fibre length is crucial, if the asbestos fibres are longer than 10–20 µm then fibrosis occurs. Macrophages are unable to phagocytose the long fibres fully, the macrophage membrane becomes damaged and there is leakage of hydrolytic enzymes and cell contents. This leakage may contribute to the aggregation of lymphoid tissue and stimulation of collagen synthesis, a prelude to the development of fibrosis. The situation is worsened by the fact that the lungs are unable to remove the fibres because of the fibre length. There is involvement of the immune system, in that there are cell surface changes and changes in the receptors for C3 complement and immunoglobulin G (IgG) antibodies. The complement pathway is also activated.

Bronchial carcinoma may also be caused by prolonged exposure to asbestos; again this depends on dose, duration of exposure and type of exposure. Mesothelioma, a cancer that affects the chest lining is also caused by exposure to asbestos, though it has a latency period of 30 years. The mechanism of action is unknown and toxic alteration of cell genetic mechanisms, have been excluded as a possible reason.

Organophosphorus compounds

Organophosphorus compounds are largely used as insecticides though they do have a use as nerve gases in chemical warfare. These compounds, e.g. malaoxon, act by phosphorylating acetylcholinesterase. This leads to an accumulation of the neurotransmitter acetylcholine and the toxic syndrome can best be described in terms of excessive cholinergic effects. By acting at muscarinic receptors, there will be a preponderance of parasympathetic effects, tightness of the chest, bronchoconstriction, bradycardia, pupillary constriction, salivation, lacrimation and sweating. Peristalsis is stimulated resulting

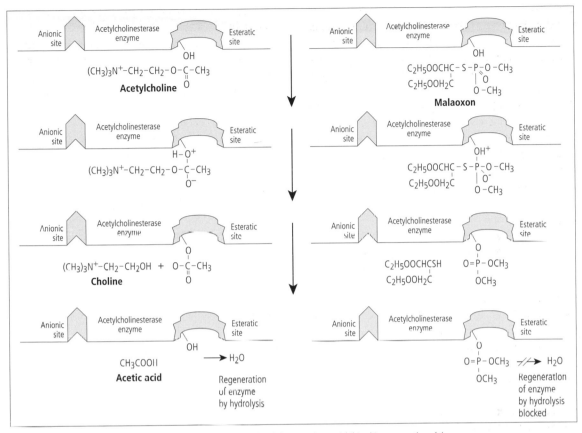

Fig. 18.2 Hydrolysis of acetylcholinesterase following acetylcholine breakdown. Malaoxon inhibits this regeneration of the enzyme.

in gastrointestinal nausea, vomiting and diarrhoea. At nicotinic receptors, the increase in acetylcholine at motor nerve endings leads to fatigue, involuntary twitching and muscular weakness, especially the muscles of respiration. By stimulating sympathetic ganglia, hypertension and hyperglycaemia ensue. In the central nervous system, tension and anxiety may be followed by ataxia, convulsions, coma and depression of central respiratory and cardiovascular control. Death usually results from respiratory failure through respiratory muscle paralysis and respiratory centre depression.

Some organophosphorus compounds may give rise to a delayed neuropathy. The delay in onset may be 10–14 days after which time the peripheral nerves begin to degenerate in a distal–proximal direction. The process involves axonal degeneration with associated myelin degeneration. The effect depends upon a covalent interaction with a membrane-bound protein, called neuropathy target esterase, and it is thought that this compound disrupts metabolism in the neuron.

However, the main acute effects are caused by the inhibition of acetylcholinesterase whereby the organophosphorus compound acts as a substrate for the enzyme rather than acetylcholine (Fig. 18.2). In the case of malaoxon, the $P = O$ group becomes bound to the serine hydroxyl group at the esteratic site of the acetylcholinesterase enzyme. Instead of the usual rapid hydrolysis of the acetylated enzyme, the phosphorylated form can only be hydrolysed very slowly, to all intents blocking the active site. Acetylcholine breakdown cannot occur, hence the accumulation of the neurotransmitter. Fifty per cent enzyme inhibition is considered sufficient for signs of toxicity to be manifested; fatalities occur at

80–90% inhibition. Acute symptoms may be treated by use of atropine to antagonize the muscarinic effects and pralidoxime, which forms a complex with the organophosphorus moiety and allows the acetylcholinesterase to be regenerated.

Summary

At the beginning of the chapter, toxicology was described as the study of poisons. The extent to which a given chemical can exert a deleterious effect, occurs in a dose-dependent manner which is governed by the exposure and distribution characteristics of the toxin. In turn this depends on the physicochemical properties of the agent and the susceptibility of the receiving organism. Toxic effects are described as acute, after single exposure to a toxin followed by a rapid onset of action. Conversely, chronic effects are the result of repeated exposures over a period of time. Toxic effects develop from perturbation at the molecular level, progressing to altered cellular function, eventually giving rise to a disturbance of tissue/organ function. The resulting influence on homoeostasis may range from mild discomfort to death.

Further reading

Aldridge W.N. (1996) *Mechanisms and Concepts in Toxicology.* Taylor & Francis Ltd., London.

Timbrell J.A. (1995) *Introduction to Toxicology* (2nd edn). Taylor & Francis Ltd., London.

Timbrell J.A. (1998) *Principles of Biochemical Toxicology* (2nd edn). Taylor & Francis Ltd., London.

Key points

1 Toxicology is the science of poisons—any chemical has the potential to exert a toxic effect. Drugs, food additives, environmental pollutants, industrial chemicals, natural toxins and household products may all be toxic agents.

2 It is the extent and size of exposure to the agent that determines its toxic effect. The common modes of entry of toxins are via the respiratory or gastrointestinal systems or through the skin. Entry and distribution depend on the physicochemical properties of the toxic agent.

3 Acute exposure refers to a single application of a substance resulting in a toxic effect that occurs within minutes or hours. Chronic exposure is repeated delivery over a longer period such that the substance accumulates in the body resulting in a toxic effect.

4 By interacting with biomolecules particularly enzymes, ion channels, nucleic acids and lipids, toxic agents can disrupt a number of cellular processes such as ATP synthesis, calcium homoeostasis and protein synthesis. In turn physiological function such as nerve conduction may be severely affected. Other consequences may comprise carcinogenic, mutagenic, teratogenic and immunotoxic effects.

Inherited Single Gene Disorders

Over the last decade there have been major advances in the diagnosis of genetic diseases. This has been brought about in part by the increased awareness of the role of a genetic component in the pathogenesis of many diseases and partly by the increased application of molecular techniques. Together these factors have resulted in genetics being one of the fastest moving fields in medicine today.

This chapter examines the different types of mutations which occur in the genes leading to some of the major inherited single gene disorders and shows how the genotypic changes lead to expression of a specific disease phenotype.

The nature of mutations

A mutation is a change in the genetic make up (*genotype*) of a cell. If mutations occur in the cells that form the *gametes*, that is the germ cells, then the mutation may be transmitted to the offspring where it will be present in every cell of an affected individual. These heritable mutations may arise as *de novo* (new) mutations in the germ cells of one or both parents or may have been inherited by the parents from previous generations.

Alternatively, mutations occurring in other body cells, termed *somatic mutations*, will not be inherited by subsequent generations but will result in genetic differences between the cells of the same organism. Somatic mutations may have consequences for the individual, since particular types of these mutations

are thought to contribute to the development of cancer (see Chapter 21).

Mutations range from rearrangements or deletions involving large sections of whole chromosomes through to single base changes. Large deletions or rearrangements of entire sections of a chromosome can be detected by the examination of chromosome morphology and are the subject of Chapter 20. Mutations involving single genes are usually the result of either the substitution of a single base with another (known as a *point mutation*), or the deletion or insertion of bases. These mutations may arise within the regions of a gene which code for protein (*exons*), within the non-coding regions (*introns*) or within nearby control elements.

Mutations arising in the exons of a gene often affect the nature of the protein product. For example, the insertion or deletion of one or two base pairs will lead to alterations in the reading frame of the DNA. Mutations arising in this way are known as *frameshift mutations*. A point mutation may alter the code in a triplet of bases (*codon*) and lead to the replacement of one amino acid by another in the protein product. This is referred to as a *missense mutation* and if it occurs in a critical region can dramatically change the function of the encoded protein. A point mutation can also change an amino acid codon to a stop codon resulting in premature termination of protein synthesis and a truncated protein product. Such a mutation is called a *nonsense mutation*.

Mutations within gene control regions can lead to a marked reduction or total lack of transcription, as seen in several forms of haemolytic anaemia (see Chapter 14). Point mutations within introns can result in defective splicing of intervening sequences. This in turn affects normal processing of messenger RNA (mRNA) and hence formation of the mature mRNA necessary for protein synthesis.

It is important to recognize that for some inherited single gene disorders (e.g. sickle cell anaemia) all affected individuals carry an identical mutation. However, for many diseases there is often more than one type of mutation which can produce the same phenotype. Beta-thalassaemia, for example, may result from many different mutations in the β-globin gene.

Testing for inherited single gene disorders

The identification of specific disease-causing genes has a number of implications. Firstly, for a severe disorder, such as Duchenne muscular dystrophy (DMD) or cystic fibrosis (CF), it is possible to offer parents the option of prenatal testing and termination of an affected fetus at an early stage in pregnancy. Secondly, in diseases where presymptomatic diagnosis is possible, e.g. in inherited cancer syn-

dromes, early treatment can lead to a substantial improvement in survival and the quality of life. Thirdly, population screening has become possible for diseases which are common in the population, e.g. cystic fibrosis. This can reduce the incidence of the disease in the population and at the same time reduce the health burden from these disorders.

Patterns of inheritance

The majority of single gene disorders show clear patterns of mendelian inheritance. Diseases can either be *X-linked* (i.e. the affected gene is on the X chromosome) or *autosomal* (the affected gene is on one of chromosomes 1–22). In addition, they may be *dominant*, requiring a mutation in only one copy of the gene, or *recessive*, where mutations in both copies are needed for expression of the phenotype. Examples of these different patterns of inheritance are shown in Fig. 19.1.

Methods of diagnosis of single gene disorders

Prenatal and presymptomatic diagnosis of genetic diseases can be indirect or direct. If the chromosomal

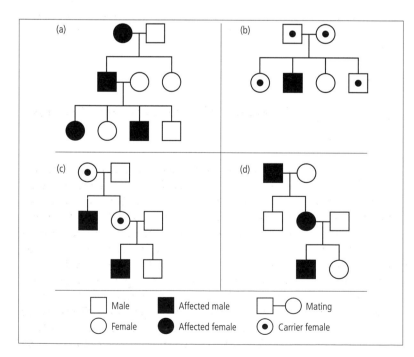

Fig. 19.1 Mendelian patterns of inheritance: (a) autosomal dominant inheritance; (b) autosomal recessive inheritance; (c) X-linked recessive inheritance; and (d) X-linked dominant inheritance.

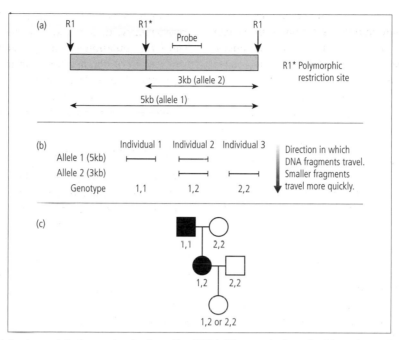

Fig. 19.2 Linkage analysis using *restriction fragment length polymorphisms* (RFLPs). This approach relies on the ability to cleave DNA at specific sites (*restriction sites*) using restriction enzymes. Restriction enzyme digestion of DNA yields a number of fragments (*restriction fragments*) of different sizes depending on the number of restriction sites and their position within the DNA. (a) Two different RFLPs known to be located on a specific chromosome near the gene of interest. If restriction site, R1* is present then restriction enzyme digestion will yield two fragments and the probe will recognize a 3 kilobase (kb) sized fragment. If R1* is absent then the probe will recognize a single 5-kb fragment. (b) Gel electrophoresis separates the restriction fragments on the basis of their size, and below the genotype results of three individuals with the three possible outcomes using the RFLP in (a). (c) Results of an RFLP entered into the pedigree. By looking at the affected individual in the first generation, it can be seen that he has allele 1 on both chromosomes, one of which carries the mutated gene. He has passed the disease to his daughter along with allele 1. If she in turn passes on the chromosome with allele 1 to her 'at-risk' daughter, the daughter will be affected. If she passes on the chromosome with allele 2 the daughter will not be affected.

location of a gene is known but the gene itself has not yet been isolated, indirect analysis, termed *linkage analysis*, is possible. This depends on the tracking of a disease gene through a family by the use of polymorphic markers, that is, markers which vary from one individual to the next, to 'tag' the chromosome carrying the disease mutation. The two most commonly used markers are restriction fragment length polymers (RFLP) or microsatellite markers, usually dinucleotide or tetranucleotide repeats. The principle of this approach for family analysis is illustrated in Fig. 19.2. Direct analysis is possible by the detection of specific mutations in the affected gene(s) and is the subject of the following sections.

Molecular basis of the single gene disorders

Deletions

Large *deletions* are a major cause of *Duchenne muscular dystrophy* (DMD). This is an X-linked recessive condition seen primarily in boys which causes muscle degeneration and eventually death. 50–60% of affected boys show deletions of one or more exons of the very large *dystrophin* gene (Fig. 19.3). These deletions occur with particularly high frequency at certain points ('hot spots') throughout the gene. The deletions cause an alteration in the reading frame of the *dystrophin* gene so that a premature stop codon is introduced and hence a truncated and unstable protein is produced. If muscle tissue from affected boys is examined it can be seen that dystrophin protein is virtually absent.

In contrast, in *Becker muscular dystrophy* (BMD), a milder disease also caused by abnormalities in the *dystrophin* gene, muscle sections show the presence of *dystrophin*. The *dystrophin* gene in BMD patients also shows large deletions but because they occur in triplets they leave the reading frame intact. Therefore, although part of the protein is missing it is still able to function at a lower level and the phenotype of the disease is consequently milder than that of DMD.

Cystic fibrosis (CF) is one of the most common autosomal recessive conditions. It is characterized by abnormally thick mucus secretions in the lungs and by pancreatic enzyme insufficiency. The observation of elevated sweat electrolytes suggested that the causative abnormality might be a defect in the regulation of chloride ion conductance. Whe the *CF* gene was isolated in 1989, it was shown to encode a transmembrane protein which functions as a chloride ion channel. The gene is now referred to as the *cystic fibrosis transmembrane regulator* (*CFTR*) gene. The CFTR protein produced by the gene has five functional domains as shown in Fig. 19.4.

Over 700 different CF mutations have so far been identified (see Fig. 19.4). These include non-sense mutations, frameshift mutations or splice site mutations. Unlike DMD, large deletions are rare. The

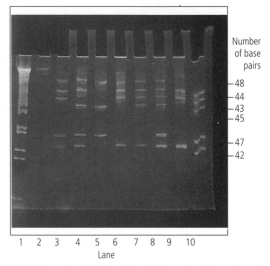

Number of base pairs

— 48
— 44
— 43
— 45

— 47
— 42

1 2 3 4 5 6 7 8 9 10
Lane

Fig. 19.3 Detection of deletions in the *DMD* gene by gel electrophoresis of amplified DNA. A normal female in lane 8 shows six bands corresponding to six exons of the *DMD* gene. Other lanes from affected boys show absence of some of the bands indicating that DNA from these exons of the gene has been deleted. Lane 1 is a molecular weight marker. Courtesy of Dr Sarah Warburton, DNA Laboratory, Regional Genetics Service, Birmingham Womens' Hospital.

majority of mutations occur at low frequency, but one, known as $^\Delta$F508, has been found on approximately 75% of CF chromosomes in the UK population. This mutation is a 3-base-pair (bp) deletion in exon 10 which causes the deletion of the amino acid

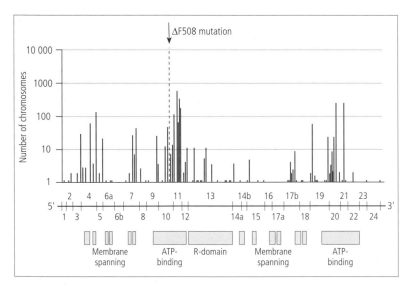

Fig. 19.4 Distribution and frequency of *CF* mutations in each of the five domains of the *CFTR* gene. Exons are numbered 1–24. From Lap-Chee Tsui (1992).

phenylalanine from the adenosine triphosphate (ATP)-binding domain of the protein.

CFTR gene mutations fall into three functional groups. Group 1 mutations, which include the ΔF508 mutation, prevent correct folding and maturation of the protein. CF proteins with the second group of mutations are processed correctly but the chloride ion channel fails to open on stimulation. Group 3 mutations are likely to produce chloride channels with slightly altered properties.

An analysis of genotype/phenotype correlations has been made in CF but many of the correlations are not clear cut. However, one group of patients, comprising between 10 and 15% of cases, have some preservation of pancreatic enzyme levels. These patients tend to have 'milder' mutations such as missense mutations and rarely have the ΔF508 mutation (see case study 27).

Point mutations

Single base changes (point mutations) are a common disease-causing mechanism. For some diseases all affected individuals carry the same point mutation, whereas for other disorders the nature of the point mutation may vary between affected individuals.

An example of a disease in which all affected individuals have the same single point mutation is sickle cell anaemia (see also Chapter 14). This autosomal recessive disease has an incidence of about 1 in 500 in the black population and carries significant morbidity and mortality. It is caused by a point mutation in codon 6 of the β-globin chain that changes the DNA sequence from GAG:CTC to GTG:CAC. This changes the mRNA triplets from GAG to GUG, resulting on translation in the substitution of L-glutamic acid by valine. The alteration in this single amino acid results in the production of insoluble haemoglobin. As soon as haemoglobin formed from mutant β-globin becomes deoxygenated, it aggregates and forms crystalline deposits in the red cell causing the cells to assume the characteristic sickle shape. Repeated sickling and unsickling damages the red cell membrane and shortens its lifespan. This leads to haemolytic anaemia, blockage of the microcirculation and associated tissue death.

Other diseases have a more complicated pattern of point mutations. One such disease is a form of inherited colon cancer called *familial adenomatous polyposis* (FAP). In this autosomal dominant disease, affected individuals develop polyps throughout their colon and rectum. By the third or fourth decade of life, at least one of these polyps will become malignant, and if left untreated, the patient will die. The ability to diagnose the disease early, means that preventative surgery can be carried out (see case study 22).

When the gene for this disease (the *APC* gene) was identified it became apparent that the majority of patients had different mutations and that most of these were either point mutations or very small insertions or deletions of a few bases. The mutations are scattered throughout the gene. Over 95% of mutations result in the introduction of a premature stop codon and a truncated protein is produced. In FAP, a mutation in only one allele of the *FAP* gene is necessary for disease. This is thought to be because the normal protein produced by the unaffected allele is inactivated by its interaction with the abnormal protein. In order to detect the mutation in a particular FAP family, it is necessary to scan each exon in turn until an abnormality is found (Fig. 19.5). Once the location of a mutation is pinpointed to a particular exon, the mutation can be confirmed by sequencing of the DNA in that region (Fig. 19.6).

As the phenotype of patients with FAP can be variable, e.g. with regard to the age of onset, it was initially believed that this would be explained by the position and nature of the mutations. On the whole this has not been the case although there are some exceptions. An attenuated form of the disease with fewer polyps and a delayed age of onset is caused by mutations in exon 3. The protein made from this mutated gene is very short and rapidly degraded. Only low levels of normal sized protein (produced by the unaffected allele) are present and the subsequent effect is a milder phenotype. Similarly, mutations at the 3' end of the gene result in a mild phenotype.

Duplications

Charcot–Marie–Tooth (CMT) syndrome is the most common inherited disorder of the peripheral

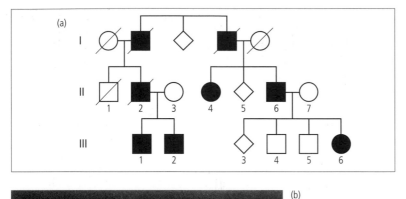

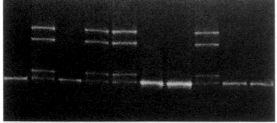

Fig. 19.5 Mutation analysis of a family with familial adenomatous polyposis. (a) Family pedigree (note that symbols with a diagonal line through them indicate that the patient is deceased). (b) Gel electrophoresis of amplified DNA from the *FAP* gene. Lanes II.1, II.3, III.3, III.4, III.5 and II.7 show only a single normal band indicating that no mutation is present. The other lanes show four bands indicating the presence of mutant DNA fragments.

nervous system affecting 1 in 2500 people and is characterized by wasting of the distal muscles of the limbs. It is subdivided into a number of types based on pathology and electrophysiology, the most common of which is type 1A. The gene for the disease has been mapped to chromosome 17 and a surprising mechanism of mutation was identified. In this disorder the phenotype is associated with a large duplication of DNA. The most likely explanation for the phenotype is overexpression of the gene encoding peripheral myelin protein (PMP) within the duplicated region. Interestingly, the CMT type 1A phenotype is also seen if point mutations occur in this gene—yet another example of the same disease occurring via a number of different mechanisms.

Expansion of trinucleotide repeats

In recent years a completely different mechanism has been identified as the cause of genetic disease. This involves the expansion of trinucleotide repeat sequences (either CAG, CTG or CGG) and has been recognized as causing several different single gene disorders to date (Table 19.1). Each of these diseases share some features in common, particularly the increasing severity of the disease with successive generations (termed *anticipation*) and a parental bias in the transmission of the severe forms of the disorder. There is, however, some variation in the way in which these repeats function at the DNA or mRNA level.

The first of these diseases to be recognized was *fragile X mental retardation*, the most common inherited form of mental retardation, affecting 1 in 4000 to 1 in 6000 males. The pattern of inheritance in fragile X is unusual for an X-linked dominant disease in that there are both carrier males and carrier females. In addition, a proportion of carrier females are affected and these affected females always inherit the disease from their mothers.

The gene causing the disease is known as the *FMR-1* gene and when it was identified, an unstable region was noted in the 5′ end of the gene. This region contains a repeat of the trinucleotide, CGG. In normal individuals, the number of these repeats varies between 10 and 45. A 'grey' area exists between 45 and 55 repeats but clinically this appears not to be significant. Carriers of the repeat have

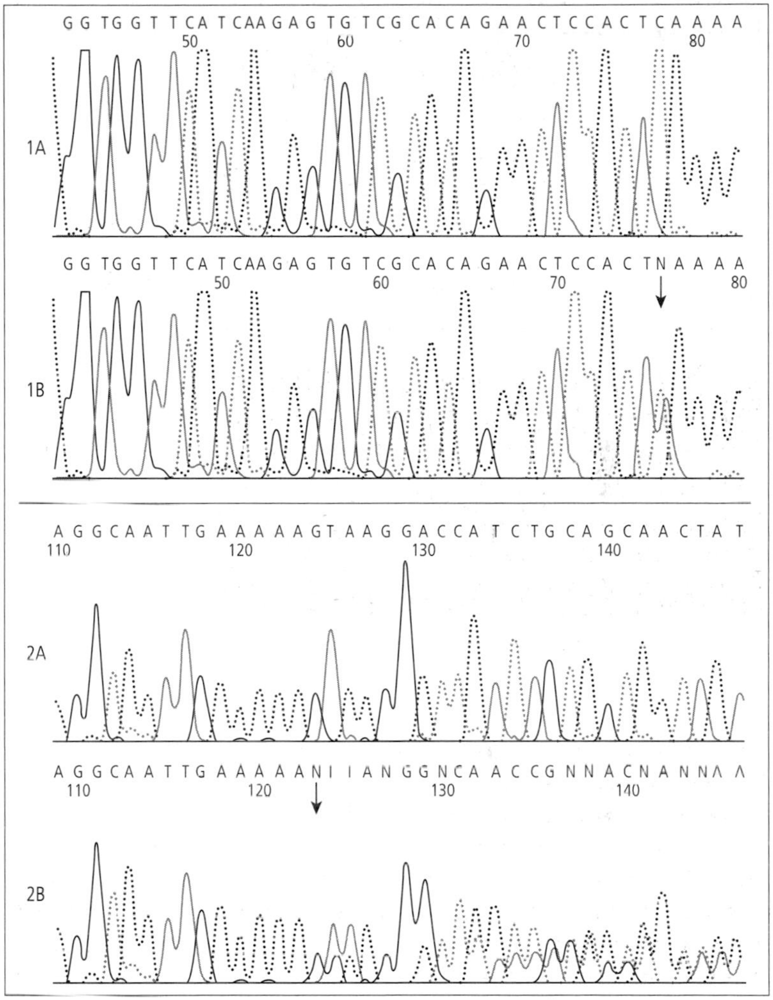

Fig. 19.6 Example of DNA sequencing using fluorescently labelled bases. (1A) The normal sequence of a section of a gene. (1B) Sequence of the same region of DNA from a patient showing the presence of a mutation indicated by the arrow. The mutation is a C to T transition. Comparison with the normal tract shows not only the presence of a mutated base but also that the peak height of the normal base is decreased as there is now only one copy of the normal allele. (2A) Normal sequence from a different section of a gene. (2B) The same region of the gene in a patient with a mutation identified from the sequence as an insertion of an A indicated by the arrow. The normal sequence can be read along with that of the mutant sequence.

between 55 and 200 copies (the so-called *premutation* for fragile X), whereas affected individuals have over 200 copies. The clinical phenotype is only seen if there are over 200 copies of the repeat.

Now that the gene has been identified the patterns of inheritance can be explained. A male carrier will transmit the premutation to all his daughters. The number of CGG repeats varies only slightly during this process but remains within the premutation range so that all of his daughters are carriers of the disease and clinically unaffected. It is only when the premutation is transmitted by a female that there is a significant increase in the number of repeats leading to expression of the full mutation.

If a carrier female transmits the mutation to her son the number of repeats will increase significantly to the full mutation range and he will be clinically affected. The premutation can also be transmitted to a daughter with a similar increase in repeat number but in this case only about 50% of females who inherit the full mutation will be mentally retarded. At the molecular level, expansion of the CGG repeat above 200 copies, results in abnormal methylation of DNA sequences at the 5' end of the gene and complete shut down of transcription of the *FMR-1* gene.

Following identification of the *FMR-1* gene, other diseases were identified where trinucleotide repeat expansion was shown to be the cause of the

Table 19.1 Diseases associated with expansion of trinucleotide repeats.

Disease	Mode of inheritance	Sex bias for transmission	Nature of repeat	Location of repeat	Mechanism of mutation	Size of repeat in normals	Size of repeat in patients
Fragile X (FraxA)	X-linked	Full mutation only if transmitted by female	CGG	5′ untranslated region	Transcription shut down	6–45	55–200 (premutation), > 200 (full mutation)
Fragile X (FraxE)	X-linked		GCC	?	?	6–25	43–200 (premutation) > 200 (full mutation)
Myotonic dystrophy	Autosomal dominant	Congenital form normally transmitted by female	CTG	3′ untranslated region	?	5–37	> 50
Huntington's disease	Autosomal dominant	Early onset transmitted by male	CAG	Protein coding	Gain of function	6–35	36–121
Dentatorubral pallidoluysian atrophy	Autosomal dominant	Mainly paternal	CAG	Protein coding	Gain of function	8–25	49–55
Spinobulbar muscular atrophy	Autosomal dominant	Increased instability if transmitted by male	CAG	Protein coding	Gain of function	11–31	40–62
Spinocerebellar ataxia 1	Autosomal dominant	Paternal bias	CAG	Protein coding	Gain of function	6–44	40–81
Spinocerebellar ataxia 2	Autosomal dominant	Paternal bias	CAG	Protein coding	Gain of function	15–29	35–59
Spinocerebellar ataxia 3	Autosomal dominant	Possibly paternal	CAG	Protein coding	Gain of function	12–41	55–84
Spinocerebellar ataxia 6	Autosomal dominant	?	CAG	Protein coding	Gain of function	4–17	20–30
Spinocerebellar ataxia 7	Autosomal dominant	Paternal bias	CAG	Protein coding	Gain of function	4–35	37 > 200
Spinocerebellar ataxia 8	Autosomal dominant	?	CTG	Untranslated region			107–127
Friedreich's ataxia	Autosomal recessive		GAA	Intron	Loss of function	7–22	110 > 900

disorder. *Myotonic dystrophy* is a progressive wasting disease of the muscles. When the responsible gene (the *DM* gene) was identified, an unstable CTG repeat was found in the 3′ untranslated region. Normal individuals have 5–37 repeats. Affected patients have between 50 and several thousand repeats (Fig. 19.7).

There are many similarities to fragile X. In general, the greater the number of repeats the more severe the disease. Again the disease increases in severity with successive generations but can be transmitted by both males and females. There is also a sex bias in transmission of the disease. There is a congenital form of myotonic dystrophy which results in the birth of a severely affected child and this only arises if the mother transmits the mutation. Unlike fragile X, expansion of the CTG repeats does not result in the shut down of transcription of the gene. Instead

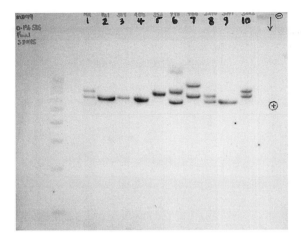

Fig. 19.7 Molecular analysis of the *DM* gene followed by gel electrophoresis. Normal individuals have either two 9-kb sized *DM* alleles, two 10-kb sized alleles, or are heterozygous. (This pattern in normals is due to an insertion of 1 kb in the gene which is not directly related to the disease.) Affected individuals have amplification of the CTG repeat which can be seen as an increase in size of the 10-kb allele. Lanes 1 and 8 show normal individuals heterozygous for the 9- and 10-kb alleles. Lanes 2–4 and 9 show normals homozygous for the 9-kb allele. Lane 5 shows a normal individual homozygous for the 10-kb allele. Affected individuals are in lanes 6, 7 and 10 and show an increase in the fragment size (bands do not travel as far to the anode) due to amplification of the CTG repeat. Courtesy of Andrea Mitchell, DNA Laboratory, Regional Genetics Service, Birmingham Heartlands Hospital.

the mechanism of action may be an abnormal gain in function of the product of the *DM* gene.

Huntington's disease is one of the most serious genetic diseases affecting the central nervous system (CNS). It was one of the first single gene disorders to be localized to a specific chromosome (chromosome 4) but it has taken longer to isolate the gene. An unstable CAG repeat sequence has been identified in the 5′ coding sequence of a gene now known as *huntingtin*. As with fragile X and myotonic dystrophy there is a variation in repeat number in the normal population and an unstable expansion of the repeat number in affected individuals. Again there is evidence of anticipation—those with early onset disease have the highest number of repeats. There is also a sex bias with juvenile onset disease seen this time with transmission from the father. The precise effect of the trinucleotide repeat in Huntington's

disease remains unclear, although it is more likely to be a gain in function of the abnormal protein as with myotonic dystrophy, rather than a shut down in transcription of the gene as with fragile X. As with the other diseases, molecular diagnosis of Huntington's disease is now possible.

The features of other diseases associated with expansions in trinucleotide repeats are summarized in Table 19.1.

Summary

Genetic diseases are a significant cause of illness and death. It is estimated that 10% of all adult admissions and up to 50% of paediatric admissions to hospital are due to a genetic cause. Molecular techniques can now be used to diagnose the more common of these diseases. In some cases it is possible to show that a fetus is affected with a disease and also to give some idea about the severity of the disease. Presymptomatic diagnosis of some genetic diseases is also possible in selected cases.

Key points

1 Mutations are changes in the genetic make-up of cells.
2 If a mutation is present in the cells that form the gametes, then the mutation may be transmitted to the offspring where it will be present in every cell of an affected individual. This mutation may arise as a new mutation in the germ cells of one or both parents, or it may have been inherited by the parents from previous generations.
3 The inherited single gene disorders are characterized by the presence of mutations involving only a single gene. These mutations may be deletions or insertions of bases, or involve the substitution of one base for another (point mutation).
4 Single gene disorders show clear patterns of mendelian inheritance. They may be either X-linked (mutation is present in a gene on the X chromosome), or autosomal (mutation is present in a gene present on one of chromosomes 1–22). In addition, they may be dominant, requiring a mutation in only one copy of the gene, or recessive, when a mutation in both copies of the gene is required.

Each month several new genes are identified. The next few years are therefore likely to be a very exciting time, enabling geneticists not only to understand more about the basic functions of cells but also to benefit individuals who are carriers of a genetic defect or are themselves affected by a genetic disease.

Further reading

Lap-Chee Tsui (1992) The spectrum of cystic fibrosis mutations. *Trends in Genetics* **8**: 392–398.

Strachen T. & Read A. (1999) *Human Molecular Genetics.* Bios Scientific Publishers, Oxford.

Chromosome Abnormalities

The previous chapter described a group of mutations which disrupt the expression of single genes. These mutations give rise to various single gene disorders (e.g. muscular dystrophy) that can now be defined using molecular techniques. This chapter describes the other clinically important group of mutations which involve changes in chromosome number or structure.

A point worth emphasizing is the difference in scale between the two groups of mutations. Single gene mutations may involve as little as a single base substitution ranging up to deletions of tens of kilobases of DNA. In contrast, the gain or loss of entire chromosomes, or the presence of microscopically visible deletions, involves relatively huge amounts of DNA, inevitably involving a large number of genes. The smallest chromosomal deletion, visible by light microscopy of suitably prepared and stained chromosomes, will remove a minimum of several megabases of DNA.

Constitutional and acquired chromosome abnormalities

Chromosome abnormalities may be broadly subdivided into two types: *constitutional* and *acquired*.

Constitutional chromosome abnormalities

Constitutional chromosome abnormalities are those that are either inherited from one or other parent, or arise as *de novo* (new) mutations during gamete development (*gametogenesis*) or during early embryogenesis. The mutation is found either in all cells of an affected individual or, less commonly, in a proportion of cells (mosaicism). Since it is usually present in the germ cells it can be transmitted to the next generation.

Acquired chromosome abnormalities

Acquired chromosome abnormalities may arise either during fetal growth, or later in cells retaining the ability to undergo cell division. Such acquired chromosomal mutations are confined to the cell in which they arise and its progeny. Non-random acquired chromosome abnormalities have now been described in a variety of leukaemias and solid tumours and are believed to contribute to the development of these lesions. This area is dealt with in more detail in Chapter 22.

Mitotic errors, resulting in gain or loss of single chromosomes at cell division, also occur at a very low rate in all individuals. Most of these errors are lethal for the cell progeny but a few are benign and may accumulate with age. Examples are the loss of the Y chromosome which occurs in a proportion of leucocytes in older men and the addition of an extra X chromosome which occurs in a proportion of leucocytes in older women.

The structure of chromosomes

Chromosomes are complex macromolecular

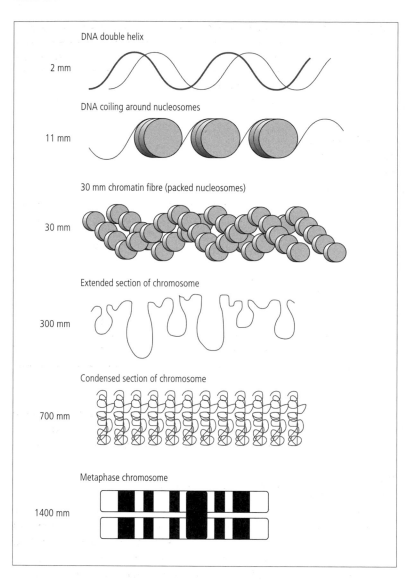

DNA double helix

2 mm

DNA coiling around nucleosomes

11 mm

30 mm chromatin fibre (packed nucleosomes)

30 mm

Extended section of chromosome

300 mm

Condensed section of chromosome

700 mm

Metaphase chromosome

1400 mm

Fig. 20.1 Schematic representation of the organization of the chromosome.

structures which are a fundamental unit of genome organization. In order to appreciate the potential phenotypic effect of chromosome abnormalities it is helpful to have some idea of the relationship between the size of a chromosome and the DNA base-pair (bp) sequence from which genes are transcribed. Human somatic cells each contain about 6000 million base pairs of DNA organized in 46 chromosomes (known as the *diploid set*) consisting of 22 pairs of autosomes and two sex chromosomes (XX in females and XY in males). At a conservative

estimate there are around 40 000 genes per *haploid set* (i.e. 23 chromosomes), this implies that each chromosome contains on average about 2000 genes.

Chromosomes are highly organized structures consisting of a single, linear, double-stranded DNA molecule which interacts with various DNA-binding proteins in a complex manner (Fig. 20.1). The overall packing ratio from DNA strand to a chromosome at metaphase is about 8000 : 1. Chromosome 1 is the largest and contains approximately 300 megabases (i.e. 300 million basepairs) of DNA, whereas chromosome 21 contains only 50 mega-bases of DNA.

Chromosome examination

'Banding' and other techniques allow unequivocal identification of chromosome pairs and detection of chromosome abnormalities. The simplest starting material for the examination of chromosomes is a small volume of blood (usually as little as 0.2 mL). This is cultured for 72 h in medium containing *phytohaemagglutinin* (PHA). PHA stimulates the lymphocytes present in the blood to divide. Addition of colchicine arrests the lymphocytes at metaphase by inhibiting the polymerization of tubulin in the formation of spindle fibres. Preparations of the lymphocytes in metaphase (so-called *metaphase spreads*) are then made on microscope slides, stained and examined.

Various stains may be employed which enable bands within each chromosome to be identified. This technique, known as *banding*, allows unequivocal identification of chromosome pairs, enabling delineation of many types of chromosome abnormality. Typically a combination of the protease *trypsin* and Leishman stain reveals 550 chromosome bands per haploid set. This approximates to about 6 megabases of DNA per chromosome band.

Newer molecular cytogenetic techniques exploit the fact that single-stranded DNA, tagged with a fluorescent label, will hybridize with its complementary strand on pretreated metaphase chromosomes. This technique, known as *fluorescence in situ hybridization* (FISH), allows the detection of sub-microsopic deletions at critical points in the genome known to be associated with genetic disease (see case study 23). This approach underlines the fact that disruption of genetic material at the chromosomal level is part of a size continuum of mutation from a single base-pair alteration to the gain or loss of whole chromosomes involving tens of thousands of kilobases of DNA.

Types of chromosome abnormalities

Chromosome abnormalities are more common than is generally supposed (Tables 20.1 and 20.2). They

Table 20.1 Frequency of chromosome abnormalities in various groups.

Group	Frequency (%)
Clinically recognized pregnancies	8
Spontaneous abortions	50
Stillbirths	5
Live births (overall)	0.5

Table 20.2 Frequency of specific chromosome abnormalities.

Chromosome abnormality	Frequency (live conceptuses)
Trisomy 21	1 : 700
Trisomy 18	1 : 3000
Trisomy 13	1 : 5000
47,XXY	1 : 750 males
47,XXX	1 : 1000 males
45,X	1 : 10 000 females
Balanced translocations	1 : 500
Unbalanced translocations	1 : 2000

generally involve either a change in chromosome number, a change in chromosome structure or abnormalities in the way chromosomes are inherited.

Numerical abnormalities

Numerical abnormalities may involve either the gain or loss of individual chromosomes (known as *aneuploidy*) or more rarely the gain of entire haploid sets of chromosomes resulting in *triploidy* ($n = 69$) or *tetraploidy* ($n = 92$). Aneuploidy may take the form of an extra chromosome, known as *trisomy* (three copies present) or loss of a chromosome, referred to as *monosomy* (one copy present). Monosomy or trisomy involving the sex chromosomes are compatible with life and are usually associated with varying degrees of phenotypic abnormalities. This is because X inactivation normally ensures that only one X chromosome is actively transcribed in each cell and the Y chromosome contains a large amount of inert, highly repetitive, DNA. Clinically, the best defined sex chromosome abnormalities are *Klinefelter syndrome* and *Turner syndrome*.

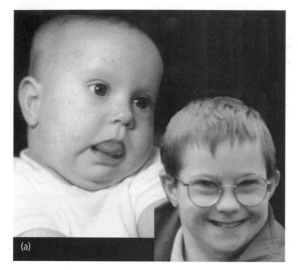

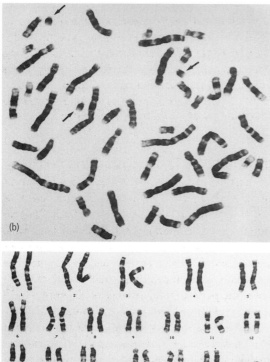

Fig. 20.2 (a) The typical facial characteristics of Down syndrome (see Table 20.4). (b) A chromosomal metaphase spread from a case of Down syndrome showing three copies of chromosome 21 (arrowed). (c) Chromosomes from the same spread organized into groups (a karyotype) to show trisomy 21 more clearly. (a) Courtesy of Down's Syndrome Research Foundation Ltd; www.dsrf.co.uk.

Klinefelter syndrome (frequency 1 in 1000 males) occurs when two X chromosomes and one Y chromosome are present (47,XXY). The clinical features may include *hypogonadism* (small reproductive organs) or *gynaecomastia* (enlargement of male breasts). Individuals are invariably infertile. Educational difficulty (partly as a result of delayed speech development) is more likely, though not invariable, compared to normal siblings.

Turner syndrome (frequency 1 in 10 000 females) results from complete or partial monosomy of the X chromosome and is characterized primarily by short stature and infertility in affected females. Intelligence is normal. In just over one half of all cases there is complete monosomy of the X chromosome (i.e. 45,X). The remainder of patients show either mosaicism or only partial monosomy, involving various structural rearrangements (e.g. deletions, rings or isochromosomes) of one X chromosome.

In contrast, monosomy or trisomy involving autosomes generally result in the loss or gain of too much important genetic information to be compatible with live birth. However, a number of autosomal trisomies may survive to birth. Trisomy 21 or Down syndrome (Fig. 20.2), trisomy 18 (Edward syndrome) and trisomy 13 (Patau syndrome) are the most common, in descending order of frequency.

Structural abnormalities

Structural abnormalities can take many forms including large deletions or insertions of genetic material, duplication of segments of a chromosome, inversions or translocations. The features of some of these structural abnormalities are illustrated in Fig. 20.3.

Many structural abnormalities produce chromosome imbalance as a result of gain or loss of genetic material. This usually results in profound physical and mental disability. Imbalance can be expressed as a percentage of the ratio of the length of the missing or additional segment over the total length of the haploid autosomal chromosome complement (% HAL). This crude measurement, takes no account of gene content. Excess material, if less than 1% of HAL, in the form of partial trisomy, may result in a viable pregnancy with frequent live birth. An excess of between 1 and 3% HAL increases the risk of

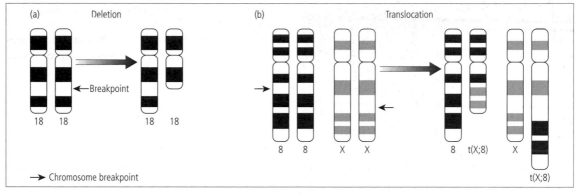

Fig. 20.3 Examples of structural chromosome abnormalities. (a) Deletion. Loss of chromosomal material, in this case from one of the chromosome 18 pair. Losses of segments of a chromosome may remove many important genes leading to severe phenotypic abnormalities. (b) Translocation. Shown here is a reciprocal translocation. Part of one chromosome 8 has been transferred to one X chromosome, and part of the X chromosome has been transferred to chromosome 8.

a severely compromised phenotype resulting in non-viability *in utero* and therefore abortion. Partial monosomy (i.e. a HAL deficit of 1–2%) is much less well tolerated than partial trisomy.

Translocation or inversion of chromosomal material may have no phenotypic effect on the individual because the rearrangement results in no gain or loss of material. However, such rearrangement of genetic material may give rise, through recombination or through segregation of translocated chromosomes during meiosis, to the production of unbalanced gametes with profound reproductive consequences for the carrier individual resulting in infertility, miscarriage or disabled offspring.

Structural abnormalities occur with high frequency in certain conditions associated with an increased sensitivity to chromosome breakage. These diseases include Fanconi's anaemia, Bloom's syndrome and ataxia telangiectasia (see also Chapter 21). The type of breakage, which is not generally site-specific, is characteristic for each disease and reflects the underlying DNA repair defect in each case.

Site-specific fragility may also occur both spontaneously and in the presence of various inducing agents. Only one site appears to be clinically important, situated towards the end of the long arm of the X chromosome at Xq27.3. Expression of this fragile site is seen in the fragile X syndrome which in affected males may result in mild to moderate

mental retardation, large ears, prominent forehead, macro-orchidism (enlarged testes), hyperflexibility of joints and perserverative speech. The underlying molecular basis for this chromosome fragility is now known to be an expansion beyond a critical threshold of the number of copies of a trinucleotide (CGG) repeat sequence (see Chapter 19).

Uniparental disomy

A third class of abnormality results when both chromosomes of a pair are inherited from one or other parent resulting in *uniparental disomy*. Such a finding implies that the parental origin of a chromosome may determine gene expression on that chromosome. This phenomenon is called *imprinting*. The best example of imprinting is the relationship between the pattern of inheritance of chromosome 15 in *Prader–Willi* and *Angelman* syndromes.

Prader–Willi syndrome (PWS) is characterized by infantile *hypotonia* (poor muscle tone), short stature, small hands and feet, almond-shaped eyes, hypogonadism, psychomotor retardation, *hypopigmentation* (pale skin) and early onset of childhood *hyperphagia* (overeating) with consequent obesity.

Angelman syndrome (AS) is characterized by severe mental retardation, seizures, inappropriate laughter, *ataxic gait* (unsteady posture, lurching walk), puppet-like upper limb movements, lack of speech and a large jaw.

Table 20.3 Phenotypic consequences of triploid chromosome complements. The phenotypic effects depend upon the parental origin of the extra chromosome set.

Syndrome	Genotype	Phenotype
Triploid conceptus	Two maternal sets, one paternal set	Small and fibrotic placenta, embryo retarded
Partial mole	One maternal set, two paternal sets	Trophoblast hyperplasia, embryo retarded and/or malformed

Table 20.4 Frequency of phenotypic abnormalities seen in Down syndrome patients

Phenotypic feature	Frequency in Down syndrome patients (%)
Oblique (up-slanting) palpebral fissures	82
Loose skin on nape of neck	81
Brachycephaly (short anteroposterior skull length)	75
Hyperflexibility	73
Flat nasal bridge	68
Short, broad hands	64
Epicanthic folds (skin folds over inner canthi)	59
Short fifth finger	58
Brushfield spots (speckled iris ring)	56
Furrowed tongue	55
Transverse palmar crease	53
Folded or dysplastic ear	50
Protruding tongue	47
Congenital cardiac defects	40

In PWS, deletions within the long arm of chromosome 15 (q11–q13) are always found on the paternally derived chromosome. Non-deletion cases can display uniparental disomy and in these cases two copies of the maternal chromosome 15 are present. These findings imply that the absence of a sequence on the paternally derived chromosome 15 at q11–q13 gives rise to the PWS phenotype.

In contrast in AS, deletions are always on the maternally derived chromosome and uniparental disomy, although much less frequent than in PWS, manifests itself in the presence of two paternal copies of chromosome 15. Another example of imprinting is seen in triploidy ($n = 69$). The phenotypic outcomes of triploid chromosome complements are listed in Table 20.3.

Chromosome abnormality and clinical syndrome

Variation is the hallmark of the relationship between a chromosome abnormality and a clinical syndrome. Using the example of Down syndrome (trisomy 21) it can be seen (Table 20.4) that there is considerable variability in the phenotype of such individuals. Indeed no single feature is considered to be *pathognomic* (i.e. specific) for Down syndrome. Such variation may well partly reflect the different genetic background, consisting of the other chromosomes that make up the diploid set, in each individual. It should also be noted that no simple correlation exists between a particular gene locus and a particular Down syndrome phenotypic trait (e.g. brachycephaly). Rather, two overlapping 'critical regions' (DS1 and DS2) have been

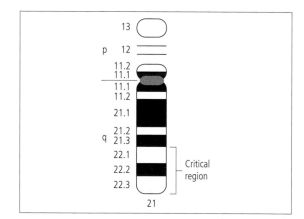

Fig. 20.4 Critical regions (DS1 and DS2) within chromosome 21 are required to be trisomic for the Down syndrome phenotype to be expressed.

identified within chromosome 21q22 which are required to be trisomic for the Down syndrome phenotype to be expressed (Fig. 20.4).

Another general consideration is that the influence of a gene or set of genes acts through a number of developmental pathways. Chromosome abnormalities therefore increase the probability of particular developmental anomalies without predetermining them.

How chromosome abnormalities arise

It is now possible to determine both the parental origin of chromosomal abnormalities and in some cases the mechanisms by which they arise. In general, maternal errors account for most aneuploidy states, whereas point mutations and structural rearrangements are more likely to result from paternal errors.

Maternal errors

By the time of birth the average human ovary contains about 2 million oöcytes in the diplotene stage of the first meiotic division. Here they remain in a resting phase until further maturation through the meiotic cycle occurs prior to ovulation.

Many trisomies arise as a result of errors in segregation at the first maternal meiotic division (M1) in oöcytes. *Non-disjunction* is the most common segregation defect. Non-disjunction occurs when an homologous pair of chromosomes fail to disjoin, resulting in two aneuploid cells. The oöcytes formed will therefore have either an extra chromosome ($n + 1$), or one less chromosome ($n - 1$). Fertilization of such oöcytes with normal spermatocytes will result in either trisomic ($2n + 1$), or monosomic ($2n - 1$) zygotes. The underlying mechanism(s) leading to non-disjunction are not known but alterations in the level of recombination between chromosomes are associated with non-disjunction. Trisomy 21, 47,XXY and 47,XXX, but not trisomy 16 and 18, have been associated with a significant reduction in recombination.

Paternal errors

'*De novo*' structural rearrangements and point mutations giving rise to a variety of inherited conditions, such as familial retinoblastoma and type 1 neurofibromatosis (see also Chapter 21), show a strong bias towards a paternal origin. In contrast to oögenesis, spermatogenesis is a continuous process of production of spermatozoa from puberty onwards. Studies in mice and *Drosophila* which closely resemble humans with respect to spermatogenesis, indicate that point mutations arise and accumulate in spermatogonia which are premeiotic cells capable of mitotic division. In contrast, in mice and *Drosophila* and by extrapolation in humans, structural rearrangements may fatally disrupt meiosis. Paternal bias is accounted for because structural rearrangements may arise during postmeiotic maturation (i.e. during spermatid and spermatozoon stages).

Summary

The ability to recognize and define chromosome abnormalities has contributed to our understanding of the nature and origin of much congenital abnormality and in many cases allows the possibility of prenatal diagnosis in subsequent pregnancies. The nature of the fundamental causes of chromosome abnormalities are still not clear.

Key points

1 Chromosome abnormalities may be defined as microscopically visible changes in chromosome morphology and represent mutations involving a large number of genes. The smallest detectable chromosomal deletions remove a minimum of several megabases of DNA.

2 Chromosome abnormalities may be either constitutional, if they are inherited from one or other parent, or acquired, if the mutation arises during fetal growth or later in cells retaining the ability to undergo cell division.

3 Chromosome abnormalities may involve either a change in chromosome number, structure or pattern of inheritance.

4 Changes in chromosome number may involve either the gain or loss of individual chromosomes (aneuploidy) or the gain of entire haploid sets (triploidy or tetraploidy). Aneuploidy of the germ cells can give rise to either trisomic or monosomic zygotes.

5 Structural abnormalities include large deletions or insertions of genetic material, duplication of segments of a chromosome, inversions or translocations.

6 A third class of abnormality arises when both chromosomes of a pair are inherited from one or other parent. This is known as uniparental disomy and implies that the parental origin of a chromosome may determine gene expression on that chromosome.

Further reading

Connor J.M. & Ferguson-Smith M.A. (1997) *Essential Medical Genetics* (5th edn). Blackwell Science Ltd., Oxford.

Gardner R.J.M. & Sutherland G.R. (1996) *Chromosome Abnormalities and Genetic Counselling* (2nd edn). Oxford University Press, Oxford.

Mueller R.F. & Young I.D. (1998) *Emery's Elements of Medical Genetics* (10th edn). Blackwell Science Ltd., Oxford.

Reilly P.A. (1999) Down syndrome. *Journal of the Association of Genetic Technologists* **25**: 65–73.

Principles of Neoplasia

Neoplasia, literally meaning 'new growth', is a disorder characterized by the abnormal and continuous growth of cells which are no longer subject to the homoeostatic controls which maintain the appropriate number of cells in normal tissues. In most cases these cells form a solid mass of tissue which is referred to as a *tumour* (literally 'swelling') or *neoplasm*. An exception to this is leukaemia in which the abnormal cells arise from precursor cells in the bone marrow and pass into the blood stream in the same way as normal blood cells.

This chapter introduces the basic principles of neoplasia. The cellular basis of neoplasia is outlined, and benign and malignant forms of this disorder are described. The role of causative influences, including both environmental and genetic factors, are considered in relation to the development and progression of neoplasia. Finally, host responses to neoplasia are reviewed.

Growth characteristics of neoplasms

Under normal circumstances the number of cells in a given tissue is subject to variation. Thus, when an increased workload demand is placed upon a particular tissue, the tissue may respond by increasing cell number, a process known as *hyperplasia*. In some settings hyperplasia may be abnormal. Cells which no longer have the capacity to divide respond to increases in workload demand by increasing cell size. This is known as *hypertrophy*. Examples of hypertrophy include the increase in skeletal muscle

size in training athletes and the 'pathological' hypertrophy of the muscle cells of the left ventricle (left ventricular hypertrophy) that occurs in long-standing hypertension (see case studies 8 and 11).

In contrast to the processes of hyperplasia and hypertrophy which are essentially reversible once the provoking stimulus has been removed, neoplastic growth is usually not reversible. Neoplastic cells are no longer responsive to the controlling mechanisms that maintain cell number in normal tissues and therefore continue to divide under circumstances in which normal cells cease proliferation. The net result is the progressive accumulation of neoplastic cells and the formation of a tumour mass. The differences in growth regulation between normal and neoplastic cells may be summarized under the following five headings.

Growth factor dependency

Stimulation of a normal cell into a proliferative state often depends upon an external signal in the form of a growth factor. *Platelet-derived growth factor* (PDGF) is an example of a growth factor. Following tissue damage, PDGF is released by platelets and stimulates adjacent fibroblasts to divide and form a fibrous scar. Many growth factors bind to receptors situated on the surface of target cells. Binding of growth factor to a receptor initiates a series of biochemical changes within the cell which ultimately leads to cell division.

Tumour cells are not as dependent on growth

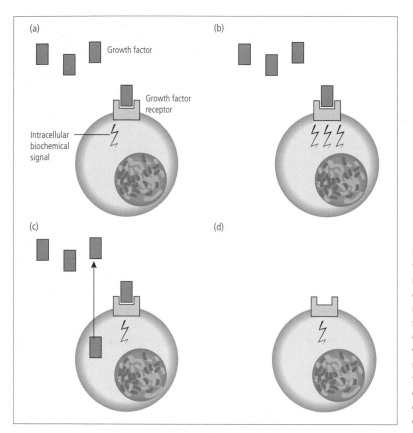

Fig. 21.1 Possible mechanisms leading to reduced growth factor dependency by neoplastic cells. (a) Normal cell. Ligation of a growth factor to a receptor on the cell membrane leads to intracellular biochemical signalling which will eventually produce cell division. (b) Neoplastic cells may respond more vigorously to growth factor ligation, or (c) they may secrete growth factors which stimulate their own proliferation. Alternatively, (d) a defective receptor may transmit intracellular growth signals in the absence of an extracellular growth factor.

factors as normal cells and are able to proliferate when concentrations of growth factors are much lower than those required by normal cells. These differences in growth factor requirements can be explained by several possible mechanisms. Tumour cells may secrete growth factors which are able to stimulate their own proliferation (*autocrine stimulation*), or they may respond more vigorously to growth factors produced by other cells. Alternatively, the tumour cells may proliferate in the absence of the usual growth factors required by normal cells. These mechanisms are outlined in Fig. 21.1.

Density-dependent inhibition of growth

Once normal dividing cells reach a finite density they stop proliferating. In contrast, neoplastic cells do not cease proliferation but continue to replicate to much higher densities than normal cells.

Anchorage dependence

Most normal cells need contact with a substratum in the extracellular environment to reproduce. Neoplastic cells are able to grow without attachment to a substratum. This is well illustrated *in vitro* by the ability of some tumour cells to form colonies when suspended as single cells in agar.

Contact inhibition of movement

When normal cells are placed in culture, they have the ability to respond to the presence of other cells. Thus, when two cells come into contact, one or both will change direction ensuring that the cells do not overlay each other, This characteristic is referred to as *contact inhibition of movement*. Neoplastic cells lack contact inhibition of movement and often grow over or under each other.

Adhesiveness

Tumour cells are less adhesive than normal cells and are less firmly attached to neighbouring cells or to the extracellular matrix. Loss of adhesiveness contributes to the invasive and metastatic properties of some neoplasms (see Chapter 24).

Tumour growth rate

Tumour growth rate is determined by various factors, including the rate at which new tumour cells are generated by cell division, and the rate at which cells are lost from the dividing cell pool, either by cell death or by differentiation. Factors other than cell kinetics can modify the rate of growth of neoplasms. An adequate blood supply, for example, is necessary for tumour growth. In experimental systems, tumours can only grow to several millimetres in diameter without provision of a blood supply. Although tumours often rely upon the host for their blood supply, tumour cells can secrete *angiogenic* (blood vessel forming) factors, which result in the proliferation of blood vessels within the tumour. Tumours secrete soluble factors that are able to stimulate vascular endothelial cell growth. One of the best studied is the vascular endothelial growth factor (VEGF). VEGF is important in the stimulation of vascular growth following hypoxia. Several VEGF-producing tumours have also been shown to express the receptor for VEGF, Flk-1, suggesting that in some settings VEGF may be mitogenic as a result of autocrine growth.

Hormones can also influence the growth rate of tumours arising in hormone-responsive cells. Some breast tumours, for example, grow very rapidly during pregnancy in response to the high oestrogen levels. Many oestrogen-dependent breast tumours are successfully treated with the use of antioestrogen drugs (e.g. tamoxifen).

The cellular basis of neoplasia

Neoplasms are believed to arise from a single *target cell* which has undergone a series of genetic changes (*mutations*) that ultimately result in its ability to escape the normal proliferative controls imposed upon normal cells. Mutations may occur spontaneously within cells or they may be induced following exposure to chemicals or radiation. Most mutations impair cell survival and ultimately result in cell death. However, in some cases a mutation may provide a cell with a growth advantage when compared to its normal counterparts. Mutations that enhance cell growth usually arise either in genes that stimulate cell division (*oncogenes*), or in those that inhibit cell division (*tumour suppressor genes*). The functions of these genes are discussed in detail in Chapter 22.

A cell bearing a beneficial mutation may continue to divide until a collection of genetically identical cells or *clone* is formed. Cells from this clone may in turn acquire new mutations which further enhance their growth potential. Eventually a point may be reached when some of these cells are able to grow in an uncontrolled fashion and a tumour results. Once a tumour is established, mutations within tumour cells may give rise to multiple subclones within the tumour, each with differing properties. This is referred to as *tumour heterogeneity* and is an important concept in relation to tumour progression (see Chapter 24).

Benign and malignant neoplasms

Neoplasms are broadly divisible into *benign* and *malignant* subgroups. *Cancer* is a term which is commonly used to describe the disease which results from the presence of a malignant neoplasm. Benign and malignant neoplasms differ in a number of important ways as outlined in the following sections.

Invasion and metastasis

Malignant neoplasms are characterized by their capacity to invade surrounding normal tissue and to spread to distant parts of the body to generate secondary growths. This latter property is known as *metastasis* and is described in detail in Chapter 24. In general, benign tumours do not invade adjacent tissues and do not metastasize.

Degree of differentiation

The tumour cells of benign neoplasms closely resemble the cell of origin and are therefore described as being *well differentiated*. Although malignant neoplasms may also be well differentiated, many are either *poorly differentiated* (cells of the tumour do not closely resemble cell of origin) or *undifferentiated* (the origin of the tumour cells cannot be determined). In general, undifferentiated tumours have higher growth rates than their well-differentiated counterparts.

Clinical outcome

Malignant neoplasms are often fatal to their host. This is primarily due to their ability to metastasize and to develop resistance to various forms of therapy (see Chapter 24). In contrast, benign neoplasms are life threatening only in the following exceptional circumstances.

• *If the tumour is present within, or impinges upon, a vital structure*. Certain benign tumours of the atrium (*atrial myxomas*) may cause valve obstruction, cardiac insufficiency and sudden death in some cases.

• *If the tumour produces a physiologically active substance in increased amounts*. Some benign tumours of the adrenal medulla (*phaeochromocytomas*) secrete excessive amounts of adrenaline leading to hypertension which can precipitate myocardial infarction or cerebral haemorrhage. Likewise, β-cell adenomas of the pancreas can secrete enough insulin to produce fatal hypoglycaemia (low blood glucose levels).

• *If the tumour is present within the central nervous system (CNS)*. Because the CNS is an enclosed system, expanding lesions can cause pressure damage to surrounding nervous tissue or produce serious complications as a result of associated rises in intracranial pressure.

Classification of neoplasia

Neoplasms are usually classified on the basis of the presumed cell or tissue of origin irrespective of the site at which the tumour is found. Thus, squamous cell carcinomas are malignant neoplasms derived from squamous epithelial cells. Since this type of epithelial cell is found in many locations within the body, squamous cell carcinoma can arise in many sites which include skin, upper oesophagus and cervix.

Some neoplasms, e.g. *chronic myeloid leukaemia* (CML, see also case study 29), arise in *stem cells*. Stem cells are present in small numbers in cell populations and have two critical functions: to generate descendants which will become differentiated and perform the function of the tissue; and to renew themselves so that a stable number of stem cells remain. CML is characterized by the accumulation of neoplastic cells of differing myeloid lineages which have all descended from a common neoplastic myeloid stem cell. Table 21.1 gives a brief classification of some neoplasms.

Causal factors in the development of cancer

Analysis of the incidence of cancer in different human populations throughout the world has lead to the identification of groups of causal factors. These are broadly divided into environmental and genetic subgroups.

Environmental factors

Chemical agents

The classic example of cancer following exposure to chemicals was described in 1775 by Percival Pott who noted that chimney sweeps had a high incidence of cancer of the scrotum which he attributed to exposure to soot. Subsequently, many hundreds of chemical carcinogens have been implicated in the causation of cancer. Examples of these are listed in Table 21.2.

Most chemical carcinogens are *electrophilic* (electron seeking) and chemically modify the DNA of exposed cells, thereby inducing mutations. Some chemical agents are not themselves carcinogenic but are converted to carcinogenic derivatives by metabolic enzymes of the body (Fig. 21.2). These are called *indirect carcinogens*. Carcinogens which do not require chemical modification for their cancer-causing properties are known as *direct carcinogens*.

Table 21.1 Some neoplasms and their cell or tissue of origin.

Tissue or cell of origin	Benign neoplasm	Malignant neoplasm
Epithelium		
Squamous epithelium	Squamous cell papilloma	Squamous cell carcinoma
Glandular epithelium includes glandular epithelium of solid organs	Adenoma	Adenocarcinoma
Mesothelium	Mesothelioma	Malignant mesothelioma
Connective tissue		
Cartilage	Chondroma	Chondrosarcoma
Bone	Osteoma	Osteosarcoma
Smooth muscle	Leiomyoma	Leiomyosarcoma
Striated muscle	Rhabdomyoma	Rhabdomyosarcoma
Lymphocytes	—	Lymphoma
Haemopoietic cells	—	Leukaemia
Melanocytes	Melanoma	Malignant melanoma

Note that there are no well-defined benign counterparts of the lymphomas and leukaemias.

Table 21.2 Examples of chemical carcinogens.

Chemical agent	Nature of exposure	Resultant cancer
Beta-naphthylamine	Chemical used in rubber industry	Bladder cancer in exposed workers
Benzo(a)pyrene	Constituent of cigarette smoke	Lung cancer
Asbestos	Inhalation of asbestos fibres	Malignant mesothelioma of pleural cavity
Aflatoxin B_1	Produced by mould *Aspergillus flavus* found on groundnuts	Hepatocellular adenocarcinoma in populations whose diet includes affected nuts
Cyclophosphamide	Drug used in the treatment of cancer	Lymphomas and leukaemias

The process of chemical carcinogenesis can be observed experimentally by monitoring the effect of chemical carcinogens on experimental animals. This has led to the concepts of *initiation* and *promotion* (Fig. 21.3).

Initiation is the acquisition of a mutation (or mutations) by a cell following exposure to a carcinogen. Initiation is rapid and irreversible but alone is not usually sufficient for tumour formation. If the initiated cell is then exposed to a second agent known as a *promoter* then a tumour may be formed. Application of a promoter without prior initiation will not lead to tumour formation. Promoters include substances such as phorbol esters and unlike *initiators* are not mutagenic but are potent mitogens. The role of promoters, therefore, is to induce clonal

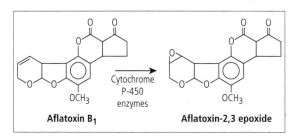

Fig. 21.2 Aflatoxin B_1 is an indirect carcinogen requiring conversion to aflatoxin-2,3 epoxide by the action of the cytochrome P-450 enzymes in the liver. This compound then reacts with guanine residues in DNA.

proliferation of initiated cells which will ultimately lead to tumour formation. It should be noted that some chemicals possess the capability of both initiation and promotion, as evidenced by their ability to

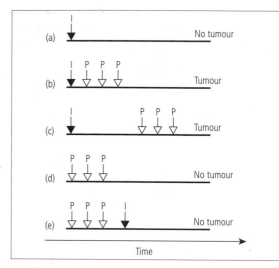

Fig. 21.3 Experiments demonstrating the initiation and promotion stages of chemical-induced skin cancer in mice. (a) Application of an initiating agent (I) alone does not result in tumour formation. (b) Initiating agent followed by promoter (P) results in tumour formation. (c) Application of promoter delayed for several months after initiation also results in tumour formation indicating that initiation has 'memory'. (d) Promotion alone and (e) promotion followed by initiation do not produce tumours.

induce tumours without any added factors. These chemicals are known as *complete carcinogens* to distinguish them from *incomplete carcinogens* which are only capable of initiation. Although these concepts are based on animal studies there is evidence that these stages are also discernible in some human cancers. Figure 21.4 gives an overview of events in chemical carcinogenesis.

Radiation

The increased risk of cancer in individuals exposed to *ionizing radiation* is well documented. Uranium miners, for example, have a 10-fold increase in the incidence of lung cancer, and mortality rates from leukaemia and other cancers are increased in survivors of the Hiroshima and Nagasaki atom bombs. Ionizing radiations are carcinogenic because they can interact with DNA and induce mutations.

Particulate radiation (e.g. α- and β-particles) can react with DNA directly, whereas *electromagnetic radiation* (X-rays, γ-rays) are indirectly ionizing by releasing energetic electrons when these rays are absorbed. These rays can either be absorbed directly by DNA or by other molecules such as water. The release of electrons from water generates *free radical species* such as the hydroxyl ion which then react with DNA. The resulting disruption of chemical bonds leads to a variety of lesions in DNA including base damage, intermolecular cross-linking and strand breaks.

Epidemiological studies have shown an increased incidence of various skin cancers following exposure to *ultraviolet radiation*. In contrast to ionizing radiation, ultraviolet rays deposit energy which is insufficient to ionize molecules but is enough to excite them temporarily and make them chemically active. Ultraviolet rays, for example, excite pyrimidine bases of DNA which then react with each other forming *pyrimidine dimers*.

DNA damage caused by exposure to chemical carcinogens or radiation is not necessarily permanent because cells have the capacity to repair DNA. *DNA repair* must take place prior to cell division to prevent the transmission of a potentially harmful mutation to the daughter cells. Cells can delay their progression through the cell cycle to allow sufficient time for DNA repair to take place prior to cell division. Many cells carrying damaged DNA have the additional option of activating apoptosis (see Chapter 4) to precipitate their self-destruction.

A key strategy used by mammalian cells to remove damaged DNA caused by ultraviolet light or other mutagens is *excision repair* (Fig. 21.5). During this process a multiprotein system locates a lesion in DNA and removes the damaged nucleotides. DNA synthesis proceeds using the remaining normal strand as a template. Finally, the newly synthesized DNA is joined to the two ends of the undamaged strand by a DNA *ligase* enzyme.

The importance of DNA repair in preventing the transmission of potentially carcinogenic mutations is highlighted by the increased cancer risk observed in patients with defects in DNA repair (Table 21.3).

Oncogenic viruses

A large number of viruses including both DNA and RNA viruses have proved to be cancer causing in a

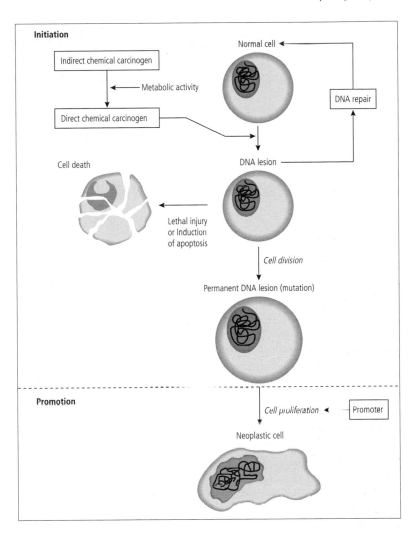

Fig. 21.4 An overview of events in chemical carcinogenesis. DNA damage following exposure of a normal cell to a chemical carcinogen may either be repaired or result in cell death. Alternatively, if the cell divides, the genetic change may be transmitted to daughter cells. Clonal expansion of mutated cells can lead to the development of a neoplasm.

wide variety of animals. There is increasing evidence that viruses are also important in the development of some human cancers. The contribution of viruses as oncogenic agents is discussed in Chapter 23.

Genetic factors

Evidence indicates that for a large number of cancers there exist not only environmental influences but also hereditary predispositions. The classical example here is *retinoblastoma*, a tumour of the retina, which is inherited in some families as an autosomal dominant disorder. Affected individuals inherit a mutation in one allele of the *retinoblastoma gene*, a known tumour suppressor gene, so that only a single somatic mutation in the second allele is required for the development of a tumour.

A defect in a tumour suppressor gene (*NF-1*) has also been shown to be responsible for the increased risk of tumours in type 1 neurofibromatosis. This autosomal dominant condition is characterized by the development of multiple benign tumours derived from Schwann's cells (*neurofibromas*), some

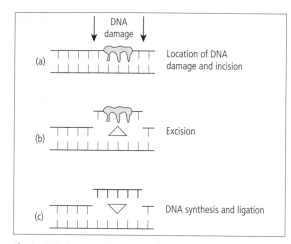

Fig. 21.5 Nucleotide excision repair pathway. During this process, DNA damage is located (a) and removed by a series of enzymes (b). New DNA is synthesized and joined to the two ends of the undamaged strand (c).

of which may become malignant in later life. *Familial adenomatous polyposis* (FAP) is another autosomal dominant condition in which affected people develop multiple adenomas of the large bowel. In adulthood there is a high risk of one or more adenomas developing a focus of carcinoma. Many of the gene defects responsible for FAP have now been identified (see Chapter 19 and case study 22). Similarly, inherited mutations in the *BRCA-1* and *BRCA-2* genes have been shown to be responsible for the increased susceptibility to breast cancer in some families (see Chapter 22 and case study

28). Other inherited conditions that predispose individuals to cancer include some DNA repair disorders (see Table 21.3) and immunodeficiency syndromes.

Clustering of cancers within families in the absence of any recognizable underlying inherited condition also occurs. Some of these familial cancers may be due to common environmental factors within the families or may have occurred by chance. However, in other families the pattern of inheritance, specific associations of certain malignancies within the familial clusters and an unusually early age at diagnosis suggest a genetic aetiology.

A particularly good example of this is the *Li–Fraumeni cancer family syndrome*. The principal features of this syndrome are soft-tissue sarcomas in children and young adults, and the early onset of breast cancer in their mothers and other close female relatives (Fig. 21.6). Osteosarcoma and leukaemia also occur to excess. An autosomal dominant pattern of inheritance is seen and there is a high incidence of multiple primary malignancies. The Li–Fraumeni cancer family syndrome is the result of the genetic transmission of mutations within the *p53* tumour suppressor gene (see Chapter 22).

Host responses to neoplasia

The concept of *immune surveillance* suggests that the immune system is able to eradicate potential cancer cells and that cancer arises because of a defect in this

Disorder	Defect	Common neoplasms
Xeroderma pigmentosum	Defect in nucleotide excision repair pathway (see Fig. 21.5)	Various skin cancers, including basal cell carcinoma and malignant melanoma
Bloom's syndrome	Defect in BLM gene leading to high mutation rate and hyper-recombination	Various, characterized by early onset
Fanconi's anaemia	Increased susceptibility to DNA cross-linking agents	Leukaemia, particularly acute myeloid type
Ataxia telangiectasia	Increased sensitivity to radiation and spontaneous chromosome translocations, impaired ability to induce p53-mediated cell cycle arrest	Leukaemias and lymphomas particularly of T-cell type, some epithelial tumours, e.g. ovaries and stomach

Table 21.3 Examples of inherited defects in DNA repair associated with an increased cancer risk. All are autosomal recessive disorders.

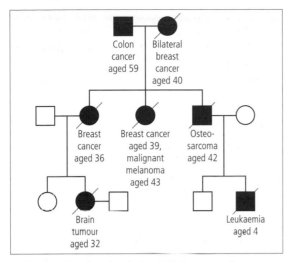

Fig. 21.6 Family pedigree for a family with Li–Fraumeni syndrome.

antigens. These antigens may be expressed only on fetal cells and not on normal adult cells, or they may be expressed at low levels on normal adult cells but at increased levels on tumour cells. An example of a tumour-associated antigen is a protein designated p97, high levels of which are found on melanoma cells. A vaccine has been developed against this protein which has been shown to protect mice from developing malignant melanoma. Results such as this highlight the potential use of tumour-associated antigens as targets for therapeutic intervention in some forms of cancer. Immune responses to tumour antigens may be mediated by a number of integrated and interdependent cell systems as described in the following sections.

surveillance process. This is supported by the observation that cancer is more common in immunosuppressed individuals. However, only certain cancers occur with increased frequency in immunosuppression, for example lymphomas, and the incidence of the more common cancers, such as lung and breast, is not significantly increased. Many of the cancers that arise in persistent immunosuppressive states are virus associated. These are discussed in more detail in Chapter 23.

Host defence systems include both *adaptive* and *innate* systems. The adaptive arm of the immune system includes antigen-specific T and B lymphocytes which have the capacity of distinguishing self from non-self. It follows that if tumours are to be recognized by T or B lymphocytes they must express non-self antigens. Non-self antigens found on tumour cells are referred to as *tumour antigens.* Experimental cancers induced in laboratory animals either by chemicals, radiation or viruses frequently express antigens which are not found on normal cells and which are often unique to individual tumours. These tumour antigens are known as *tumour-specific antigens.* In contrast, spontaneous tumours in animals are weakly, if at all, immunogenic.

The majority of antigens present on human cancers are not unique to tumour cells but are also present on normal cells and are called *tumour-associated*

B cells

For antibodies to have an antitumour effect, the tumour must express an antigen recognizable to B cells. In most cases the antigen must also be recognized by T-helper cells that are capable of secreting lymphokines including the interleukins (IL)-4, IL-5 and IL-6 which are necessary for B-cell proliferation and differentiation. Once antibody has bound to the target cell it may induce *antibody-dependent cellular cytotoxicity* (ADCC) or *complement-mediated lysis* (see Chapter 6).

T cells

Cytotoxic T cells (CTLs) recognize antigen in association with major histocompatibility complex (MHC) class I molecules and are important in the recognition and elimination of virus-infected tumour cells. This is supported by recent studies showing that infusion of virus-specific CTLs into patients with Epstein–Barr virus-associated lymphoproliferative disease produces dramatic regression of these tumours. T-cell secretion of interferon-γ (IFN-γ) activates macrophages and increases expression of MHC molecules on tumour cells. The precise role of T cells, however, is unclear since some T-cell depletion syndromes, for example Di George syndrome (see case study 23), do not show a significant increase in spontaneous malignancies.

Natural killer cells

The importance of natural killer (NK) cells in tumour immunity is highlighted in the beige mouse strain and in *Chediak–Higashi syndrome* in humans. In both cases there is a marked impairment of NK function and an increase in the incidence of certain types of cancer. Although it is not known how NK cells recognize tumour cells, recognition does not require processing or presentation and is not MHC restricted. NK cells possess neither surface immunoglobulin nor T-cell receptors. However, NK cells do have Fc receptors and can participate in antibody-dependent cell-mediated cytotoxicity (ADCC).

Macrophages

Activated macrophages also have Fc receptors and can participate in ADCC. They can also induce tumour cell lysis by the release of a variety of extracellular factors which include tumour necrosis factor α (TNF-α).

Summary

Neoplastic cells differ from normal cells because they do not respond to normal growth control mechanisms. In most cases this subversion of growth control is the result of mutations in important growth control genes. These mutations may be the result of a variety of environmental insults (including exposure to carcinogenic chemicals or radiation), or they may be inherited. Other inherited conditions, such as disorders of DNA repair and some immunodeficiency states, may predispose individuals to cancer.

Key points

1 Neoplasia, literally meaning 'new growth' is a disorder characterized by the accumulation of cells which are no longer responsive to the controlling mechanisms that maintain cell number in normal tissues.

2 Neoplasms or tumours are the tissue masses which result from the accumulation of these abnormal cells. Neoplasms may be either benign or malignant. Malignant neoplasms are almost always life threatening, whereas benign neoplasms rarely are.

3 Neoplasms are usually classified on the basis of the presumed cell of origin, irrespective of where they are found.

4 Neoplasms are believed to arise from a single target cell which has undergone a series of mutations. These mutations enable the cell to escape the normal proliferative constraints imposed upon normal cells.

5 These mutations may arise spontaneously, as a result of exposure to a variety of environmental agents including chemicals and radiant energy, or they may be inherited.

6 The incidence of some forms of cancer, particularly virus-associated tumours, is increased in a number of immunodeficiency states. This suggests that the immune system is important in preventing the development of these forms of cancer.

Further reading

Taunock I.F. & Hill R.P. (1998) *The Basic Science of Oncology.* McGraw Hill, Maidenhead.

Vogelstein B. & Kinzler K.W. (1999) *The Genetic Basis of Human Cancer.* McGraw Hill, Maidenhead.

Weinberg R.A. (1998) *One Renegade Cell: how cancer begins* (Science Masters Series).

CHAPTER 22

The Molecular Basis of Cancer

A fundamental characteristic of malignant cells is that they continue to divide under circumstances in which normal cells cease proliferation. It is now clear that this is due to the aberrant expression of genes that regulate cell proliferation. There are different kinds of these regulatory genes: some called *oncogenes* promote cell growth and division and others, termed *antioncogenes* or *tumour suppressor genes*, suppress growth. This chapter examines how changes in the expression of these regulatory genes can lead to the development of cancer.

Oncogenes and viruses

The concept that there are genes capable of causing cancer (oncogenes) is based largely on studies carried out on tumours arising in animals. In 1911, Peyton Rous described a transmissible sarcoma in chickens. The original tumour found in an adult bird could be transmitted to other chickens by injection of a cell-free filtrate of the tumour. Later, similar observations were made for tumours arising in other animals.

The causative agents for these transmissible tumours were found to be *retroviruses*. When a retrovirus infects a cell it uses the enzyme reverse transcriptase to generate a double-stranded DNA copy of its RNA genome (see Chapter 9). This DNA copy, known as the *provirus*, integrates into the host cell DNA. The structure of a typical retrovirus genome is shown in Fig. 22.1a.

Retroviruses are responsible for a variety of diseases in humans and other animals although not all

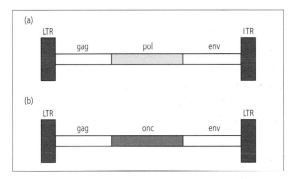
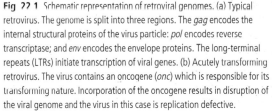

Fig. 22.1 Schematic representation of retroviral genomes. (a) Typical retrovirus. The genome is split into three regions. The *gag* encodes the internal structural proteins of the virus particle; *pol* encodes reverse transcriptase; and *env* encodes the envelope proteins. The long-terminal repeats (LTRs) initiate transcription of viral genes. (b) Acutely transforming retrovirus. The virus contains an oncogene (*onc*) which is responsible for its transforming nature. Incorporation of the oncogene results in disruption of the viral genome and the virus in this case is replication defective.

of them are able to cause cancer. The cancer-causing (oncogenic) retroviruses may be divided into those that are able to induce tumours in infected experimental animals after very short latency periods, generally days or weeks (*acutely transforming*) and those which induce tumours over a much longer period of time, often many months or even years (*slowly transforming*). The mechanisms of tumour formation in both groups are different, and are discussed below.

Acutely transforming retroviruses

Dissection of the genome of acutely transforming

193

Table 22.1 Examples of acutely transforming retroviruses

Acutely transforming retrovirus	Species affected	Tumour type	Oncogene present in viral genome
Rous sarcoma virus	Chicken	Sarcoma	v-*src*
Avian myelocytomatosis virus	Chicken	Sarcoma	v-*myc*
Simian sarcoma virus	Monkey	Sarcoma	v-*sis*
Avian erythroblastosis virus, ES4	Chicken	Erythroblastosis, sarcoma	v-*erbA* and v-*erbB*

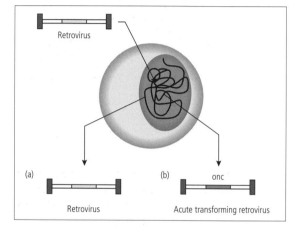

Fig. 22.2 Proposed evolution of acutely transforming retroviruses. A retrovirus infects a cell and its complementary provirus integrates into the host cell DNA. (a) Normal lifecycle; new virus is produced which contains intact genome. (b) Viral sequences are lost and replaced by sequences derived from a cellular oncogene. The new genome is packaged into viral particles. The new virus released henceforth is an acutely transforming variant of the original infecting virus.

the v-*oncs* were created when a retrovirus captured genetic information from the host cell in the form of whole or part of the cellular oncogene sequence (Fig. 22.2). In most cases, the incorporation of the oncogene into the virus resulted in the deletion of important viral sequences, thus rendering the virus defective for replication. Such viruses require coinfection with a helper virus, which provides the structural proteins and enzymes necessary for the propagation of the acutely transforming virus. The single exception to this is the *Rous sarcoma virus*. Incorporation of *src*, the oncogene present within this virus, did not disrupt the viral genome, and the virus is therefore able to replicate without the need for a helper virus.

Although acutely transforming retroviruses are responsible for many neoplasms in experimental animals, to date no members of this group have been shown to cause cancer in humans.

Growth control in normal cells

The identification of cellular oncogenes prompted intensive investigation of the function of these genes in normal cells. What is now clear is that the protein products of cellular oncogenes are involved in pathways controlling cell division.

Stimulation of a cell into a proliferative state depends upon an external signal in the form of a growth factor. In order for a growth factor to alter cell function, it must transmit its message through the cell membrane. Some growth factors, e.g. the steroid hormones, are lipid soluble and readily pass through the cell membrane. Once inside the cell they bind to intracellular receptors. These receptors then bind to DNA and regulate the transcription of important cellular genes.

retroviruses revealed that they possessed genes that were responsible for their transforming properties (Fig. 22.1b). These genes were therefore called oncogenes (*onc*). Each oncogene was given a three-letter name derived from the virus in which the oncogene was identified (Table 22.1). Most acutely transforming retroviruses contain only one oncogene, although some (e.g. the avian erythroblastosis virus ES4) contain two.

Later, studies showed that these viral oncogene sequences were almost identical to endogenous sequences in the DNA of the animal species in which the virus was isolated. These cellular sequences were designated *cellular oncogenes* (c-*onc*) or *proto-oncogenes* to distinguish them from their viral counterparts (v-*onc*). It is now generally accepted that

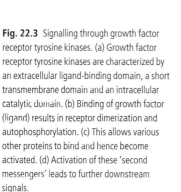
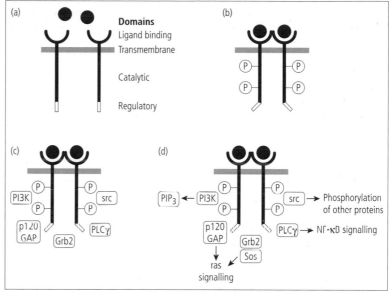

Fig. 22.3 Signalling through growth factor receptor tyrosine kinases. (a) Growth factor receptor tyrosine kinases are characterized by an extracellular ligand-binding domain, a short transmembrane domain and an intracellular catalytic domain. (b) Binding of growth factor (ligand) results in receptor dimerization and autophosphorylation. (c) This allows various other proteins to bind and hence become activated. (d) Activation of these 'second messengers' leads to further downstream signals.

Most growth factors do not enter the cell but instead bind to receptors situated within the cell membrane. These membrane receptors have a cytoplasmic domain, which becomes activated once the growth factor has bound. Activation of the receptor in this way allows the signal to be transferred to other proteins situated within the cytoplasm.

This is well illustrated in the case of *growth factor receptor tyrosine kinases* (growth factor receptors that have the ability to phosphorylate themselves or other proteins on the amino acid, tyrosine) such as epidermal growth factor (EGF) receptor and platelet-derived growth factor (PDGF) receptor. These receptors typically have an extracellular ligand binding domain, a single transmembrane domain and an intracellular catalytic domain (Fig. 22.3). Binding of growth factor results in receptor dimerization and activation of the catalytic domain, which then phosphorylates tyrosine residues within the receptor. This *autophosphorylation* event allows the receptor to bind other proteins, notably those containing so-called *src*-homology 2 (SH2) domains. These include proteins such as phospholipase C γ (PLC-γ), phosphatidyl inositol 3 kinase (PI3K) and the guanosine triphosphatase (GTPase) activating protein for p21 ras (p120^{GAP}), growth factor receptor bound protein-2 (Grb2) and the c-src protein itself.

Binding of these proteins to the receptor results in their activation. For example, c-src is itself a tyrosine kinase and once bound to a receptor is able to phosphorylate other downstream proteins.

Phosphorylation is a key event in signal transduction and serves two basic purposes. Firstly, it can change the conformation of the phosphorylated protein and induce enzymatic kinase activation. Secondly, phosphorylation may generate docking sites that recruit other proteins, which the activated kinase may then phosphorylate.

Growth factor receptor tyrosine kinases also activate the *ras* pathway. The *ras* family of oncogenes encode a group of highly conserved cytoplasmic proteins of 21 000 Da (p21^{ras}). They are guanine nucleotide binding proteins (G proteins). Activated ras protein recruits raf, a serine threonine kinase (a protein that phosphorylates other proteins on serine/threonine residues) (Fig. 22.4). Activation of raf stimulates the mitogen-activated protein (MAP) kinase pathway which ultimately leads to the phosphorylation and activation of the transcription factors, fos and jun.

The net result of the activation of these signalling pathways is the activation of transcription factors. These proteins regulate the expression of growth control genes by binding to specific DNA sequences.

195

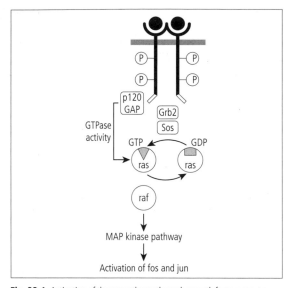

Fig. 22.4 Activation of the ras pathway through growth factor receptor tyrosine kinases. Autophosphorylation of the growth factor receptor tyrosine kinase enables the Grb2 protein to bind. Grb2 then recruits the nucleotide exchange factor, son of sevenless (Sos). Grb2 is an adapter protein, i.e. it serves as a link between the receptor and the Sos protein. Sos catalyses the exchange of GDP for GTP on ras, converting ras from an inactive to an active form. Active ras interacts with and recruits raf, a serine threonine kinase. Activation of raf stimulates the MAP kinase pathway leading to the activation of fos and jun, which together make up the mammalian transcription factor, AP-1. A GTPase-activating protein (GAP) which also binds to the receptor via an SH2 homology domain terminates activation of the ras–GTP complex.

There are two groups of transcription factors: those that only interact with DNA when bound together with other molecules in a complex (heterodimers); and those that have the ability to bind to DNA as monomers.

The myc family of proteins are examples of transcription factors that form heterodimers. Myc proteins form heterodimers with a protein known as Max. Myc–Max heterodimers bind to specific DNA sequences and initiate the transcription of genes that will directly stimulate cell division. Max also bind two other proteins, Mad and MxI1. Heterodimers comprising Max–Mad or Max–MxI1 bind to the same sequences as Myc–Max heterodimers but inhibit transcription from these sites.

Many of the genes transcribed in response to transcription factor activation are components of the cell

cycle machinery and promote progression through the restriction point in G1 (see Chapter 4). For example, cyclin D1 when complexed with a cyclin-dependent kinase (CDK4/6) phosphorylates the retinoblastoma protein (pRb, see Chapter 21). Hyperphosphorylation of pRb releases the E2F transcription factor and enables it to activate the transcription of genes necessary for cell cycle entry.

In addition to the presence of extracellular growth factors, cell proliferation often also requires attachment to the extracellular matrix (ECM). Cell surface integrin receptors (see Chapter 4) promote the attachment of cells to the ECM. Following this attachment, the receptors utilize the same signalling pathways as growth factor receptors. For example, integrin-mediated adhesion to the ECM stimulates the MAP kinase pathway. This pathway involves the progressive cascade of signal transduction from receptor-dependent activation of Ras, to the kinase Raf, through several MAPK/ERK enzymes, finally culminating in the induction of cyclin D1. Cyclin D1 begins the phosphorylation of pRb, which will ultimately lead to entry to S phase. Several recent studies have shown that growth factor receptor and integrin receptor activation are jointly required for efficient stimulation of these growth signalling cascades. Furthermore, cells that are not allowed to spread on their ECM are growth arrested. Thus, the integrity of the actin cytoskeleton, which is the key to cell spreading and determines cell shape, is critical to G1 progression. Actin disruption leads to downregulation of cyclin D1 and upregulation of p27 and cell cycle arrest.

Thus, the emerging concept is that normal cells have several mechanisms to prevent uncontrolled growth, including the restriction of growth factors, stabilization of cell–cell and cell–ECM contacts, and the maintenance of cell shape. We know that cancer cells often grow in the absence or in lower concentrations of growth factors, proliferate in an anchorage-independent fashion and do not restrict their growth when they are unable to spread (see Chapter 21).

Oncogenes encode many of the proteins involved in growth control

Oncogenes encode many of the proteins involved in

the transduction of growth signals described above. In normal cells, as we might expect, their expression is tightly regulated. In malignant cells, however, this is not so and the expression of one or more oncogenes is either quantitatively or qualitatively different from that seen in normal cells. It is these changes in oncogene expression, which are in part responsible for the subversion of growth control, which is so characteristic of malignant cells.

Growth factors

Several oncogenes encode growth factors. For example the c-*sis* gene encodes the β-chain of PDGF. PDGF is normally released by platelets and stimulates the growth of a number of cell types, including fibroblasts. Certain connective tissue tumours, such as sarcomas and glioblastomas, have been shown to express c-*sis*, whereas their normal counterpart cells do not. Production of PDGF by the tumour cells of sarcomas would be expected to stimulate an autocrine growth loop since these cells also express the PDGF receptor on their surface. The molecular mechanisms responsible for expression of c-*sis* in these tumours have yet to be fully elucidated.

Growth factor receptors

Oncogenes encode many growth factor receptors. In cancer cells structural changes in the receptor appear to deregulate the receptor kinase activity so that these proteins induce transformation by delivering a continuous ligand-independent signal. For example, the retrovirus gene v-*erbB* is transforming because there is a deletion of the ligand-binding domain and the negative regulatory domain so that the catalytic domain is constitutively active in the absence of the ligand (Fig. 22.5). Likewise, a single amino acid substitution as a result of a *point mutation* (see Chapter 21) in the *HER-2/neu* receptor oncogene is sufficient for ligand-independent activation. This mutation promotes receptor dimerization and hence kinase activation in the absence of ligand.

In addition to these structural changes, growth factor receptors are frequently overexpressed as a result of *gene amplification*. Gene amplification is an increase in the number of copies of an oncogene often resulting in its overexpression. The amplified genes may be seen on cytogenetic analysis where

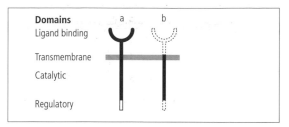

Fig. 22.5 Structure of the epidermal growth factor (EGF) receptor. (a) Normal EGF receptor showing ligand-binding domain, the catalytic domain responsible for tyrosine kinase activity, and the regulatory domain. The regulatory domain exerts a negative influence on tyrosine kinase activity. (b) Truncated receptor encoded by v-*erbB*. Ligand-binding and negative regulatory domains are absent and the receptor has constitutive tyrosine kinase activity.

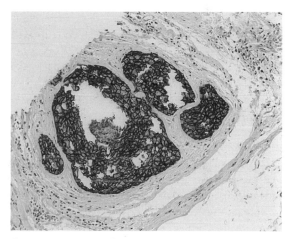

Fig. 22.6 Overexpression of HER-2/neu in breast cancer. Immunohistochemistry has been used to detect overexpression of the HER-2/neu protein that localizes to the breast cancer cells in a typical 'basket-weave' pattern. Courtesy of G.M. Reynolds, University of Birmingham.

they are represented by *homogeneously staining regions* (HSRs) or *double minutes*. The *HER-2/neu* gene, for example, is frequently over-expressed in adenocarcinomas of the breast, stomach and ovary (Fig. 22.6). In many cases high copy numbers of an amplified oncogene correlates with an unfavourable prognosis and predicts a poor response to treatment. In other cases, the overexpressed oncogene protein has served as a useful target in immunotherapy. For example, a monoclonal antibody directed to the HER-2/neu protein, known as Herceptin has

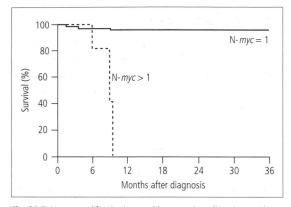

Fig. 22.7 N-*myc* amplification in neuroblastoma. Overall, patients with amplified N-*myc* (N-*myc* > 1) have a poorer survival when compared to those patients without amplified N-*myc* (N-*myc* = 1).

been used successfully to treat some patients with advanced breast cancer.

Signal transducers

Mutations within the *ras* gene are a particularly common abnormality in many types of cancer. These mutations result in amino acid substitutions that 'lock' the ras protein in its active GTP-bound state (see Fig. 22.4), through an increased exchange of guanosine diphosphate (GDP) for GTP or through an inability of ras to interact with the GAP proteins. Consequently, downstream ras signalling is prolonged (see Fig. 22.4). Transformation of cells by an oncogenic *ras* also requires the activity of members of the Rho family of GTPases, Rho and Rac. These proteins are involved in rearrangements in the actin cytoskeleton and are thought to regulate the morphological changes associated with *ras* transformation.

The abl tyrosine kinases constitute a separate family of non-receptor tyrosine kinases that are localized to both the nucleus and the cytoplasm and are important transducers of growth signals. In chronic myeloid leukaemia (CML, see case study 29) a reciprocal *chromosome translocation* (transfer of part of one chromosome to another, see Chapter 20) involving chromosomes 9 and 22 leads to the production of a *fusion protein* (i.e. a single protein transcribed from two genes that have become fused, usually when they are juxtaposed following a trans-

location). Parts of the *bcr* gene and elements of the *abl* gene encode this fusion protein. The bcr region of this new protein promotes constitutive activation of the abl kinase and the stimulation of downstream signalling molecules. Furthermore, the bcr–abl fusion protein is excluded from the nucleus and this also prevents its interaction with substrates within the nucleus that are able to negatively regulate cell growth.

The 9;22 translocation is also observed in some patients with acute lymphoblastic leukaemia where it is associated with a poor prognosis.

Transcription factors

Oncogenes also encode many of the transcription factors identified as being important in cell growth. A number of these are aberrantly expressed in tumour cells either as a result of gene amplification or by chromosome translocation. In *Burkitt's lymphoma*, for example, a neoplasm of B lymphocytes, there is typically a reciprocal exchange of chromosomal material between chromosomes 8 and 14. In this translocation the c-*myc* gene, normally located on chromosome 8, moves to the immunogloblin heavy chain (IgH) locus on chromosome 14, and part of the IgH locus migrates to chromosome 8. The effect is constitutive expression of the c-*myc* gene and continuous cell proliferation. In some cases the change in c-*myc* regulation is due to the presence of potent transcriptional enhancer elements of the IgH locus which are now located next to the c-*myc* gene, whereas in others it is the result of the loss of c-*myc* regulatory sequences which remain on chromosome 8.

The N-*myc* gene (a member of the myc family of proteins) is frequently overexpressed as a result of gene amplification. N-*myc* amplification is common in neuroblastomas, retinoblastomas and gliomas. Neuroblastomas are tumours of the peripheral nervous system that almost exclusively occur in children. In children with neuroblastoma increasing N-*myc* copy number is associated with a poor prognosis (Fig. 22.7).

Cell cycle regulators

The gene encoding cyclin D1, known as *CCND1* or *PRAD1*, is overexpressed by gene amplification in gastric, breast and oesophageal cancer. As a result the cell is driven into cell cycle beyond G1 in the absence of the normal growth factor stimulation. Constitutive expression of *CCND1* also results from the t(11;14) chromosomal translocation that is commonly observed in some B-cell lymphomas, B-cell chronic lymphocytic leukaemias and multiple myelomas.

Oncogenes as antiapoptosis genes

Some cancer cells are resistant to programmed cell death, or *apoptosis* (see Chapter 4). It is now known that this is due in part to the aberrant expression of genes that control apoptosis. For example the follicular B-cell lymphomas are characterized by a translocation in which the *bcl*-2 oncogene moves from its normal position on chromosome 18 to the IgH locus on chromosome 14. The result of this translocation is an increase in *bcl*-2 expression. Expression of the *bcl*-2 oncogene has been shown to protect cells from apoptosis. Consequently, follicular lymphomas are characterized by an accumulation of B lymphocytes, which are resistant to apoptosis and are therefore long lived. *Bcl*-2 overexpression is observed in many other forms of cancer (Fig. 22.8) and in a number of these tumours correlates with a poor prognosis. Since many anticancer drugs work by inducing apoptosis in tumour cells, failure to undergo apoptosis may protect cells from these drugs and lead to drug resistance and treatment failure.

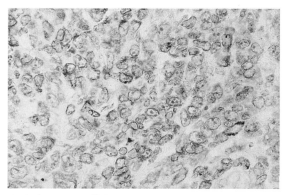

Fig. 22.8 Expression of bcl-2 in a high grade non-Hodgkin's lymphoma. In these tumours expression of bcl-2 is associated with a poor prognosis.

Retroviral oncogenesis

Although retroviruses are a rare cause of human cancer their study has been indispensable in the discovery and analysis of oncogenes. The oncogenic retroviruses are divided into the following two groups.

Acutely transforming retroviruses

These retroviruses transform cells by virtue of the fact their genomes contain oncogenes. Once they infect a cell, expression of the v-*onc* is initiated. In contrast to its normal cellular partner, the v-*onc* is expressed constitutively and at relatively higher levels since its transcription is under the control of the viral long terminal repeats (LTRs). In addition, the v-*onc* often represent modified forms of their cellular progenitors that have been truncated, mutated or fused to viral coding sequences, and as a result the encoded proteins are often more active than their normal counterparts (e.g. the v-*erbB* oncogene, see Fig. 22.5).

Slowly transforming retroviruses

Unlike their acutely transforming counterparts, the slowly transforming retroviruses do not possess oncogenes, but induce tumours by other means. A common mechanism is *insertional mutagenesis*. This involves integration of the retrovirus into close proximity of a cellular oncogene. In this position the retrovirus can alter the expression of the cellular oncogene. A good example is the *avian leukosis viruses* (ALVs) which are responsible for B-cell lymphomas in chickens. In most tumours the ALV provirus is integrated within or near to the normal c-*myc* gene, usually between the normal promoters for c-*myc* and exon 2 (Fig. 22.9). This divorces the body of the c-*myc* gene from its promoters, and hence its normal transcriptional control. Expression of c-*myc* is now initiated from the viral LTRs resulting in a considerable increase (20–100-fold) in the levels of c-*myc* mRNA.

The long latency period between infection with these retroviruses and the development of a tumour is in part due to the low probability that the

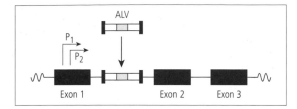

Fig. 22.9 Structure of the c-*myc* gene showing a typical insertion point for ALV provirus. The c-*myc* gene is composed of three coding regions (exons). Normal promoters are shown (P1 and P2). ALV commonly inserts between the promoters and exon 2 of c-*myc*, effectively divorcing c-*myc* from its normal transcriptional control. Transcription of c-*myc* is now controlled by the viral LTRs.

retrovirus will integrate into or adjacent to host cellular oncogenes.

The human T-lymphotropic virus 1 (HTLV-1) is an example of a slowly transforming retrovirus that is implicated in the development of human adult T-cell leukaemia. The molecular mechanisms by which HTLV-1 transforms cells are different to that described above and are outlined in Chapter 23.

Tumour suppressor genes

Oncogenes code for proteins which when present in abnormal form or amount may induce malignant growth by upregulating or turning on cell division. Genes with the opposite function are called *antioncogenes* or *tumour suppressor genes*. The proteins of tumour suppressor genes downregulate cell proliferation, and their inactivation may produce a neoplastic cell in which the effect of a growth-promoting factor goes unopposed. Many tumour suppressor genes are said to act recessively since abnormalities in both alleles are often necessary for loss of function. Inactivation of one allele alone is usually insufficient since the normal allele continues to produce protein, which can suppress cell proliferation. Thus, two 'knockout' mutations in tumour suppressor genes are required to contribute to tumorigenesis. This is often referred to as Knudson's 'two-hit' hypothesis. Some known and candidate tumour suppressor genes are outlined in Table 22.2. Some are discussed briefly below.

The retinoblastoma gene

Abnormalities in the retinoblastoma (*pRb*) gene were first detected in retinoblastoma, a neoplasm of the retinal precursor cells (*retinoblasts*) and subsequently in other tumours, notably osteosarcomas. Normal pRb product inhibits cell cycle progression.

In retinoblastoma, both alleles of the *pRb* gene on chromosome 13 are inactivated, either by deletion or point mutation. This results in neoplastic growth since pRb product can no longer suppress cell division. The majority of cases of retinoblastoma arise in a sporadic fashion in the population. In these cases, defects in both alleles of the *pRb* gene occur *somatically* (i.e. postconception) in the same retinoblast. However, as many as one-third of retinoblastomas arise from a genetic predisposition. In these cases a mutation is already present in one allele at conception (and consequently present in all cells of the developing retina), whereas the second occurs as a

Table 22.2 Some known and candidate tumour suppressor genes

Gene	Tumour(s)	Function of encoded protein
pRb	Retinoblastoma, osteosarcoma	Transcriptional regulator
p53	Common cancers, e.g. breast, colon, lung	Transcription factor
NF-1	Neurofibroma	GTPase-activating protein
APC	Colon cancer	?Regulator of β-catenin
BRCA1	Breast, ovarian cancer	?DNA repair
BRCA2	Breast cancer	?DNA repair
p16	Melanoma, pancreatic cancer	Cdk inhibitor
WT1	Wilms' tumour (nephroblastoma)	Transcription factor
DPC4	Pancreatic cancer	TGF-β signalling

somatic event. This model explains the observed single focus of tumour formation in sporadic cases, since the tumour arises following the convergence of two rare genetic events on a single target retinoblast.

Multiple tumour foci in both eyes are usually seen in heritable retinoblastoma. This can be explained by the fact that one of the two mutations is already present in the retinal cells and only a single mutation is required to complete the triggering process.

The *p53* gene

One of the most common defects in human cancer involves the tumour suppressor gene, *p53*. Abnormalities in this gene have been detected in many common cancers including those of the colon, breast and lung. The p53 protein is a transcription factor that exists as a complex composed of four molecules (*tetramer*) of p53 and normally stimulates the expression of a number of genes, including *Bax* (a promoter of apoptosis; see Chapter 4), *GADD45* (a DNA repair gene) and *p21*$^{\text{CIP1/WAF1}}$ (a gene involved in cell cycle arrest). Following a range of cellular stresses, including DNA damage, p53-induced expression results either in cell cycle arrest until the damage is repaired, or cell death by apoptosis. In this way potentially harmful DNA lesions are not transmitted to daughter cells and thereby do not become permanent heritable mutations. For this reason the *p53* gene has been referred to as the 'Guardian of the Genome'.

The way in which p53 is induced following DNA damage is not well understood although it appears that certain kinases such as *DNA activated protein kinase* (DNA-PK) and the *ataxia telangiectasia mutated* (ATM) protein phosphorylate particular residues within p53. This prevents degradation of p53 by a protein known as mdm2 leading to stabilization of p53 and subsequent transcriptional activation

Recent evidence suggests that *p53* is of central importance in a second pathway distinct from the DNA damage pathway outlined above and points to a route by which organisms avoid neoplasia following the inappropriate stimulation of oncogenes or other growth stimuli. Activation of oncogenes

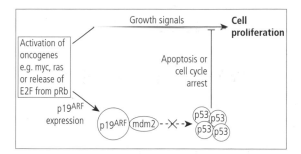

Fig. 22.10 *p19^{ARF}* provides a mechanism by which the inappropriate activation of oncogenes leads to apoptosis. Activity of oncogenes such as *myc* or *ras*, or release of pRb from E2F normally stimulates cell proliferation. However, these oncogenes also stimulate expression of *p19^{ARF}*. This gene encodes a protein that binds to mdm2 preventing it from degrading *p53*. This leads to stabilization of *p53*, which can then induce apoptosis or cell cycle arrest.

such as *myc* or *ras*, or release of pRb from E2F, would normally stimulate cell proliferation. However, these oncogenes also stimulate expression of *p19^{ARF}*. This gene encodes a protein that binds to mdm2 preventing it from degrading p53. This in turn leads to stabilization of p53, which can then induce apoptosis or cell cycle arrest (Fig. 22.10). Thus, cells have evolved a 'fail safe' mechanism for controlling inappropriate cell proliferation by inducing apoptosis.

There are a number of ways in which normal function of *p53* may be lost in cancer cells.
• Deletion of one or both *p53* alleles, which reduces the concentration of p53 below that required for normal function.
• Missense mutations (see Chapter 19). These are common in the region of *p53* that interacts with DNA.
• In tumours in which one allele remains normal, activity of the normal protein may be inhibited due to its participation in inactive tetramer formation. In some cases therefore, abnormalities in only one allele may be sufficient for inhibition of normal *p53* function.
• Inactivation of *p53* through binding to other proteins. Some of the DNA tumour virus genes, including *SV40* T antigen, the *E1B* gene of adenoviruses and the *E6* gene of the human papillomaviruses (see Chapter 23), encode proteins that bind to and

inactivate *p53*. As described above mdm2 targets *p53* for degradation. Mdm2 is amplified in some human sarcomas, which in turn leads to the inappropriate degradation of *p53* by increased quantities of mdm2 protein.

Recently two homologues of *p53*, known as *p63* and *p73*, have been identified. Thus, *p53* may be just one member of a *p53* family. The exact role of these homologues in the pathogenesis of cancer remains to be determined, although the *p73* gene maps to chromosome 1p36, a region frequently deleted in neuroblastoma.

The neurofibromatosis 1 gene

Abnormalities in the neurofibromatosis gene (*NF-1*) have been detected in neurofibromatosis type 1; a disorder characterized by the development of multiple benign neurofibromas, some of which may become malignant in later life. The *NF-1* gene codes for a GAP called *neurofibromin*, which negatively regulates active ras protein (see Fig. 22.4). Most neurofibromatosis type 1 sufferers have loss of function mutations in the *NF-1* gene.

There is evidence that in some cases, mutations in tumour suppressor genes are due to the activity of carcinogenic agents. For example, when exposed to aflatoxin B1 cells show specific *p53* mutations (at codon 249). These same mutations are seen in aflatoxin-induced hepatocellular carcinoma.

Genomic imprinting and cancer

Genomic imprinting is parental-specific expression of certain genes. Thus, in normal tissues some genes are preferentially expressed from either the maternal or paternal copy of the gene, but not from both alleles. Often the way in which one allele is silenced is by *methylation* of the gene concerned which prevents its transcription.

Loss of imprinting (LOI) has been shown to be important in the development of some cancers. For example in Wilms' tumour (nephroblastoma), a tumour of the kidney that arises predominantly in young children, LOI is one of several factors, which include alterations in the *WT1* gene (see Table 22.2), that are thought to contribute to the development of

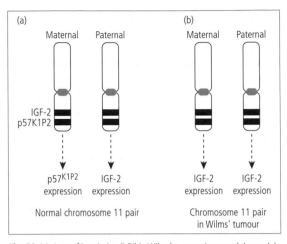

Fig. 22.11 Loss of imprinting (LOI) in Wilms' tumour. In normal tissues (a) genomic imprinting results in selective expression of insulin growth factor type 2 (*IGF-2*) gene from the paternal chromosome and *p57KIP2* expression from the maternal chromosome. However, in Wilms' tumour (b) this part of the maternal chromosome switches to a paternal pattern of expression. Expression of *IGF-2* is now twofold higher and *p57KIP2* expression is lost.

this tumour. In Wilms' tumour LOI involves a region on chromosome 11. In normal tissues, expression of two genes, the insulin growth factor type 2 (*IGF-2*) gene and *p57KIP2* gene, are imprinted on this chromosome such that expression of *IGF-2* is limited to the paternal chromosome and *p57KIP2* expression only occurs from the maternal chromosome (Fig. 22.11). However, in Wilms' tumour there is LOI so that the maternal chromosome switches to a pattern of paternal expression. This means that expression of *IGF-2* is initiated from both alleles and is therefore twofold higher, whereas *p57KIP2* expression is lost altogether.

Previous studies have shown that *IGF-2* contributes to tumour cell growth and so this explains why an increase in expression of this gene may be important. Likewise *p57KIP2* is a *cdk* inhibitor that arrests cell division. Its loss in Wilms' tumour may represent an important early event in the development of this tumour.

Methylation may represent a generally important mechanism that silences tumour suppressor genes. Thus, in some cancers lacking *p16* tumour suppressor gene expression but in which 'knockout' mutations cannot be demonstrated, it has been shown that methylation is responsible for the lack of expression.

Multistep transformation

Much experimental and epidemiological evidence argues that malignant change is a process which results from multiple genetic alterations involving both growth-promoting and growth-inhibiting genes. Experiments with mice, for example, show that the activation of a single oncogene is usually not sufficient to cause a tumour, and that changes in at least two oncogenes or tumour suppressor genes are required.

If tumours arise as a result of multiple events then an important question arises over which stage of malignant transformation a particular oncogene or tumour suppressor gene becomes involved. From studies on the experimental activation of c-*ras* in carcinogen-treated animals, it has been shown that *ras* gene activation is an early initiating event in carcinogenesis. Likewise, mutations in the *p53* gene constitute an intermediate or late step in tumour development. For example, mutations in *p53* usually occur around or during the transition of benign tumours of the colonic epithelial cells (*adenomas*) to their malignant counterparts (adenocarcinomas) (see case study 34). Similarly, they are found in the *blast crisis* of CML, but not in the earlier chronic phase (see case study 29).

Summary

At the beginning of this chapter, oncogenes were described as the genetic material carried by acutely transforming retroviruses that results in malignant transformation of infected cells. It is now clear that oncogenes represent normal cellular genes that function at key points in the transduction of growth signals within cells. They may contribute to the development of a malignant cell if their expression is altered through mutation, amplification or some other mechanism. In contrast, tumour suppressor genes inhibit cell growth and their inactivation can also lead to neoplastic growth. It appears that the development of cancer is a multistep phenomenon and that at least two or more changes in oncogenes or tumour suppressor genes are necessary.

Key points

1 Oncogenes were first identified as the genetic material carried by acutely transforming retroviruses that were responsible for their ability to induce tumours in animals.

2 Subsequently, similar genes were identified in the DNA of normal mammalian cells—these were termed cellular oncogenes (c-*onc*) to distinguish them from viral oncogenes (v-*onc*).

3 In normal cells, cellular oncogenes function to promote cell growth and division. Oncogenes that function at each step of the transduction of growth signals within cells have been identified. In normal cells, the expression of cellular oncogenes is tightly controlled.

4 Malignant cells show changes in oncogene expression. These changes are partly responsible for the subversion of cell growth and division which is characteristic of neoplasia. These changes commonly involve amplification of the oncogene, a point mutation within an oncogene or a chromosome translocation, which involves an oncogene.

5 Virus infection can also affect oncogene expression. Acutely transforming retroviruses carry viral oncogenes, which are often abnormal forms of their cellular counterparts. Once infection occurs, v-*onc* expression by the host cell can lead to the development of malignancy.

6 Slowly transforming retroviruses do not possess oncogenes. They are able to induce tumours by integrating near to cellular oncogenes (insertional mutagenesis). In this position they can upregulate the expression of the cellular oncogene.

7 Tumour suppressor genes suppress cell growth. Usually loss of function of both alleles of a tumour suppressor gene is required to contribute to malignant transformation.

8 The development of a tumour is a multistep process and alterations in the expression of at least two or more oncogenes or tumour suppressor genes are required.

Further reading

Klein G. (1999) The tale of the great cuckoo egg. *Nature* **400**: 6744, 515.

Vogelstein B. & Kinzler K.W. (1999) *The Genetic Basis of Human Cancer*. McGraw Hill, Maidenhead.

Wallis Y.L. & MacDonald F. (1999) Demystified, oncogenes. *Journal of Clinical Pathology: Molecular Pathology* **52**: 55–63.

Tumour Viruses and Human Cancer

The association between virus infection and the development of cancer has been recognized for over 90 years. However, it was not until 1964 that the first human tumour virus, the Epstein–Barr virus (EBV), was isolated from tumour samples of patients with African Burkitt's lymphoma (BL). Subsequently, EBV has been linked to the development of other forms of cancer. In the 36 years since the discovery of EBV other tumour viruses have been identified and their association with a variety of human cancers determined (see Table 23.1). This chapter will consider the major human tumour viruses and review their role in the causation of human cancers.

Tumour virus epidemiology

The development of cancer is an infrequent consequence of viral infection and often occurs many years after any initial infection. Therefore, tumour viruses often infect individuals without adverse effects. For example, approximately 95% of the world's adult population are infected with EBV. The majority of these individuals carry the virus asymptomatically and will not develop cancer as a consequence of EBV infection. Likewise, tumours associated with the human T-lymphotropic virus 1 (HTLV-1) arise infrequently in populations where the virus is endemic. These findings may be explained by the fact that alone tumour viruses are usually insufficient to cause full malignancy. A survey of the epidemiology of non-viral cancers suggests that between four and six independent

causal events are required to induce malignancy (see Chapter 22). Therefore, virus infection probably represents only one of these causal events.

Although virus infection may be linked epidemiologically to a particular cancer type, in order to establish a clear association between the virus and the development of a tumour it is usually necessary to identify the presence of the virus within the tumour cell population.

Immunosurveillance and viral oncogenesis

Virus-associated cancers occur in both immunocompetent and immunodeficient patients. However, the latter group has a particularly high risk for the development of these tumours, suggesting that the immune system plays an important role in preventing the development of virus-associated cancers. There is evidence that CD8+ cytotoxic T cells (CTLs) are particularly important in the recognition and elimination of virus-infected cells (see Chapter 6). CTLs recognize virus-derived peptides that are presented by the infected cell in association with major histocompatibility complex (MHC) class I. The development of virus-associated cancers in immunocompetent individuals suggests that in these individuals the virus-infected tumour cell is able to escape immune recognition.

Tumour viruses

There are a number of different viruses that have been associated with the development of cancer.

Table 23.1 Some oncogenic viruses.

Virus family	Virus	Natural host	Host in which virus is oncogenic	Tumour produced	Oncogenic protein
Adenovirus	Human adenoviruses A, B, D	Humans	Hamster, rat	Various	E1A, E1B
Papovavirus	Polyoma	Mouse	Mouse	Various	Middle T antigen, Large T antigen
	SV40	Monkey	Hamster, rat	Various	Large T antigen
	HPV16, -18	Humans	Humans	Skin cancer, cervical cancer, anal cancer	E6, E7
Herpesvirus	EBV	Humans	Humans	Burkitt's lymphoma Nasopharyngeal carcinoma, Hodgkin's lymphoma	EBNA2, LMP1
Hepadnaviruses	Hepatitis B virus	Humans	Humans	Hepatocellular carcinoma	Hepatitis B x antigen
Retroviridae	HTLV-1	Humans	Humans	Adult T cell leukaemia	Tax

The acutely transforming retroviruses cause cancer in animals but to date none have been associated with the development of human tumours. The following sections consider the important human tumour viruses.

The herpesviruses

The major oncogenic herpesviruses are the EBV and the Kaposi's sarcoma herpesvirus (KSHV).

Epstein–Barr virus

EBV is a double-stranded DNA virus of the γ herpesvirus family. EBV infects the majority of the world's adult population and following primary infection the individual remains a life-long carrier of the virus. In poorly developed countries, primary infection with EBV usually occurs during the first few years of life and is often either asymptomatic or produces only a mild febrile illness. However, in developed populations primary infection is frequently delayed until adolescence or adulthood, in many cases producing the characteristic clinical features of infectious mononucleosis (also known as glandular fever) including sore throat, fever, malaise, lymphadenopathy and mild hepatitis. EBV is often transmitted from one individual to another in saliva and the oropharynx is believed to be both

the primary site of infection and where virus replication occurs. Virus replication in the oropharynx ensures the production of new virions for salivary transfer to other susceptible hosts. Because EBV is transmitted in this way infectious mononucleosis is often referred to as the 'kissing disease'.

EBV infects B lymphocytes, usually by the interaction of the viral envelope glycoproteins, gp350/220, with the CD21 molecule found on B cells, which is the EBV receptor. EBV does not usually replicate in B lymphocytes but instead establishes a latent infection during which no new virions are produced and only a subset of viral genes are expressed. As a consequence of the host immune response, the number of latently infected B lymphocytes in the peripheral blood falls to approximately 1 in 10^6 during the months following primary EBV infection. This low number is maintained in healthy carriers by the continual elimination of proliferating EBV-transformed B lymphocytes by virus-specific CTLs (Fig. 23.1).

Within the host cell the EBV genome usually exists as an extrachromosomal piece of circular DNA, known as an *episome*. During latency only a limited number of viral gene products are made, including six nuclear proteins, referred to as the Epstein–Barr nuclear antigens (EBNA1, -2, -3a, -3b, -3c and EBNA-LP), two proteins found in the cell

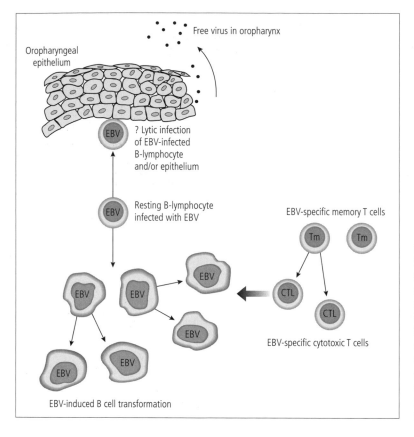

Fig. 23.1 Natural history of EBV infection. EBV is believed to replicate in the oropharynx but the exact site of replication has yet to be determined. Lytic infection of B lymphocytes may be the most likely source of free virus. Resting B lymphocytes infected by EBV may become transformed if they express the full complement of latent viral genes. In this case they may be eliminated by EBV-specific cytotoxic T cells reactivated from EBV-specific memory T cells. Thus, in normal asymptomatic EBV carriers, the potentially harmful effects of EBV are usually subjugated.

Table 23.2 Three forms of viral latency are associated with EBV infection.

Latency	Viral genes expressed
I	EBERs, EBNA1
II	EBERs, EBNA1, LMP1, LMP2A and LMP2B
III	EBERs, EBNA1, EBNA2, EBNA3a, EBNA3b, EBNA3c and EBNA LP, LMP1, LMP2A and LMP2B

membrane of infected cells known as the latent membrane proteins (LMPs), and non-translated RNA molecules known as the Epstein–Barr early RNAs (EBERs). Three forms of viral latency are identifiable dependent upon which combinations of these latent genes are expressed (Table 23.2).

The purpose of the expression of latent genes is to ensure the maintenance of virus infection within the host cell. To this end the coordinated expression of the latent viral genes induces cell proliferation and protects the host cell from apoptosis, e.g. by increasing levels of the antiapoptosis protein, BCL-2 (see Chapter 4). However, the subversion of cell growth induced by the virus may also occasionally lead to the development of malignancy.

Of the latent genes, LMP1 has been shown to be one of the most important for EBV-induced transformation. LMP1 is a transmembrane protein in infected cells and appears to mimic a constitutively activated tumour necrosis factor receptor (TNFR). TNFRs include TNFRI, TNFRII, CD30 and CD40. In normal cells binding of the appropriate ligand to these receptors causes intracellular signalling and a

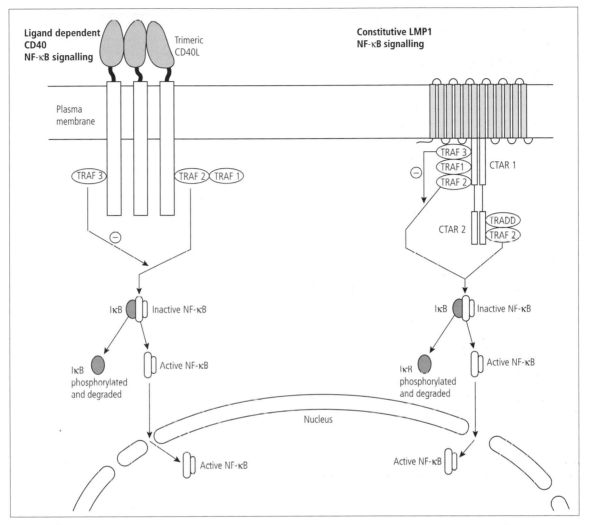

Fig. 23.2 CD40 and the EBV-encoded protein, LMP1, signal via common pathways. CD40 molecules aggregate upon ligation with trimeric CD40 ligand (CD40L). This allows the association of tumour necrosis factor-associated factors (TRAFs) leading to degradation of the inhibitory protein, IκB, release of NF-κB and its nuclear translocation. NF-κB then switches on expression of important genes. In this normal situation signalling only occurs when the appropriate ligand, CD40L, is present. The EBV-encoded LMP1 constitutively aggregates within the plasma membrane. Two regions within the C-terminus, CTAR1 and CTAR2, interact with either TRAFs alone (CTAR1) or TRADD (tumour necrosis factor associated death domain protein)/TRAF2 complexes (CTAR2) causing constitutive activation of NF-κB signalling in the absence of any ligand. The NF-κB signalling pathway is just one example of signalling pathways shared by CD40 and LMP1.

number of effects including either proliferation or apoptosis, depending upon the nature of the signal and the cell type involved. In contrast, LMP1 requires no ligand for its activation and delivers constitutive intracellular signals leading to cell transformation (Fig. 23.2).

The malignant diseases associated with EBV in-

clude BL, nasopharyngeal carcinoma, certain forms of Hodgkin's disease (HD) and a variety of other cancer types. Some of these associations are reviewed below.

Burkitt's lymphoma

BL is an aggressive tumour of B lymphocytes. There

are two main types of BL. The endemic (African) type occurs with high frequency (5–20 cases/ 100 000 children/year) in equatorial Africa and Papua New Guinea and with a distribution that matches that of holoendemic malaria. Almost all cases of endemic BL are EBV positive. Conversely, sporadic BL occurs worldwide with a much lower incidence and only around 15% of cases are EBV positive. A third form of BL occurs in patients with acquired immunodeficiency syndrome (AIDS) and approximately one-third of these tumours harbour EBV.

The cells of EBV-infected BL tumours display a latency 1 phenotype, i.e. they only produce the EBNA1 viral protein and the EBER RNAs (which are not made into protein). Although infected BL tumour cells could potentially process peptides from the EBNA1 protein and present them to specific CTLs, a number of studies have shown EBNA1 is able to inhibit the antigen-processing machinery. Therefore, in practice EBNA1 cannot be recognized by CD8+ CTLs. This, together with the downregulation of MHC class I and adhesion molecules that is a feature of BL cells, contributes to the ability of BL to evade immunodetection. This is a good example of how virus-infected tumour cells are able to survive in the face of an apparently competent immune system.

BL is characterized by reciprocal translocations that result in deregulation of the c-*MYC* gene (see Chapter 22). In endemic BL, EBV-driven proliferation of B lymphocytes, together with a general polyclonal stimulation of B cells induced by malarial infection, is thought to increase the chances of one of these specific translocations occurring in the B lymphocytes that will eventually give rise to BL. BL is one of the fastest growing tumours in humans with a doubling time of around 24 h. However, it responds well to chemotherapy and is often treated successfully using this approach.

Nasopharyngeal carcinoma

Nasopharyngeal carcinoma (NPC) is an epithelial tumour of the nasopharynx that is rare in the West but endemic in China, South-East Asia and North Africa. There are three main types of NPC: undifferentiated, non-keratinizing and squamous NPC.

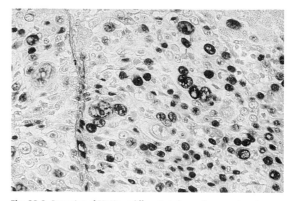

Fig. 23.3 Detection of EBV in undifferentiated nasopharyngeal carcinoma (UNPC). EBV can be detected in the majority of UNPC tumours. Here *in situ* hybridization has been used to detect the EBERs within the nuclei of EBV-infected UNPC tumour cells (see text).

EBV is strongly associated with the undifferentiated type (UNPC) (Fig. 23.3). UNPC is an aggressive tumour that metastasizes early to bone, liver and lung, and to the lymph nodes of the neck. Although the transforming LMP1 gene is expressed in around two-thirds of these tumours, the exact contribution of EBV to the pathogenesis of this tumour is not known. A study involving Chinese and Malays living in Singapore has shown that only the Chinese developed UNPC. This suggests that genetic, cultural or dietary factors (possibly nitrosamines from preserved fish), as well as EBV, are important risk factors for UNPC.

Hodgkin's disease

HD is characterized by relatively low numbers of malignant, so-called Hodgkin–Reed–Sternberg (HRS) cells surrounded by a mass of 'reactive' non-malignant cells (see also case study 31). HD is classified into four major subtypes on the basis of the relative proportions and morphology of the HRS cells, the nature of the reactive component, and the degree of fibrosis. In most cases the malignant HRS cell is derived from germinal centre B lymphocytes.

The frequency of the EBV association in HD is dependent upon a number of factors. EBV is most often associated with the mixed cellularity form and less commonly with the other subtypes. In North America and Europe fewer (20–40%) HD tumours are EBV associated, compared to developing

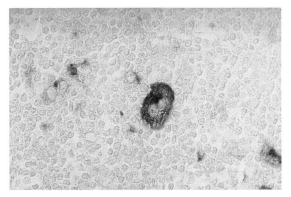

Fig. 23.4 The transforming LMP1 protein is expressed by HRS cells of EBV-associated HD. In all EBV-associated cases of HD the EBV encoded LMP1 protein is highly expressed by the malignant HRS cells. In this slide immunohistochemistry has been used to demonstrate LMP1.

countries where the association approaches 100%. Males also seem to be more at risk than females for EBV-positive HD. In EBV-positive cases the HRS cells express EBNA1, LMP1 (Fig. 23.4) and LMP2 (latency 2 pattern, see Table 23.2). In contrast to EBNA1, epitopes from both LMP1 and LMP2 are effectively processed and presented to CTLs by infected cells. Thus, at least in theory, EBV-infected HRS cells should be recognized by EBV-specific CTLs and eliminated. However, the very fact that these tumours can survive in immunocompetent patients suggests that, like BL, they have evolved some mechanism of immune escape. EBV-infected HRS cells are known to produce excessive quantities of interleukin 10 (IL-10). This cytokine inhibits CTL activity and therefore probably protects the HRS cells from EBV-specific CTL responses that otherwise might destroy them. This inhibitory effect is limited to the tumour itself and is an example of local (intratumour) immunosuppression.

Lymphoproliferative disease in immunosuppressed patients

We have seen examples of how EBV-infected tumour cells are able to evade the immune system in apparently immunocompetent individuals. However, in immunosuppressed patients the lack of EBV-specific CTLs can lead to an increase in the numbers of EBV-infected B lymphocytes. In persist-ent immunosuppressive states, such as in patients immunosuppressed for transplant surgery or with AIDS, these infected B lymphocytes can proliferate to produce tumour-like masses. Later, the acquisition of other genomic changes, such as those that affect *p53*, c-MYC or BCL-*6* (see Chapter 22), can lead to the formation of a classic lymphoma (Fig. 23.5). Therefore, these so-called lymphoproliferative diseases constitute a spectrum of disorders ranging from relatively benign atypical lymphoproliferations which will regress if the immunosuppressive therapy is withdrawn through to highly aggressive lymphomas which do not respond to immune reconstitution (see also case study 12).

Other tumours

EBV is associated with a number of other tumours. For example some T-cell lymphomas, particularly nasal T/natural killer cell lymphomas which are consistently EBV-genome positive. EBV is also associated with some gastric cancers and more recently with smooth muscle tumours that arise in some immunodeficient patients. Thus EBV is apparently able to infect and contribute to neoplastic growth in a number of different cell types.

Kaposi's sarcoma herpesvirus

Kaposi's sarcoma (KS) was originally described in 1872. It is a tumour of endothelial cells that usually presents as a brown/purple skin tumour with more aggressive forms involving the lungs, lymph nodes and gastrointestinal tract. Until the advent of the AIDS epidemic it was a relatively rare disease the aetiology of which remained obscure. KS occurs frequently in human immunodeficiency virus (HIV)-positive individuals, particularly in homosexual/bisexual males. Suspicions that KS might be due to an infectious agent were confirmed when a new human herpesvirus, known as KSHV (also referred to as human herpesvirus 8, HHV8), was discovered in KS tumours from patients with AIDS. In fact, viral sequences are present in all types of KS including KS that arises in HIV-negative individuals. Serological assays to detect antibodies to KSHV were developed and showed a higher prevalence of infection in those groups at high risk for the development of KS. KSHV is also associated

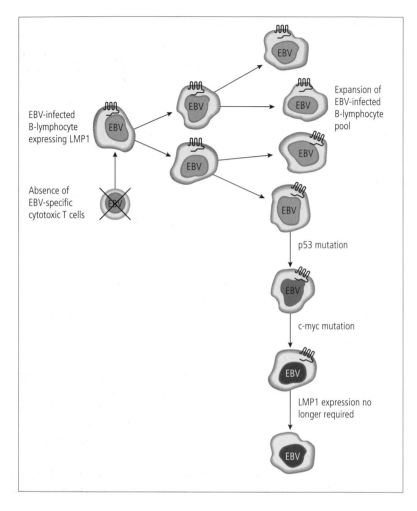

EBV-infected B-lymphocyte expressing LMP1

Expansion of EBV-infected B-lymphocyte pool

Absence of EBV-specific cytotoxic T cells

p53 mutation

c-myc mutation

LMP1 expression no longer required

Fig. 23.5 The development of post-transplant lymphoproliferative disease. The lack of EBV-specific CTLs in immunosuppressed patients leads to expansion of the EBV-infected B lymphocytes which are shown here expressing LMP1. The LMP1 protein (see text) drives the transformation of these cells. In persistent immunosuppressive states, such as in organ transplant recipients these EBV-positive B lymphocytes can produce tumour-like masses. Immune reconstitution at this stage may sometimes result in tumour regression. Later, the acquisition of other genetic changes in these cells, e.g. in the *p53* and c-*MYC* genes, provides further stimulation of cell proliferation. At this stage the tumour represents a classic lymphoma and will not regress following immune reconstitution. LMP1 expression is no longer required for cell proliferation and may be switched off.

with pleural effusion lymphomas and a rare lymphoproliferative disease known as multicentric Castleman's disease.

KSHV is a double-stranded DNA virus that is closely related to EBV. The genome contains 81 potential coding regions known as open reading frames (ORFs), some of which show homology to known human genes. A number of these genes are expressed in KSHV-associated tumours. For example, KSHV encodes a cyclin D gene (v-cyclin D) which activates cyclin-dependent kinase 6 (CDK6). The active protein kinase then phosphorylates Rb and releases the cell from G1 arrest (see Chapter 4). An IL-6 homologue (vIL-6) encoded by the virus in infected cells may contribute to autocrine growth in KSHV-associated tumours (Fig. 23.6). Similarly a viral homologue of bcl-2 is also produced in KSHV-infected cells. This homologue known as v-bcl-2 may, like cellular bcl-2 (see Chapter 4), protect infected cells from apoptosis. KSHV ORF74 encodes a protein with homology to the human IL-8 receptor; a member of the G-protein coupled receptor family (see Chapter 22). These proteins activate the phosphatidylinositol signal transduction pathway. The KSHV homologue is able constitutively to activate this pathway leading to continuous cell division.

Some of the important KSHV proteins are outlined in Table 23.3. The exact contribution of each of these in KSHV-associated lesions remains to be established.

The papovaviruses

The papovavirus family includes the polyoma and papillomaviruses. The polyoma group include the polyoma virus, simian virus 40 (SV40), and the human polyomaviruses, BK and JC. With the exception of the polyomavirus, these viruses do not cause cancer in their natural hosts but do induce tumours in newborn animals, including hamsters and rats. Proteins produced by each of these viruses interact with host-derived proteins to bring about transformation. The so-called large T antigen (tumour antigen), a protein produced by SV40, is able to bind to and inactivate Rb and p53 proteins. The large T antigen produced by polyomavirus can bind Rb protein, but not p53. The src protein (see Chapter 22) activates other proteins by phosphorylating their tyrosine component (tyrosine kinase activity). By complexing to src protein, polyoma middle T antigen enhances this tyrosine kinase activity.

Human papillomaviruses

Human papilloma viruses (HPVs) are small DNA viruses that commonly infect epithelial tissues. There are over 70 subtypes of HPV and the majority are responsible for benign lesions of the genital, upper respiratory and digestive tracts. However, some HPV subtypes are associated with malignant diseases including skin and cervical cancer.

Skin cancer

Cutaneous HPV infection normally results in the

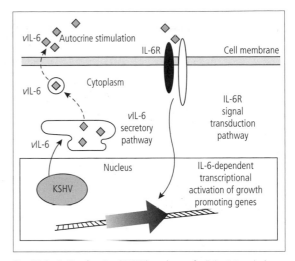

Fig. 23.6 vIL-6 is a functional KSHV homologue of cellular IL-6 and when secreted may potentially act on IL-6 receptors (II-6R) expressed on the same cell. In this way secretion of IL-6 may contribute to autocrine growth of KSHV-infected cells. From M.L. Gillison & R.F. Ambinder (1997) Human herpesvirus-8. *Current Opinion in Oncology* **9**: 440–449.

appearance of benign warts, however, in the rare but life-long skin disease epidermodysplasia verruciformis (EV) these multiple benign warts can convert to malignant squamous carcinoma when exposed to ultraviolet (UV) light. The tumour cells often contain HPV5 or -8. These two HPVs are also associated with the type of skin carcinoma observed in long-term immunosuppressed renal transplant patients.

Cervical cancer

The majority of cervical cancers are HPV positive. HPV may be sexually transmitted and the associ-

Table 23.3 KSHV encodes many homologues of cellular proteins, some of these viral proteins and their effects upon the infected cell are summarized.

Cellular gene	KSHV gene	Effect of virus gene expression
Cyclin gene	v-*cyclin D*	Phosphorylates Rb and releases cell from cell cycle arrest
IL-6	v*IL-6*	Autocrine stimulation of cell growth
IL-8R	v*GPCR*	Constitutive activation of phosphatidylinositol pathway leading to cell division
FLICE inhibitor protein (*FLIP*)	v*FLIP*	Inhibits CD95-mediated apoptosis
IRF	v*IRF*	Inhibits interferon-β signal transduction
Bcl-2	v*Bcl-2*	Protects infected cell from apoptosis

ation of HPV with cervical cancer explains many of the risk factors for this disease including early age at first sexual encounter and multiple sexual partners. HPV subtypes 16 and 18 are most commonly associated with cervical cancer and in these cases the virus often integrates into the host cell DNA. HPV16 DNA is also commonly detected in cancers of the vulva, vagina, anus and penis. Although anal cancer is predominantly a female tumour, the incidence of this disease is increasing in both sexes, particularly amongst homosexual males. Individuals with one type of anogenital cancer also have an increased risk of developing others. An increased incidence of HPV-positive tumours, including cervical cancer, is observed under conditions of immunosuppression, e.g. in HIV infection (see case study 4).

Two HPV proteins appear to be particularly important for oncogenesis and these are the E6 and E7 proteins. E6 binds to and inhibits p53, a tumour suppressor protein whose activity is essential to prevent the transmission of mutations during cell division (see Chapter 4). Mutations of the *p53* gene are not generally seen in HPV-positive cervical tumours, further supporting the role of E6 as an inactivator of p53 at the protein level. The E6 produced by low risk HPVs binds to *p53* less efficiently than that from high-risk HPVs. E7 protein binds to phosphorylated Rb protein preventing it from blocking the cell cycle and hence allowing cells to enter the S phase (see Chapter 4). E7 proteins from the high- and low-risk HPV groups also show different binding affinities for Rb.

The hepadnaviruses

Hepatitis B virus

The hepatitis B virus (HBV) is associated with the development of hepatocellular carcinoma (HCC) where integrated HBV DNA can be detected in the tumours. The exact role of HBV in the development of HCC is yet to be established. However, there is evidence that the HBV X protein may be important. The X protein seems to induce a number of cellular changes that contribute to transformation, including the activation of several intracellular

signalling pathways, including NF-κB (see Fig. 23.2).

Other factors in addition to HBV status contribute to the risk of developing HCC and these include smoking, dietary components such as aflatoxin (see Chapter 21) and exposure to other hepatotoxic agents. Hepatitis C virus is also associated with the development of HCC.

The retroviridae

Acutely transforming and slowly transforming viruses are described in Chapter 22 in relation to the development of cancers in animals. HTLV-1 is the only retrovirus that has been directly associated with the development of human cancer.

The human T-lymphotropic virus 1

HTLV-1 is a retrovirus that infects CD4-positive T lymphocytes and is associated with the development of adult T-cell leukaemia/lymphoma (ATLL).

The transforming functions of HTLV-1 have mainly been assigned to one protein, Tax. Tax is a 42-kDa nuclear phosphoprotein that initiates transcription of cellular genes by activating various transcription factors that are important for cell division, e.g. NF-κB (see Fig. 23.2). NF-κB activates genes which are potentially important for cellular transformation, e.g. granulocyte–macrophage colony-stimulating factor (GM-CSF), tumour necrosis factor β and the receptor for IL-2 (IL-2Rα). Tax functions by binding inhibitors of NF-κB resulting in dissociation of the inhibitor–NF-κB complex and nuclear translocation of NF-κB (see Fig. 23.2).

HTLV-1 is thought to initiate clonal expansion of CD4+ T lymphocytes which is later followed by the acquisition of other genomic changes in these cells leading to the development of ATLL.

Summary

In most cases viruses produce at least one transforming protein which contributes to the subversion of cellular growth. In addition, many virus-infected tumour cells are able to evade immune detection. These mechanisms of growth subversion and immune evasion are increasingly well understood and should contribute to the development of novel therapies for virus-associated tumours.

Further reading

Arrand J.R. & Harper D.R. (eds) (1998) *Viruses and Human Cancer*. Bios Scientific, Oxford.

Fields B.N., Knipe D.M. & Howley P.M. (eds) (1996) *Virology*. Lippincott–Raven, Philadelphia.

McCance D.J. (ed.) (1998) *Human Tumor Viruses*. American Society for Microbiology, Washington DC.

Key points

1 Most transforming viruses are ubiquitous within human populations. However, only a fraction of infected individuals develop a virus-associated malignancy. This is explained by the fact that virus infection accounts for only one of the genetic events required for full transformation.

2 Virus-associated cancers are more common in immunodeficient patients. There is evidence that CD8+ cytotoxic T lymphocytes are important for eliminating virus-infected cells.

3 Virus-associated cancers also occur in immunocompetent patients. In these situations the virus-infected tumour cells have developed immune evasion strategies.

4 Most tumour viruses encode at least one protein which is responsible for the subversion of cell growth.

Cancer: Invasion and Metastasis

Previous chapters have described the process of cellular transformation that results in neoplasia. This transformation process is caused by genetic mutations that cause inappropriate protein expression, resulting in the loss of tight mitogenic regulation that exists in non-transformed cells. If the mutations result in neoplasms that grow in a defined restricted space the tumour is defined as benign. These types of growth are rarely life threatening except in the cases where the growth compresses vessels or ducts obstructing fluid flow or when it occurs in a confined space such as the skull, again causing compression. However, since mutations occur most frequently during DNA replication the continuation of cell division seen in neoplastic cells means that such cells are more likely to accumulate genetic mutations. Furthermore, as described in Chapter 22, loss of function of the product of the tumour suppressor gene *p53*, is the most common mutation in human cancers. Loss of *p53* activity results in an increased frequency of cells with genetic mutations and chromosomal translocations surviving to divide. These combined effects contribute to the observation that tumour cells have a higher frequency of somatic mutations than non-transformed cells. If, by chance, these mutations or translocations result in the production of aberrant proteins or proteins with modified activity the affected cell may acquire novel properties regulated by these proteins. Should these acquired properties allow the cells to break away from the tumour and invade into the surrounding tissue (this process is termed *invasion*) or to escape entirely from the bounded confines of the tumour and spread to distant sites in the body (*metastasis*) the tumour is termed malignant (Fig. 24.1). This chapter outlines some of the important factors involved in the spread of malignant (cancer) cells.

Micrometastasis and dormancy

Cancers are thought to shed a large number of cells from the main tumour mass, many of which are not capable of setting up a secondary metastatic tumour. Some are carried along in groups with other cells or are released aberrantly as a result of the turnover of the tissue architecture during the rapid growth of the tumour. Only very few of the released cells evade immune surveillance, attach to a vessel wall and escape into a new tissue compartment (Fig. 24.2). Having done so the metastatic tumour cell must associate itself with a blood vessel to survive. All cells in the body have to maintain relatively close contact with the vascular compartment in order to allow rapid gaseous exchange, nutrient uptake and waste removal. Metastatic cells manage this by migrating to blood vessels and then growing as a micrometastasis limited to a few cells deep around the vessel. This micrometastasis can remain 'dormant' for many years. In this case dormant means that the cell number stays relatively constant. However, the cells are dividing at a rate comparable to the primary tumour and the reason why the cell number stays relatively constant is that programmed cell death (apoptosis, see Chapter 4) occurs at a very similar rate to cell division. After a

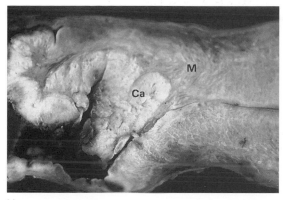

(a)

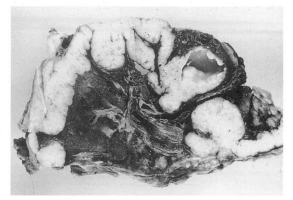

(b)

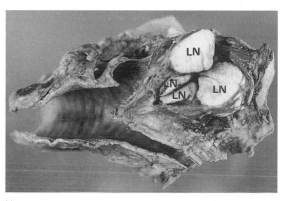

(c)

Fig. 24.1 Examples of cancer invasion and metastasis: (a) local invasion of cervical carcinoma (Ca) upwards from the cervix into the deep tissues of the myometrium (M); (b) local invasion of malignant mesothelioma from pleural cavity into the lungs, much of the normal lung tissue is replaced by pale tumour. (c) Two bisected lymph nodes (LN) beneath the bronchi. Both lymph nodes have been replaced by pale tumour from a nearby bronchogenic carcinoma. This is an example of metastatic spread to lymph nodes. (d) Chest radiograph showing at least two well-defined metastatic deposits within the lungs (MD), the original primary tumour was a malignant smooth muscle tumour (leiomyosarcoma) of the uterus.

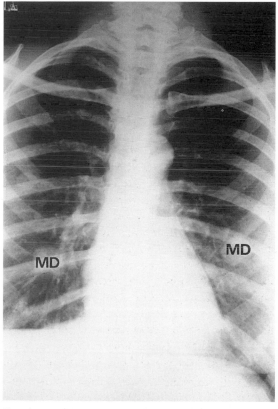

(d)

variable period of dormancy the micrometastasis may develop its own blood supply. Vascular endothelial growth factor (VEGF) and fibroblast growth factor (FGF) mediate this angiogenic event. It is not known what causes the release of these growth factors but it is clear that following the ensuing generation of new blood vessels that tumours can grow in size. The cells are thought to divide at the same rate in the growing tumour as in the dormant micrometastasis. The increased blood supply results in a decrease in apoptosis such that cell death no longer occurs at an equivalent rate to cell division, resulting in an increase in cell number and tumour mass. This concept is very important to our understanding of cancer since the recurrence of disease months or years after the initial tumour has been

215

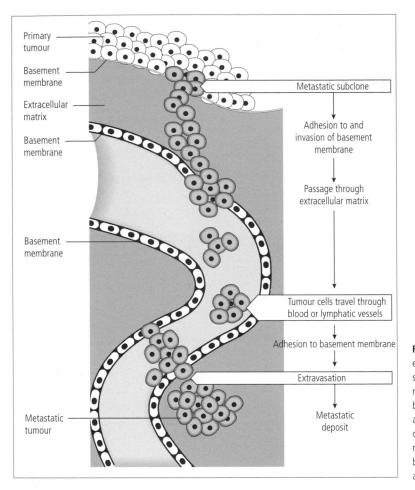

Primary tumour

Basement membrane

Extracellular matrix

Basement membrane

Basement membrane

Metastatic tumour

Metastatic subclone

Adhesion to and invasion of basement membrane

Passage through extracellular matrix

Tumour cells travel through blood or lymphatic vessels

Adhesion to basement membrane

Extravasation

Metastatic deposit

Fig. 24.2 Steps in the metastasis of a typical epithelial cancer (carcinoma). A metastatic subclone develops within the primary tumour mass. Metastatic tumour cells eventually breach the underlying basement membrane and enter connective tissues. In order to complete the metastatic process they must move through the connective tissue, enter blood or lymphatic vessels, leave the vessel and grow within a distant tissue.

successfully treated is one of the most distressing aspects for patients suffering from this disease.

As outlined above, cells must escape from their tissue of origin and migrate to a vessel in order to disseminate around the body. Some cells are able to migrate from one body compartment to another because they normally express the proteins required to do so. For example, lymphomas (tumours derived from lymphocytes) frequently spread to other lymphoid tissues. Normal lymphocytes must be able to respond to the presence of an antigen in the tissues. Consequently, lymphocytes possess receptors that enable them to 'home' to particular tissues (see Chapter 6). Thus, the spreading of lymphomas is in part due to normal tissue specificities. In fact there

is tissue specificity in the metastatic process and experiments have shown that tumours contain cells capable of metastasizing to distinct tissues (Fig. 24.3).

However, the majority of cells are not able to circulate in the same way as lymphocytes, since they are bound to each other and to the extracellular matrix (ECM). Thus, the tissue architecture and the basement membrane that surrounds cells effectively acts as a barrier to cell movement. Also cell motility is usually a tightly regulated process organized by members of the Rho family of guanosine triphosphate (GTP)-binding proteins (see Chapter 22) and in order to move out of a tissue the cell may need to overcome this tight regulation. Clearly then, transformation is associated with the modi-

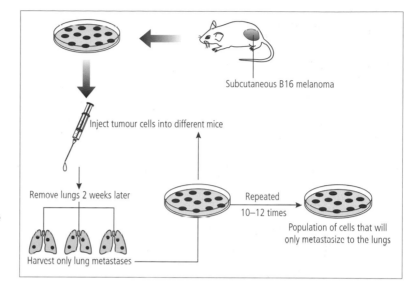

Fig. 24.3 Experiments showing that there are site-specific metastatic subclones within tumours. Subcutaneous B16 melanoma cells harvested from a single tumour will generate further tumours in mice after injection. These tumours will produce metastatic deposits in a variety of tissues, including the lungs. Only the lung metastases are harvested and reinjected into further mice. If this is repeated a number of times, a population of cells will be obtained that will only metastasize to the lungs.

fication of several highly regulated cellular processes (detachment, motility and degradation of barriers) that facilitate the migration of normally non-motile cells.

The importance of the stroma

Tumours can be crudely considered to consist of two distinct cell types, the transformed cancerous cells and the stromal cells (e.g. endothelial cells and fibroblasts) that form the supporting matrix. The stroma can constitute up to 90% of the tumour mass in some cancers, and supplies the nutrients and oxygen, and removes metabolic waste products by providing the tumour with a blood supply. As tumour size is restricted by the extent of vascularization of the tumour the process of new blood vessel production (*angiogenesis*) is closely associated with cancer-related fatality. Angiogenesis requires endothelial cells to divide and to form blood vessels within tissues. In a manner analogous to the migration of malignant cells, this process is restricted by the barrier effect of the ECM and stromal cells. Angiogenesis therefore requires remodelling of the ECM. It is thought that the physiological process of angiogenesis and migration/metastasis of tumour cells are closely related events.

Matrix metalloproteinases

The ECM is largely made of proteins secreted by cells that act as the supporting infrastructure of an organ. The cells of an organ associate with the collagens, laminin and other fibrous proteins that constitute the ECM and in this way the ECM acts as the scaffolding that holds tissues together. Remodelling of the ECM as an organ grows is a normal and necessary process. Members of a group of proteinases termed matrix metalloproteinases (MMPs) carry out this physiological role. The metalloproteinase family has some 200 members of which less than 10% are MMPs. Within tumours, the expression of MMPs that contributes to remodelling of the ECM may not be a feature of the tumour cell population, but rather occurs in the stromal fibroblasts. Tumour cells can, and sometimes do, produce and secrete MMPs themselves but this only tends to occur in the very advanced stages of a tumour. The destruction of the ECM requires the concerted action of several MMPs as each MMP only degrades specific substrates. This is important because secretion of MMPs by tumour cells is usually restricted to one or two types of enzyme but fibroblasts tend to secrete a wider variety of MMPs. Again this emphasizes the role of the stromal fibroblasts in the progression of neoplasia.

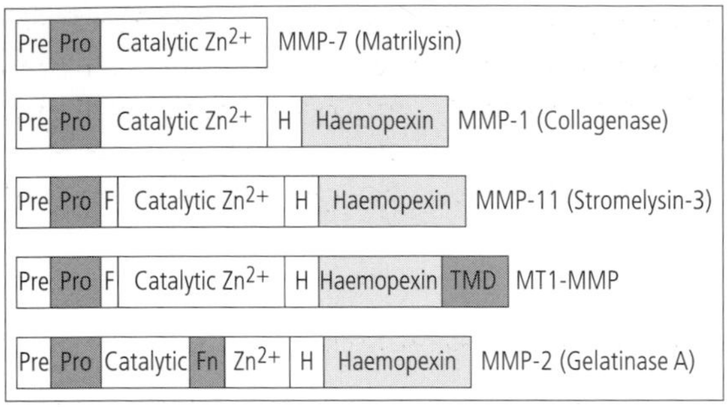

Fig. 24.4 Examples of the domain structures of some matrix metalloproteinases. Abbreviations: F, furin cleavage site; Fn, fibronectin recognition site; H, hinge region; TMD, transmembrane domain. The roles of the various domains are outlined in the text.

The primary sequences (amino acid sequences) of the MMP family members are quite similar and share significant homology within certain domains. Fig. 24.4 shows the domain structure of some MMP family members. An MMP containing all the possible domains has never been detected but matrilysin (MMP-7) contains the minimal three domains required for MMP activity. The domains and a brief description of their functions are given below.

Pre-domain

This is a sequence that is found at the N-terminus (amino terminus) of many proteins that are destined for secretion from the cell. Typically, this sequence is termed the 'signal peptide' and is 17–20 amino acids in length and contains a high proportion of hydrophobic residues. As the polypeptide chain is translated the signal peptide acts as a signal for the protein to be taken up into the lumen of the endoplasmic reticulum (ER). Once inside the ER, the signal peptide is cleaved by an endopeptidase and the cell processes the remaining sequence for secretion.

Pro-domain

The pro-domain follows the pre-domain in the newly synthesized MMPs and following cleavage of the pre-domain the pro-domain is found at the N-terminus of the secreted protein. This domain is about 80 amino acids long and has an important role in regulating the activity of the enzyme. A

highly conserved cysteine residue located in the C-terminal region of the pro-domain binds to the active site zinc molecule rendering the active site inaccessible resulting in the MMP being maintained in an inactive state. Activation occurs by releasing the binding of the zinc molecule to the cysteine by either cleavage of the pro-domain from the MMP by a protease or displacement of the zinc from the cysteine by organomercurials. This activation process is thought to be important in the regulation of MMP activity *in vivo* and is discussed below.

Catalytic domain

The catalytic domain is approximately 160–170 amino acids in length. Located within the C-terminal portion of the catalytic domain is a highly conserved sequence containing three histidine residues that ligate the active site zinc (the cysteine residue found in the pro-domain makes the fourth bond).

Other domains found in various MMPs are listed below (and see Fig. 24.4). MMPs can clearly display activity without these sequences but they appear to have roles in the regulation of the MMP activity and others confer specific properties on the proteases.

Haemopexin domain

The haemopexin domain, which is found in every MMP except MMP-7, is approximately 200 amino acids long and, with the exception of the membrane-spanning region of the membrane-type MMPs, is located at the C-terminus of the molecule. This sequence has homology to the heme-binding protein, haemopexin (and vitronectin, a component of the ECM). The function of the haemopexin domain appears to vary from protease to protease. For example, substrate recognition by the MMP-3 and -10 require the haemopexin domain, as does the activation of MMP-2 by membrane-type MMPs (MT-MMP; see below).

Hinge region

The hinge is a highly variable region that often contains several proline residues located between the catalytic and haemopexin domains.

Transmembrane domain

The MT-MMPs have a C-terminal extension of about 80–110 amino acids that anchors the protein to the membrane. This localization is thought to be important since the MT-MMPs play a role in activating other MMPs (e.g. MMP-2) at the surface of cells (see below).

Furin cleavage site

This eight amino acid conserved sequence located at the C-terminal end of the propeptide domain of the MT-MMPs and MMP-11 (stromelysin-3) is a consensus site for cleavage by a group of endoproteases. One protease implicated in this process is furin, a protease involved in the secretory pathway of cells. It is possible that this domain is important in the intracellular activation of MT-MMPs. In this way the fully processed form of the protease can be produced and tethered to the surface of cells by the transmembrane domain.

Activation of MMPs

MMPs are secreted as inactive zymogens. The *in vivo* activation process is mediated by cleavage of the pro-domain which releases zinc from a cysteine residue allowing it to take part in the catalytic mechanism. This means that the MMPs are themselves activated by proteases, some of which could also be other MMPs. It is possible that cascades of protease activation exist resulting in the key MMPs being switched on, allowing the metastatic process to progress.

This activation process is not a simple matter of cleaving the pro-domain. The initial cleavage of a portion of the pro-domain results in a partial activation of the MMP, which then removes the remainder of the pro-domain generating the fully processed, activated protein. Plasmin initiates this series of events for several MMPs.

Proteolytic activation of MMP-2 is carried out by MT-MMP. This process requires the participation of the endogenous MMP regulator, tissue inhibitor of metalloproteinase-2 (TIMP-2). The TIMPs are proteins that regulate MMP activity and were originally

discovered as endogenous inhibitors of MMPs. However, their role is more complicated than merely to inhibit MMP activity. For example, the activation of MMP-2 requires the formation of a trimeric complex of MT-MMP, TIMP-2 and pro-MMP-2 on the cell surface.

Cell adhesion and movement

Cells within a tissue are normally attached to neighbouring cells and the surrounding matrix by specific adhesion molecules. A decreased ability of malignant cells to adhere to each other and the ECM may facilitate the detachment of cells from the primary tumour and their subsequent spread. Some of the specific proteins that have been implicated in this process are discussed below.

E-cadherin

This molecule is a glycoprotein found on the surface of epithelial cells that mediates a Ca^{2+}-dependent cell-to-cell adhesion. Experiments with cell lines and animal tumours suggest that downregulation of E-cadherin expression is associated with loss of differentiation and a more invasive phenotype. Analysis of tumour cell lines has established an association between loss of E-cadherin expression, acquisition of a fibroblast-like morphology and an ability to invade collagen gels.

A number of studies on human carcinomas have demonstrated an inverse correlation between E-cadherin expression and both differentiation status and invasiveness (e.g. in breast carcinoma and head and neck squamous cell carcinoma). Thus, the downregulation of E-cadherin expression appears to correlate with the grade and histological type of a tumour and may have prognostic significance.

Integrins and CD44

Other aspects of cell adhesion may also influence the invasion and metastasis of tumour cells. Integrins (see Chapters 4 and 5) have a central role in mediating the interactions of cells with the ECM. *In vitro* evidence suggests that increased expression of certain integrins can facilitate metastasis presumably by enhancing the ability of tumour cells to adhere to certain substrates. Whilst upregulation of integrins is not an inevitable consequence of tumour progression, increased levels of certain integrins have been observed in some tumours (e.g. melanoma). Many aspects of tumour metastasis resemble the normal trafficking and migration of lymphocytes. Thus, molecules involved in the adhesion of lymphocytes to endothelial cells may have a role in tumour cell adhesion and also in the organ-specific patterns of metastasis.

CD44 is a lymphocyte-homing molecule that mediates binding to specialized lymph node endothelium. Work on rodent tumours originally identified a variant form of CD44, generated by differential mRNA splicing, which appeared to metastasize. The expression of variant CD44 isoforms by human tumours, such as breast and colon carcinomas, may increase the metastatic potential of these malignancies.

Scatter factor

The movement of cells can be stimulated by a variety of factors which may also influence the invasion and spread of tumours. These factors include the so-called motogenic cytokines such as autocrine motility factor, migration-stimulating factor and scatter factor (SF). SF is of particular interest as it induces de-differentiation and increased motility of epithelial cells. SF has been shown to be identical to hepatocyte growth factor which is a potent mitogen for many normal cells including keratinocytes, melanocytes and endothelial cells. *In vitro* experiments have shown that SF can induce the progression of epithelial cells to a more motile and invasive phenotype. SF is produced by fibroblasts and exerts in its effects on target cells by interacting with a specific receptor which has been identified as a transmembrane tyrosine kinase encoded by the c-*MET* oncogene. Thus the process of cell movement in tumour cells is linked with a known oncogene.

Genetic basis of metastasis

Most tumours are not homogenous cell populations but are composed of subpopulations of cells with differing properties. This phenomenon is referred to as tumour heterogeneity and is the result of somatic mutations occurring within tumour cells. Thus, a given tumour will contain subpopulations of cells which vary in their level of antigen expression, their degree of differentiation or some other characteristic. Likewise, tumours contain clones of cells with varying propensities for metastatic spread. Experiments also show that there are subpopulations of tumour cells within a primary tumour that have tissue-specific metastatic potential (Fig. 24.3).

That metastatic potential is derived and enhanced by progressive somatic mutations occurring within tumour cells has prompted the search for gene products involved in metastasis. Much of this work has relied on comparisons of metastatic variants derived from primary tumour cells. In this way the *nm23* gene, a potential metastasis suppressor gene, was discovered.

The *nm23* gene was identified on the basis of its reduced expression at the mRNA level in highly metastatic variants of a single murine melanoma. Loss of *nm23* expression correlates with poor survival in breast cancer while good prognosis is associated with increased expression. The *nm23* gene product is homologous with the abnormal wing disc (*awd*) gene of the fruit fly *Drosophila* that is involved in the postmetamorphosis development and differentiation of multiple tissues. A role for *nm23* in the signal transduction pathways responsible for cell-cell communication has been suggested and may explain why loss of *nm23* expression is associated with aberrant development or tumour progression.

Clues as to the proactive function of *nm23* came from the demonstration that cDNAs for nucleotide diphosphate (NDP) kinases, isolated from different species, encoded proteins that were highly homologous to the *nm23/awd* genes. Indeed, the *awd* gene product can function as an NDP kinase. The role of NDP kinases in microtubule assembly/disassembly and in G protein coupled signal transduction may

Key points

1 Local spread by tumour cells and their ability to spread to distant sites (metastasis) are the hallmarks of malignancy.
2 Metastasis is mediated by a number of key proteins. Some of these are enzymes important in the degradation of the ECM. These include proteases known as MMPs.
3 Angiogenesis (the formation of new blood vessels) is an integral part of tumour progression and is necessary for tumours to grow to a large size.
4 The stromal cells as well as the tumour cells are responsible for the production of angiogenic and prometastatic factors.

explain the function of *nm23* in metastasis. In particular it is likely that aberrant NDP kinase activity may affect the cell adhesion and motility pathways which are critically important in the metastatic process.

Summary

Knowledge of the complex processes of tumour invasion, metastasis and angiogenesis are critical to an understanding of why tumours are so often lethal. In fact, various inhibitors of these processes are in clinical trials. Consequently, there is much promise that successful therapies will emerge that target angiogenesis and metastasis.

Further reading

Michiels F. & Collard J.G. (1999) Rho-like GTPases: their role in cell adhesion and invasion. *Biochemical Society Symposium* **65**: 125–146.

Nelson A.R., Fingleton B., Rothenberg M.L. & Matrisian L.M. (2000) Matrix metalloproteinases: biologic activity and clinical implications. *Journal of Clinical Oncology* **18**: 1135–1149.

Westermarck J. & Kahari V.M. (1999) Regulation of matrix metalloproteinase expression in tumor invasion. *FASEB Journal* **13**: 781–792.

Case Studies

Neurotic symptoms following a road traffic accident

Clinical features

A 25-year-old woman complained of an inability to drive or travel by car, lack of concentration and distressing palpitations of the heart. A cardiologist had reassured her that nothing was wrong with her heart, and she had been told to 'pull herself together'.

The symptoms dated back 6 months, to when she had been injured in a car crash due to a tractor being carelessly driven out in front of her. Her head had impacted against the steering wheel and she was briefly knocked out; on recovering consciousness she had been terrified to discover that she was trapped in the wreck. On admission to hospital she was noted to have lost her memory for the first few minutes after impact (*post-traumatic amnesia*). A skull radiograph and neurological examination were normal, and she was discharged home the next day.

Two weeks after the car accident the family doctor was summoned as she had apparently become totally paralysed. Neurological examination was again completely normal and the family doctor diagnosed a 'hysterical reaction', noting that she was suing the tractor driver for compensation. Although the paralysis responded to strong reassurance, over the next few weeks other non-specific symptoms took its place. She complained of dizziness, short-temperedness and headaches (*post-concussional syndrome*). She was constantly tense (*generalized anxiety*). Attempting to drive made the anxiety worse, and at the sight of tractors she would panic, her heart thumping uncontrollably (*phobic anxiety*).

The patient had always been a worrier, although at the same time this had made her a cautious driver with an excellent safety record. It was noted that 2 years previously she had been very upset when a friend had been permanently paralysed by a spinal injury.

Further enquiry disclosed that she came from a family of high achievers, some of whom had a personality trait towards anxiety. Her brother, a company director, had developed hypertension which was successfully treated by β-blockers.

Investigations

Physical examination revealed a pale, tense woman with *tachycardia* (an elevated heart rate, usually defined as greater than 100 b.p.m.), who was hyperventilating and tremulous. Blood pressure was normal at 120 mm systolic, 82 mm diastolic. Results of laboratory investigations are shown in Table CS1.1.

Blood film examination showed a normal white cell differential count. Erythrocyte morphology revealed some microcytic hypochromic cells. This finding usually indicates early iron deficiency anaemia, but in patients of Asian or Mediterranean origin could also indicate a thalassaemia syndrome (see Chapter 14). Thyroid function tests and gammaglutamyl transferase concentration were normal.

Table CS1.1 Blood investigations.

Analyte	Value	Reference range
Total white cell count	7.45×10^9/L	4.0–11.0
Red cell count	4.26×10^{12}/L	3.8–5.8
Haemoglobin	11.2 g/dL	11.5–16.5
Haematocrit	0.338	0.37–0.47
Mean cell volume	79.5 fl	82–92
Mean cell haemoglobin	26.29 pg	27.0–32.0
Platelet count	260×10^9/L	150–400
Erythrocyte sedimentation rate	12 mm/h	0–20
Serum gammaglutamyl transferase	15 U/L	7–32
Free thyroxine	12.2 pmol/L	9.0–24.0
Thyroid-stimulating hormone	2.3 mU/L	0.4–4.0

Diagnosis

Anxiety neurosis with postconcussional syndrome.

Discussion

Unlike symptoms of physical disease, there is an unfortunate tendency for neurotic symptoms to be held to be the fault of the sufferers, who are told to 'pull themselves together'. This attitude is only partly based on prejudice, as even modern enlightened treatments presume that neurotics are capable of taking some responsibility for their difficulties, and tend to emphasize self-help and self-understanding.

Hysteria provides an example of symptoms mimicking organic disease, which on closer examination turn out to correspond to the patient's ideas or fears about what is wrong with him or her, rather than the actual physical pathology. Such fears may be suggested to the patient, in this case by her friend's injury. There is often an element of 'secondary gain', in the form of extra attention and sympathy, the avoidance of an intolerable situation or (as here) financial compensation. However, it is characteristic that the hysteric, in contrast to the malingerer, is completely unaware of such motives.

These concepts, expounded by Freud at the turn of the twentieth century, have coloured our understanding of neurosis and delayed the appreciation of the biological aspects. In the case of closed head injury, sophisticated methods of brain imaging (applied to boxers, for example), have demonstrated significant structural damage to the brain from relatively minor blows. Such diffuse damage may be insufficient to produce gross neurological signs, but may be manifest in the more sensitive area of emotional change. Here it probably contributed to the patient's postconcussional syndrome, and may have increased her vulnerability to develop a hysterical reaction. Another determinant of this reaction may have been her friend's injury. The glib assumption of financial compensation as the main cause should be viewed with caution, however.

The aetiology of this case is a typical combination of *heredity* (her worrying disposition) and *environment* (the accident). Genetic factors play a more prominent role than once assumed; note that they are expressed in her relatives as a beneficially high drive towards success, as well as a tendency towards hypertension.

Anxiety symptoms have *psychological* (fear, apprehension) and *physical* (tremor, tachycardia) aspects. Treatment should reflect this dual nature.

Treatment and prognosis

The patient was reassured that her postconcussional symptoms had a definite physical explanation and were not 'all in her imagination'. Her current difficulties in concentration, however, were caused by anxiety and not permanent brain damage, as she feared. Mild iron deficiency anaemia, which was confirmed by estimation of serum ferritin, is quite common in females of this age group (see Chapter 14), and was thought to be an incidental finding. This was treated with oral iron preparations.

Once it was explained to the patient that hyperventilation was worsening her anxiety, she felt more confident that she could overcome her symptoms by breathing control exercises. Instruction in relaxation techniques enabled her to contemplate tractors whilst remaining calm (*desensitization*). Prescription of the β-blocker propranolol, also helped considerably, by preventing the sympathetic overstimulation which had been causing her tremor and cardiac palpitations. Throughout, she was encouraged to practise driving rather than avoiding it (*exposure therapy*). After

4 months she was driving confidently again but it was some years before she was entirely comfortable as a passenger.

Neurotic symptoms following trauma were highlighted during both world wars (shell shock, battle fatigue). These days they are often labelled as *post-traumatic stress disorder*, and frequently feature in litigation following public disasters (e.g. Hillsborough Stadium, Kings Cross fire or the Mont Blanc tunnel disaster), as well as in personal injury claims.

This case illustrates the complex interplay between biological and psychological factors which makes the evaluation of neurosis so fascinating, and so controversial. Symptoms which appear explicable in psychological terms may also have a subtle biological basis.

Questions

1 Why were haematological investigations and thyroid function tests performed on this patient?
2 Why were gammaglutamyl transferase (γ-GT) levels measured?

Answers on p. 302.

CASE STUDY 2

Depressive illness in pregnancy

Clinical features

A 23-year-old woman was referred for a psychiatric opinion when 30 weeks pregnant. She was suffering from the typical features of a severe depressive illness (see Chapter 2), including agitation and insomnia. She ruminated for most of the day and well into the night on a number of morbid ideas. The most distressing of these was that she had wanted members of her family killed to attract attention to herself.

The patient had a history of depression. She had previously been prescribed fluoxetine, a specific presynaptic 5-hydroxytryptamine uptake inhibitor, which had been discontinued when she became pregnant.

Investigations

Full blood count and routine tests of thyroid, liver and renal function were performed. All were normal. Laboratory investigations have no special role in establishing the diagnosis of depressive illness but simple screening tests to exclude systemic physical illness should be done in all psychiatric inpatients; they are essential if electroconvulsive therapy (ECT) is to be used.

Diagnosis

Severe depressive episode with psychotic symptoms.

Treatment and prognosis

Two ways of treating her depression were discussed with the patient: *antidepressant drugs* and *ECT*. Initially she was treated with doxepin, a tricyclic antidepressant drug which inhibits presynaptic uptake of both noradrenaline and 5-hydroxytryptamine. It also has sedative and hypnotic properties, useful in this case, because of the patient's agitation and insomnia.

After 5 days on this treatment the patient was still deeply depressed and requested ECT. Five days is not long enough for tricyclic antidepressants to relieve symptoms, but in view of her 'serious suffering' (to use a phrase from the Mental Health Act, 1983), she was given a course of ECT.

The patient required a course of five treatments for full recovery. After the first application she enjoyed a respite from her distressing ideas which then gradually returned before the next treatment. With successive treatments the period of respite from depressive symptoms lengthened.

Discussion

One of the reasons for believing that depressive illness is 'biological' is its remarkable response to ECT. A course of ECT consists of a succession of electrically induced fits given between two and three times a week. Patients vary in the number of fits required, a few recovering after three or so but most needing six to eight; it is rarely worth giving more than 12. The fit is induced by an electrical stimulus consisting of a rapid succession of very brief pulses applied between the temples. The electrical impedance of the human skull varies considerably between individuals. Modern ECT machines adjust the voltage accordingly to ensure that peak current is near constant.

Strictly speaking ECT is a misnomer, because there is no convulsion, only muscle twitching. Succinyl choline, a muscle relaxant, is given to prevent convulsions. It does so by briefly depolarizing the muscle end-plate, making it unresponsive to its neurotransmitter, acetylcholine. A brief-acting anaesthetic, thiopentone, is also given to render the patient oblivious, not to ECT, itself an anaesthetic, but to the respiratory paralysis induced by the succinyl choline. ECT is safe in the third trimester of pregnancy (Royal College of Psychiatrists CR39), but it is important to ensure adequate muscle relaxation. Using modern equipment the incidence of adverse effects is very low. Of these effects, memory impairment has caused the most public concern. It may take the form of retrograde amnesia, that is, amnesia for events before the course of ECT. Thus it has been found that shortly after a course of bilateral ECT there may be some impairment of memory over the preceding 3 years for TV programmes, a rather contrived but nevertheless verifiable material for assessing memory. Such impairment gradually subsides and is not detectable 6 months after treatment. However, memory for events which occur shortly before treatment may never be restored. During the first few hours after treatment patients have some difficulty in learning new material. Once the course of ECT is finished this capacity returns. Indeed a successful course of ECT may improve the ability to learn, probably because depression itself impairs this ability.

Questions

1 Why should caution be exercised when treating patients with drugs during pregnancy and lactation?
2 What are the clinical indications for ECT?

Answers on p. 302.

CASE STUDY 3

Fever, vomiting and neck stiffness in a child

Clinical features

A 10-month-old boy presented with a short history of fever, persistent vomiting and marked drowsiness. On examination he was febrile (temperature: 38.5°C), with photophobia and neck stiffness. Kernig's sign (see below) was positive.

Table CS3.1 Investigations performed.

Analyte	Value	Reference range
CSF		
White cell count	4600×10^9/L, 90% neutrophils	Less than 5×10^9/L, no neutrophils
Glucose	0.7 mmol/L (blood glucose was 2.6 mmol/L)	CSF glucose levels are normally greater than two-thirds of blood glucose levels

Investigations

A specimen of cerebrospinal fluid (CSF) was taken by lumbar puncture and the investigations shown in Table CS3.1 were performed.

A Gram stain was performed on the CSF and showed the presence of Gram-positive diplococci. Culture of the CSF revealed the presence of *Streptococcus pneumoniae* organisms which were sensitive to penicillin.

Diagnosis

The cardinal clinical features of bacterial meningitis are fever, depression or disturbance of the level of consciousness, and vomiting. Other features which are more specific but appear later include photophobia (aversion to light) and neck stiffness. A specific clinical test for meningitis is Kernig's sign. This is elicited by attempting to straighten the knee while the hip is held flexed. This manoeuvre pulls the spinal nerves where they penetrate the meninges, and therefore stretches the meninges themselves. Because the meninges are inflamed in meningitis this is exquisitely painful and the muscles go into spasm to prevent it from happening.

Diagnosis: Bacterial meningitis.

Discussion

Meningitis is inflammation of the meninges (the membranes around the brain). It can be caused by infections with bacteria, viruses, protozoa or fungal organisms. Viral meningitis is not usually serious, unless the brain itself is also affected (viral encephalitis) when brain damage can ensue. Fungal and protozoal meningitis are essentially confined to those individuals who are immunosuppressed or immunodeficient.

Seventy per cent of cases of bacterial meningitis occur in childhood. Three organisms—*Haemophilus influenzae*, *Neisseria meningitidis* and *Strep. pneumoniae*—are responsible for the majority of cases. In most developed countries meningitis due to *H. influenzae* has now virtually disappeared due to the recent development and use of an effective vaccine. All of these organisms have a carbohydrate (polysaccharide) capsule that is essential for virulence (see Chapter 7). The ability to mount an immune response to this capsule is an important protective mechanism. Antibodies to carbohydrate antigens, unlike antibodies directed to many protein antigens, are thymus independent (that is they do not require T-cell help, see Chapter 6) and do not show 'memory' from previous exposure to antigen. More importantly, the immune responses to carbohydrate antigens mature relatively late in development. Therefore, children under 2 years of age are particularly susceptible to infection with the organisms listed above.

The low level of glucose in the CSF is characteristic of bacterial meningitis. This was originally explained by bacterial metabolism of the CSF glucose. However, probably more important is the finding that neurones and glial cells switch from aerobic to anaerobic metabolism. The inflammatory response produced by infection leads to the local accumulation of fluid (oedema) and compression of blood vessels with subsequent impairment of blood supply. This is compounded by blood clotting in the local microcirculation. Under conditions of reduced oxygen the cells switch from aerobic to anaerobic metabolism, with increased consumption of glucose and the production of lactate. It is not surprising, therefore, that the lower the CSF glucose and the higher the CSF lactate, the poorer the prognosis in bacterial meningitis.

Much of the tissue damage in bacterial meningitis is the result of the inflammatory response rather than a direct effect of the organism. Lipopolysaccharide (LPS, endotoxin) is a structural component of the cell wall of Gram-negative bacteria and is a potent stimulator of the inflammatory response. Gram-positive organisms have a similar component known as lipoteichoic acid. These cell wall molecules stimulate host cells (particularly macrophages) to secrete cytokines, including tumour necrosis factor α (TNF-α) and interleukin 1 (IL-1). These cytokines act on a wide variety of cells to initiate inflammation (see Chapter 5) leading to increased capillary permeability (with associated local oedema), an ingress of neutrophils and stimulation of the complement and coagulation cascades. Cerebral oedema in turn can lead to an increase in intracranial pressure and impairment of cerebral blood flow.

Treatment and prognosis

Antibiotics are the cornerstone of management of bacterial meningitis. They need to be given intravenously, at least during the acute stages of the illness, since vomiting, impaired consciousness and possible shock make oral administration impossible. In addition, many antibiotics do not cross the blood–brain barrier effectively, and thus have very poor penetration into CSF. Currently, third-generation cephalosporins are drugs of choice, but as more organisms are detected with resistance to these antibiotics, others are replacing them. In some areas of the world, antibiotic resistance in meningitis is a serious problem.

Over the last few years, the addition of dexa-

methasone (a corticosteroid) has become widespread as adjunct treatment. If given early, i.e. at the same time as the initial dose of antibiotic, dexamethasone can reduce the release of pro-inflammatory cytokines and limit the inappropriately severe host inflammatory response. There is some clinical and laboratory evidence that this improves the long-term prognosis.

Despite modern antibiotic therapy, the overall mortality remains around 10% in bacterial meningitis. Of the survivors, 10% will be deaf due to direct cochlear damage. There is a small canal (the cochlear aqueduct) connecting the cochlea directly with CSF, and bacteria can thus pass directly to the inner ear and damage it, even in the early stages of the disease. Other complications include epilepsy and other neurological damage, and up to 30% of survivors of meningitis are left with long-term sequelae.

Questions

1 In some cases of bacterial meningitis there is marked clinical deterioration within hours of starting appropriate antibiotic therapy. Can you suggest why this is?
2 Despite the inability of infants to mount an antibody response to carbohydrate antigens, they can still be successfully immunized against *H. influenzae* capsular material. Do you know how this is achieved?

Answers on p. 302.

CASE STUDY 4

Shortness of breath and vaginal discharge

Clinical features

A 28-year-old woman presented with a 3-day history of fever, shortness of breath on exertion and a

dry cough. She denied chills, night sweats, nausea, vomiting, diarrhoea or abdominal pain. She had no headache, change in vision, muscle weakness or change in sensation. She had lost 10 pounds in the last 3 months despite eating what she described as a 'healthy' diet. She had noted a new vaginal discharge accompanied by itching, as well as some burning in her mouth when she drank coffee.

She was not on any medication. She had no history of contact with homosexual or bisexual men, but had used intravenous drugs from the age of 18 to 23 and had traded sex for drugs during this period. In the last 2 years, she had had one steady male partner with whom she continued to have a sexual relationship. There was no other significant past medical history, no allergies, and all members of her family were in good health.

Investigations

On physical examination the patient was thin, in moderate respiratory distress and febrile (temperature: 39.4°C). Blood pressure was 100/60. Pulse was regular at 100 b.p.m. Respiratory rate was 24/min.

Examination of the oral cavity revealed three discrete white patches on the hard palate, but was otherwise normal. There was no apparent lymphadenopathy (enlargement of lymph nodes). Pulmonary examination revealed bilateral, diffuse end-inspiratory rales (see below), but no rhonchi (wheezes) and no sign of consolidation or pleural effusion (fluid in the pleural cavity). Cardiovascular examination was normal. Abdominal examination showed no hepatomegaly (enlargement of the liver) or splenomegaly (enlargement of the spleen), and no masses or tenderness. Neurological examination revealed normal mental status, no muscle wasting and no focal weakness or sensory abnormalities. On pelvic examination a thick white vaginal discharge was noted. There was no cervical tenderness and no cervical discharge. A cervical smear was performed.

Laboratory investigations are reported in Table CS4.1.

Initial laboratory work-up included an enzyme-linked immunosorbent assay (ELISA) test for the presence of antibodies to HIV which was positive. This was confirmed by Western blot analysis. A CD4+ cell count revealed 150 cells/mm^3 (reference range, 800–1200 cells/mm^3). CD8+ cell count was 300 cells/mm^3 (reference range, 400–600 cells/mm^3). Microbiological cultures of blood were negative.

Table CS4.1 Investigations performed.

Analyte	Value	Reference range
Blood		
Haemoglobin	9.8 g/dL	11.5–16.5
White blood cell count	1.2 × 10^9/L	4.0–11.0
Urea	5.2 mmol/L	2.5–6.7
Creatinine	120 µmol/L	60–120
Sodium	140 mmol/L	135–146
Potassium	4.8 mmol/L	3.5–5.0

A chest radiograph (Fig. CS4.1) showed bilateral interstitial infiltrates, no cavities, consolidation or pleural effusion.

No sputum was available for analysis and so sputum induction was performed. Microscopic examination of the specimen obtained revealed the presence of *Pneumocystic carinii* organisms. Microscopic examination of swabs taken from the oral cavity lesions and the vagina revealed the presence of fungal forms consistent with *Candida albicans*. The cervical smear showed a grade 3 cervical intraepithelial neoplasia (CIN 3) reflecting infection with the human papillomavirus (HPV).

Diagnosis

The patient has *P. carinii* pneumonia and *C. albicans* infection of the vaginal and oral cavities. An HIV antibody test was positive. Center for Disease Control (CDC) classification was used as a reference for clinical categorization of HIV/AIDS (Table CS4. 2).

Diagnosis: acquired immunodeficiency syndrome (AIDS).

Discussion

HIV infection is currently the most common cause of immunodeficiency. The risk factors associated with acquisition of the virus in the case of this patient include multiple sexual partners and the use of intravenous drugs. Although HIV can infect a wide variety of cell types it most efficiently binds the CD4 receptor and enters CD4+ helper T cells. Destruction of the CD4+ helper T cell results in an

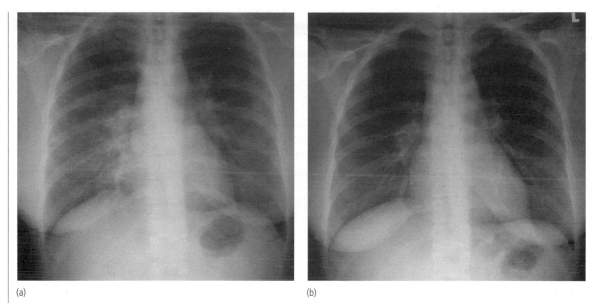

(a)   (b)

Fig. CS4.1 Clinical features of *Pneumocystis carinii* pneumonia (a) Chest radiograph from the case patient showing bilateral interstitial lung disease, which is worse in the right lung. These features are characteristic of *P. carinii* pneumonia (PCP). (b) Chest radiograph from the same patient taken 6 weeks later showing clearing of the disease after therapy.

extensive cascade of immunological abnormalities since this cell is central to almost every function of the immune system (see Chapter 6).

During the early stages of HIV infection much of the virus load is concentrated within the lymphoid system, including the spleen. With time there is a steady decline in the CD4+ helper T-cell population and with increasing destruction of this population, as well as other components of the immune system, opportunistic infections may occur. An opportunistic infection is infection by an organism which is ubiquitous in the environment and which rarely establishes an infection in an immunocompetent host.

P. carinii infection of the lungs is one of the most common opportunistic infections seen during HIV infection and may rapidly progress to pneumonia. The clinical features of *P. carinii* pneumonia (PCP) include fever, a dry cough and progressive dyspnoea (breathlessness). On examination the lungs often sound normal or end-inspiratory rales may be heard. Rales or 'crackles' are short explosive sounds that are thought to represent the equalization of pressure within collapsed small airways as they open during inspiration. Rales heard at the end of inspiration suggest fibrosis or the accumulation of

fluid (oedema) within the lungs. Untreated patients with PCP become incapacitated from dyspnoea and eventually die of hypoxaemia (reduced blood oxygen levels). Vaginal and oral infections with the fungal organism *C. albicans* (see Chapter 7) are also common in the immunocompromised host.

The decline in the CD4+ cell count is a useful indicator of the severity of immune dysfunction and is measured frequently in HIV-positive individuals. Clinically the decline in immune function can be charted through a number of distinct stages, these are summarized in Table CS4.2. The increased frequency of CIN lesions in HIV-positive females is becoming increasingly well recognized. CIN refers to premalignant transformation of the squamous epithelium of the uterine cervix. In CIN, the transformed cells are retained within the epithelium by the underlying basement membrane. CIN 3 is at the most severe end of the spectrum of these disorders and, if left untreated, frequently progresses to invasive squamous carcinoma of the cervix. In invasive squamous carcinoma, the cells comprising the CIN lesion breach the basement membrane and spread into surrounding connective tissues causing local tissue destruction. Extensive spread throughout

Table CS4.2 1993 revised classification system for HIV infection and AIDS (Center for Disease Control, USA) in adolescents (aged 13 and above) and adults. Persons with AIDS indicator conditions (i.e. categories C1–C3) as well as those with CD4+ T-lymphocyte counts less than 200/µl (i.e. categories A3 and B3) are reportable as AIDS cases.

CD4+ T-cell count	Clinical categories		
	(A) Asymptomatic, acute HIV infection or PGL	(B) Symptomatic but not (A) or (C) conditions	(C) AIDS indicator conditions
Greater than 500/µL	A1	B1	C1
200–499/µL	A2	B2	C2
Less than 200/µL	A3	B3	C3

The clinical categories are defined in the following sections.

Category A consists of one or more of the conditions listed below with documented HIV infection. Conditions listed in category B or C must not have occurred.

- Asymptomatic HIV infection.
- Persistent generalized lymphadenopathy (PGL) (lymph node enlargement).
- Acute (primary) HIV infection with accompanying illness or history of acute HIV infection.

Category B consists of symptomatic conditions in HIV infection that are not included in category C and that meet at least one of the following criteria:

- the conditions are attributable to HIV infection or are indicative of defective cell-mediated immunity.
- the conditions are considered to have a clinical course or require management that is complicated by HIV infection.

Examples of conditions in clinical **category B** include:

- oral candidosis
- constitutional symptoms, such as fever (> 38.5°C) or diarrhoea lasting for more than 1 month
- cervical intraepithelial neoplasia (CIN)
- herpes zoster (shingles) involving at least two distinct episodes or more than one site.

Category B conditions take precedence over those in category A (e.g. a patient who is now asymptomatic but has previously had a condition listed under category B should be classified under category B).

Category C conditions are AIDS indicator conditions. Examples of conditions in this category are:

- oesophageal candidosis
- invasive cervical cancer (see text)
- Kaposi's sarcoma
- Burkitt's lymphoma
- immunoblastic lymphoma
- primary lymphoma of brain
- *Mycobacterium avium* complex or *M. kansasii*, disseminated or extrapulmonary
- *M. tuberculosis*, any site
- *Pneumocystis carinii* pneumonia
- toxoplasmosis of brain.

the connective tissues and lymphatics has serious consequences for the patient and can lead to the blockage of vital pelvic organs.

The severity of CIN in immunosuppressed females may be explained in part by the association of HPV with CIN (see Chapter 23). Certain subtypes of HPV (particularly subtypes 16 and 18) are believed to contribute to the development of CIN. Immunosuppression allows outgrowth of HPV-infected tumour cells whose proliferation might otherwise be efficiently controlled by a competent immune system.

Treatment and prognosis

Unfortunately no cure exists for AIDS or HIV infection. Patients are encouraged to lead a normal healthy life and to have all associated infections treated promptly. Highly active anti-retroviral therapy (HAART), including protease inhibitors, has been shown to prolong life in many patients.

When treated early, PCP responds well to therapy with trimethoprim and sulphamethoxazole. These agents may also provide effective prophylaxis for HIV-positive individuals who have not yet developed PCP. Many clinicians continue PCP prophylaxis while the patient has a CD4+ count of 200 per mm^3 or less. If the CD4 count increases above 200 per mm^3 as a result of HAART, some clinicians would discontinue prophylaxis.

Active agents such as nystatin and fluconazole may be used to treat C. albicans infections. Treatment is also available for many other opportunistic infection such as cerebral abscesses due to Toxoplasma gondii and meningitis due to Cryptococcus neoformans. Patients who complete treatment for an opportunistic infection frequently remain on the

same medication at a lower dose for the rest of their lives as prophylaxis.

There is no specific treatment for HPV. Rather, the infected cervical tissue must be removed through any number of approaches, including freezing the tissues, electrocautery or surgical removal.

Questions

1 This patient presented with CIN 3 which is regarded as a precursor to invasive carcinoma of the cervix. Is the incidence of other types of tumour increased in HIV-positive individuals?
2 AIDS-associated tumours are often treated less aggressively than the same tumours arising in immunocompetent individuals. Why do you think this is?

Answers on p. 302.

CASE STUDY 5

Fever with chills and rigors

Clinical features

A 28-year-old male presented to hospital with fever, headache, backache and nausea of 10 days duration. No regular pattern of fever was noted during the first 3–4 days but later the fever recurred every other day. A brief chill that progressed to rigors preceded each episode of fever that terminated after 3–6 h with a bout of profuse sweating. The patient revealed that he visited a malaria-endemic area the previous month; symptoms appeared about 2 weeks after returning home. No previous experience of similar symptoms was recorded. On examination he looked ill, was pale but was not jaundiced. Oral temperature was 100.4°F. He was conscious, rational and there was no neck stiffness. Spleen was just palpable. Liver was not enlarged.

Investigations

The results of laboratory investigations are shown in Table CS5.1. The moderately raised erythrocyte sedimentation rate (ESR) indicates the presence of a disease process. Reduced haemoglobin, haematocrit and red cell count, but with other red cell indices within normal range, indicate a normocytic-normochromic anaemic state. The increased reticulocyte count supports a haemolytic condition. Malaria parasites in the blood film indicated a diagnosis of malaria due to *Plasmodium vivax* (Fig. CS5.1a).

Diagnosis

Both the clinical picture and the haemolytic, normochromic and normocytic anaemia are consistent

231

Table CS5.1 Investigations performed.

Investigation	Value	Reference range
Erythrocyte sedimentation rate (ESR)	48 mm 1st hr	0–10
Haemoglobin	9.5 g/dL	13–18
Red cell count	3.47×10^{12}/L	4.5–6.5
Haematocrit	0.295	0.40–0.54
Mean cell volume	85.1 fl	72–92
Mean cell haemoglobin	27.3 pg	27–32
Mean cell haemoglobin concentration	32.1 g/dL	30–35
Serum bilirubin	5.0 µmol/L	< 17
Reticulocyte count	3.1/100 red cells	0.5–2.5
Total white cell count	4.0×10^9/L	4.0–11
Urine examination	No pus cells seen	

Blood film
Malaria parasites seen
Plasmodium vivax—parasitaemia = 0.24%
White blood cell differential count:

Neutrophils	50%	
Lymphocytes	44%	
Eosinophils	2%	
Monocytes	4%	
Platelet count	178×10^9/L	150–400
Direct Coombs test	Negative	

with a diagnosis of malaria for which the identification of *P. vivax* parasites in a blood film is definite evidence.

Diagnosis: malaria due to *P. vivax* infection.

Discussion

Malaria is a mosquito-borne disease caused by a protozoan parasite of the genus *Plasmodium*. Four species of *Plasmodium* can cause human malaria: *P. vivax*, *P. falciparum*, *P. malariae* and *P. ovale*. Malaria remains prevalent in many tropical and subtropical parts of the world. Most infections are due to either *P. vivax* or *P. falciparum*. Following the bite of an infected mosquito, the parasites first invade cells of the liver; they multiply by the process of 'schizogony' and 6–12 days later parasites are released and invade red blood cells where they continue to multiply. The clinical features of malaria are due to the

blood stage parasites and the cyclical nature of their development results in the classical periodicity of symptoms described. *P. vivax* infection is characterized by febrile paroxysms, i.e. distinct episodes of fever associated with chills and rigors (Fig. CS5.2) typically occurring every third day (tertian pattern). This periodicity is often not apparent in the initial stages of disease due to asynchronous development of parasites. In addition, headache, myalgia, arthralgia, nausea and abdominal pain are symptoms frequently seen. Although distressing to the patient, clinical manifestations of *P. vivax* infections are almost always medically uncomplicated and the disease is hardly ever fatal.

In malaria due to *P. falciparum* (Fig. CS5.1b), fever periodicity is not so regular as with *P. vivax* and the paroxysms are less prominent. Any organ or system of the body can be affected, the brain and the circulatory system being two important sites leading to severe, often fatal, complications which can manifest, for example, as cerebral malaria, severe anaemia, renal failure and severe hypoglycaemia (reduced blood glucose levels). The anaemia that is common in malaria is due to the rupture of infected red cells but probably also to destruction of uninfected red cells and bone marrow suppression. Mild enlargement of the spleen is common in acute malaria and is due to increased blood flow to the immunologically activated spleen causing congestion of the red pulp. Massive enlargement of the spleen can be seen in chronic infections in malaria-endemic areas. This once common, but now generally rare, condition is referred to as tropical splenomegaly syndrome.

Malaria should be suspected in all cases with fever in an endemic region. Diagnosis of malaria in an area where there is no local transmission of the infection requires a high degree of clinical suspicion. Detailed history of clinical symptoms is important and travel history imperative, as would be a history of a recent blood transfusion. A patient's occupation may indicate the diagnosis, especially in areas of low malaria transmission, as outdoor workers are more likely to be exposed to mosquitoes. While a temperature chart may show the typical malaria fever pattern, fever with chills and rigors are seen in other conditions, e.g. viral infections,

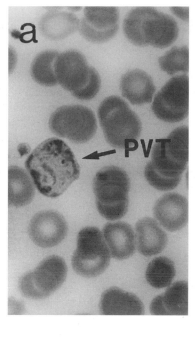 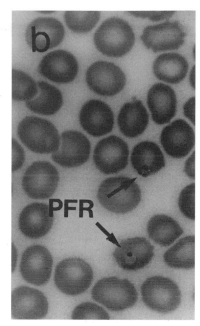

Fig. CS5.1 Photomicrographs of blood from patients with infections of (a) *Plasmodium vivax* and (b) *P. falciparum* malaria. In the *P. vivax* patient an infected red blood cell contains growing asexual trophozoites of the parasite (PVT). In the *P. falciparum* patient the infected red cells contain only the very young trophozoites, or ring stages (PFR). This is because the more mature forms of *P. falciparum* become sequestered in deep tissues of the body and are no longer present in the circulating blood from which blood smears such as these are prepared.

bacterial septicaemias and urinary tract infections. However, anaemia is infrequent in viral infections, elevated white cell counts with polymorphonuclear leucocytosis characterizes bacterial septicaemia and urinary tract infections will be marked by symptoms such as dysuria (painful passing of urine). Anaemia and splenic enlargement are common in haemolytic conditions but are also seen in leukaemias although other haematological changes will be apparent in the latter condition. Reticulocytes appear in larger than normal numbers during regeneration of red cells in the bone marrow, e.g. following haemolysis or haemorrhage. *P. falciparum* infections may be complicated by the involvement of one or more organs or systems. In such cases further investigations may be needed to exclude conditions such as meningitis, encephalitis or leptospirosis.

The presence of malaria parasites in a blood smear confirms the diagnosis of malarial infection. A thickly spread blood film is useful for spotting the parasites; whereas thinly spread films enable accurate species identification (see Fig. CS5.1) and quantification of the parasitaemia. It is recommended to make blood film examination on at least two consecutive days before malaria is excluded as

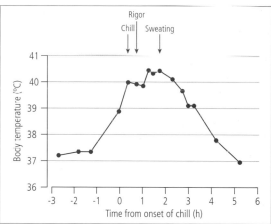

Fig. CS5.2 The course of fever during a paroxysm in a patient with a *Plasmodium vivax* infection.

the cause of fever in a probable case. Diagnostic tests, dipsticks detecting soluble parasite antigens, are also available for *P. falciparum* and *P. vivax*. Because of the acquisition of immunity to malaria in endemic areas, malaria parasites may be present in the blood without causing obvious symptoms. The association of any clinical symptom with a diagnosis of malaria is more difficult in these circumstances.

Treatment and prognosis

Antimalarial drugs are used primarily to eliminate the asexual blood parasites, which are responsible for the clinical disease, but also to destroy the sexual stages (gametocytes) which transmit the parasites through mosquitoes. With *P. vivax* and *P. ovale*, treatment also aims to eliminate the persisting liver stage parasites (hypnozoites) that could give rise to relapse infections. In *P. vivax*, *P. ovale* and *P. malariae* infections, the drug of choice is chloroquine. Relapse is prevented with primaquine daily for 14 days following the course of chloroquine. Anaemia in malaria, unless severe, does not need specific treatment and is corrected following parasite elimination.

Treatment of *P. falciparum* infections will depend on the prevalence of specific patterns of drug resistance shown by the parasites in the area where the infection was acquired and also on disease severity. If the parasites in an area are known to be sensitive to chloroquine then that would be the drug of choice and given as for *P. vivax*. Primaquine is given as a single dose following the course of chloroquine to destroy *P. falciparum* gametocytes. If drug-resistant *P. falciparum* is prevalent then alternatives should be used either singly or in combination, e.g. sulphadoxine–pyrimethamine, quinine, mefloquine or artemisinin derivatives, depending on the type of resistance. For seriously ill patients parenteral quinine, artemether or artesunate is recommended for rapid elimination of parasites, combined with other supportive therapy. Because of possible treatment failure, patients with *P. falciparum* should be followed on blood film up to 4 weeks after completion of treatment to ensure successful parasite elimination.

Complete recovery occurs following effective treatment in uncomplicated malarial infections. Early diagnosis and effective treatment usually prevent severe and complicated disease in *P. falciparum* infections. Once complications develop, case fatality rates rise to around 10–20%.

Questions

1 Why do *P. falciparum* parasites, when compared to other species, cause a more virulent form of disease with possible fatal complications?
2 How does one suspect treatment failure in a patient?

Answers on p. 303.

Fever, confusion and breathlessness

Clinical features

A 70-year-old man with a history of prostatic hypertrophy (benign enlargement of the prostate gland) was admitted to hospital with fever, confusion and breathlessness, which had developed over the past 12 h.

On examination he appeared slightly breathless, drowsy and was unable to give a coherent history of events. He was pale with cold extremities, although a raised core temperature of 38.5°C was recorded. His heart rate was regular but increased at 100 b.p.m. and blood pressure was lower than normal (hypotension) at 100/60 mmHg. Examination of his abdomen revealed an enlarged bladder, and rectal examination confirmed the presence of prostatic hypertrophy.

Table CS6.1 Investigations performed.

Analyte	Value	Reference range
Blood		
Total white cell count	4.6×10^9/L	4.0–11.0
Red cell count	5.0×10^{12}/L	4.50–6.50
Haemoglobin	14.2 g/dL	13.0–18.0
Platelets	210×10^9/L	150–400
Urea	35 mmol/L	2.5–6.7
Sodium	142 mmol/L	135–146
Potassium	4.1 mmol/L	3.5–5.0
Blood film		
White blood cell differential		
Neutrophils	51%	
Lymphocytes	40%	
Monocytes	6%	
Eosinophils	3%	
Basophils	0%	
Arterial blood gases		
P_{O_2}	12.0 kPa	10.0–13.3
P_{CO_2}	3.5 kPa	4.8–6.1
Hydrogen ion conc.	31 nmol/L	35–45
Bicarbonate	32 nmol/L	22–30
Urine microscopy		
White blood cell count	> 100/mL	< 5
Red blood cell count	20/mL	< 5
Chest X-ray	No abnormality detected	

Investigations

The results of initial laboratory investigations are shown in Table CS6.1.

Although the total white cell count is within the normal range, the proportion of neutrophils is towards the lower end of normal. This may occur in some states of immunosuppression, but may also occur in overwhelming infections. The urea is raised, consistent with mild renal failure, which may be due to dehydration but is most likely due to the chronic obstruction of urine flow caused by prostatic hypertrophy. Blood gases indicate a mild respiratory alkalosis consistent with hyperventilation.

Urine microscopy shows an increased white cell count, most commonly indicating a urinary tract infection.

Diagnosis

The patient is pyrexial, confused, hyperventilating and hypotensive, with a low neutrophil count. He has evidence of urinary tract infection and a degree of urinary tract obstruction as indicated by the palpable bladder and raised urea, which would predispose him to infection.

These findings are typical of systemic sepsis caused by Gram-negative bacteria. Results of blood and urine cultures, available on the day after admission revealed the presence of *Escherichia coli* in both.

Diagnosis: *E. coli* septicaemia secondary to urinary tract infection in a patient with partial urinary tract obstruction.

Discussion

Gram-negative bacteria form a major component of the normal human microbial flora. Apart from the anaerobic bacteria, *E. coli* predominates among the Gram-negative flora of the large intestine, although many other species may also be found. By virtue of its fimbriae, *E. coli* frequently colonizes mucosal surfaces, but rarely becomes invasive. Several strains, however, possess specific P fimbriae which bind to the P blood group antigen which is present, not only on red blood cells, but also on the epithelial cells of the urinary tract. These *uropathogenic* strains also possess a variety of other virulence factors and are the most common cause of urinary tract infections. *E. coli* bacteraemia is most commonly associated with urinary tract infection, particularly where there is obstruction to the flow of urine.

It is believed that most of the clinical features associated with Gram-negative sepsis result from cytokine-mediated responses to the presence of bacterial endotoxin. Cytokines are biochemical substances produced by immune cells (see Chapter 5) which trigger pathways involved in host defence. Exposure to endotoxin releases many cytokines, the most important of which is tumour necrosis factor (TNF). This cytokine activates the complement, clotting, fibrinolytic and kinin pathways (see Chapter 6) to the detriment of the host.

Initial signs of Gram-negative sepsis include fever, hyperventilation, relative neutropenia and changes in the mental state, but, unchecked, complications rapidly occur, including hypotension, disseminated intravascular coagulation (simultaneous features of bleeding and clot formation) and multiorgan failure. It is important that samples of blood, urine and material from other possible sites of infection are taken for culture as early as possible in the illness; ideally before the start of antimicrobial therapy.

Treatment and prognosis

The treatment of Gram-negative sepsis has three principal components: (a) primary antimicrobial therapy; (b) general supportive measures; and (c) treatment of the factor(s) predisposing to infection.

In most septic patients, the initial choice of antimicrobial agent is made 'blind', because the results of culture or antimicrobial susceptibility are usually not available at the time. A 'best guess' is therefore made on the basis of the clinical findings and the most likely source of infection. Usually, a broad-spectrum antibiotic or combination of antibiotics, which cover a wide variety of Gram-positive and Gram-negative organisms, will be chosen. This initial therapy may be modified once culture results are known, which is usually 24–48 h later. It is important that the agent chosen is bactericidal and achieves good levels at the site of infection. Intravenous administration of the antibiotic is therefore usually required.

General measures are essential in supporting the patient while the infection is brought under control. Their precise nature and duration will depend on the condition of the patient, but will be directed primarily to maintaining adequate perfusion of the tissues, particularly the brain and other vital organs.

Treating the factors predisposing the patient to Gram-negative sepsis can usually wait until the acute infective episode is over and the patient is in better condition. Examples of such treatments include prostatectomy for obstructive prostatic hypertrophy, cholecystectomy (removal of the gallbladder) for those patients with gallstones and improved control of diabetes mellitus where appropriate.

The prognosis of a patient with Gram-negative sepsis depends largely on their age and general condition—the very young and very old and those with significant underlying disease having a much higher mortality (50–60% in some studies) even with appropriate treatment. A worse outcome is also seen in those who have already developed complications or where appropriate treatment is delayed.

Questions

1 How might Gram-negative septicaemia be distinguished clinically from infection due to a Gram-positive organism?
2 Although *E. coli* is the most common cause of both hospital and community-acquired Gram-negative sepsis, *Pseudomonas aeruginosa* frequently causes life-threatening infections in immunocompromised patients. Why should this be so and what is the likely source of the infection?
3 What factors are thought to result in *E. coli* being the most common cause of Gram-negative septicaemia?

Answers on p. 303.

CASE STUDY 7

Coughing up of blood by a retired coal miner

Clinical features

A 65-year-old retired coal miner was admitted to hospital after coughing up blood (haemoptysis) on several occasions over the past 3 days. He described the amounts as ranging from a teaspoonful to a cupful.

He had worked as a miner for 20 years, but had been forced to retire early due to worsening chronic bronchitis and emphysema. He regularly produced copious amounts of white or yellowish sputum and required antibiotics for chest infections several times a year.

On examination, he was slightly breathless when speaking, and had clubbing of the fingernails. Examination of his chest confirmed the presence of features consistent with chronic bronchitis and emphysema, but no obvious signs of other acute disease. He did not appear anaemic and all other aspects of his examination were normal.

Investigations

The results of laboratory investigations are shown in Table CS7.1.

The haemoglobin concentration is within normal limits, suggesting that any blood loss had been of a minor nature.

The chest X-ray revealed a rounded shadow in the left upper lobe of the lung, with a crescent of air above. This appearance is typical of a fungal ball in the lung, colonizing an emphysematous cyst. Sputum culture showed a heavy growth of *Moraxella catarrhalis* a commensal organism of the upper respiratory tract, which is often associated with colonization or infection of the bronchi in patients with chronic lung disease. A moderate growth of *Aspergillus fumigatus* was also isolated which may indicate colonization of the sputum, but is not a diagnostic finding when taken alone.

Diagnosis

Apart from his episodes of haemoptysis, the patient's history and examination are entirely consistent with his chronic lung disease. However, the chest X-ray findings, coupled with the isolation of *A. fumigatus* from sputum suggest the presence of a fungal ball (aspergilloma) colonizing an old emphysematous cyst. The aspergilloma has eroded

Table CS7.1 Investigations performed.

Analyte	Value	Reference range
Blood		
Total white cell count	7.6×10^9/L	4.0–11.0
Red cell count	5.9×10^{12}/L	4.50–6.50
Haemoglobin	16.5 g/dL	13.0–18.0
Sputum microscopy		
Pus cells	Moderate numbers seen	
Culture	Heavy growth *Moraxella catarrhalis*	
	Moderate growth *Aspergillus fumigatus*	

a pulmonary blood vessel leading to the blood loss which was coughed up.

Diagnosis: aspergilloma eroding a pulmonary blood vessel in a patient with pre-existing chronic lung disease.

Discussion

Aspergillus is a ubiquitous environmental mould which is found predominantly in decaying vegetable matter. Its spores (conidia) can often be detected in the air, and their small size (2.5–3.0 μm) allows them to be inhaled deep into the respiratory tract. It is likely that all humans have been exposed to *Aspergillus* at some time, and many have continuing, frequent exposure, although few will become ill as a result. It is not surprising therefore that *Aspergillus* may often be isolated from sputum samples without being of clinical significance. *A. fumigatus* is the species most frequently associated with human disease, while *A. flavus* is associated with infection in the immunocompromised host.

There are three principal respiratory syndromes associated with *Aspergillus*.
• Allergic bronchopulmonary aspergillosis. Some patients who already suffer from asthma may develop hypersensitivity to *Aspergillus* spores, leading to varying degrees of lung damage.
• Invasive pulmonary aspergillosis. Profoundly immunocompromised patients may develop a life-threatening and rapidly progressive necrotizing pneumonia which may be difficult to diagnose antemortem as sputum may not be produced for culture. Such patients may also develop aspergillosis in other sites, e.g. bone and sinuses.
• Pulmonary aspergilloma. As illustrated by the case above, *Aspergillus* spores may be inhaled into cavities in previously damaged lung where they grow to form a ball of hyphae (aspergilloma). While some may resolve without treatment, others may become secondarily infected leading to abscess

formation or may erode into adjacent structures such as the pleural space or blood vessels resulting in haemoptysis.

In all of the pulmonary conditions described above, *Aspergillus* may be detectable in the sputum from time to time, but is not invariably present and will only aid diagnosis when considered as part of the overall clinical picture.

Treatment and prognosis

Essentially, the prognosis of pulmonary aspergilloma is the same as the pre-existing lung disease, and conservative management is appropriate. Small amounts of haemoptysis will usually subside spontaneously. However, if complications should arise, e.g. severe haemoptysis, lung abscess, etc., surgical excision of the lobe of the lung or drainage of the abscess may be indicated. Antifungal therapy is usually ineffective as the causative organism is protected within a cavity and inaccessible to systemically administered drugs.

In other forms of aspergillosis where antifungal drugs may be indicated, e.g. invasive disease in the immunocompromised, the two most useful compounds are amphotericin B and itraconazole; other agents having little or no activity against this organism.

Questions

1 What is the most common form of *Aspergillus* infection seen in clinical practice?
2 What preventive measures may be used to protect severely immunocompromised patients from acquiring aspergillosis?
3 Why can the presence of *Aspergillus* in foods be dangerous?

Answers on p. 303.

CASE STUDY 8

Persistent coughing up of blood and ankle swelling

Clinical features

A 24-year-old man with a 3-week history of persistent haemoptysis (the coughing up of blood) was admitted via casualty after coughing up obvious blood. He had passed only a small volume of blood-stained urine over the last 48 h.

On examination the patient was hypertensive (blood pressure: 160/90 mmHg). There was some swelling of the ankles which he had only noted over the previous 2 days.

Investigations

The results of laboratory investigations are shown in Table CS8.1.

The clinical features and laboratory results established two immediate clinical problems

- Haemoptysis.
- Significant impairment of renal function. This is indicated by the reduced urine output, raised

Table CS8.1 Investigations performed.

Analyte	Value	Reference range
Blood		
Urea	8.2 mmol/L	2.5–6.7
Creatinine	181 µmol/L	60–120
Creatinine clearance	29 ml/min	75–140
Sodium	148 mmol/L	135–146
Potassium	6.5 mmol/L	3.5–5.0
Haemoglobin	10.2 g/dL	13.0–18.0
Albumin	30 g/L	34–48
Urine		
Protein (dipstick)	2+*	0–trace

* Corresponds to an approximate protein excretion of between 1.5 and 7.5 g per 24 h.

blood urea and creatinine and reduced creatinine clearance.

A renal biopsy was performed. Histological analysis of this biopsy revealed that the patient had glomerulonephritis (inflammation of the renal glomeruli) of rapidly progressive type. This form of glomerulonephritis is characterized by infiltration of neutrophils and macrophages within the glomerulus which form 'crescent' shapes leading to the alternative designation of 'crescentic' glomerulonephritis. Immunofluorescent analysis of the tissue showed the presence of immunoglobulin G (IgG) distributed in a uniform linear pattern along the glomerular basement membrane. A chest radiograph revealed diffuse interstitial and alveolar infiltrates.

Diagnosis

The presence of haemoptysis and glomerulonephritis suggests either Goodpasture's syndrome or a systemic vasculitis such as Wegener's granulomatosis, polyarteritis nodosa or systemic lupus erythematosus (SLE). Antinuclear antibodies could not be detected in this patient and SLE is therefore an unlikely diagnosis. The detection of uniform and linear deposits of IgG within the glomerular basement membrane is a specific feature of Goodpasture's syndrome and is not seen in other forms of glomerulonephritis.

Diagnosis: Goodpasture's syndrome.

Discussion

Goodpasture's syndrome is an autoimmune disease in which autoantibodies are directed towards the α-domain of type IV collagen. Type IV collagen is a major constituent of basement membranes and is therefore present in many tissues. However, in

Goodpasture's syndrome these autoantibodies appear only to react with glomerular and alveolar basement membranes. The autoantibodies, which are predominantly IgG, may be visualized within these basement membranes by immunofluorescence on tissue sections. They may also be detected in the serum of affected individuals and will induce a condition similar to Goodpasture's syndrome when injected into monkeys.

It is now clear that the autoantibodies evoke a type II hypersensitivity reaction (see Chapter 10), and that this is responsible for the characteristic inflammation and tissue damage. The precise stimulus for the formation of these antibodies is unclear, although it may involve modification of a self-antigen found within basement membranes by viruses, hydrocarbon solvents or cigarette smoke, since exposure to these agents has been documented prior to the development of Goodpasture's syndrome. In keeping with the genetic predisposition to autoimmunity (see Chapter 11), there is a high prevalence of the DR2 haplotype in patients with Goodpasture's syndrome.

The clinical course of Goodpasture's syndrome is dominated by recurrent or even life-threatening haemoptysis which is the result of pulmonary haemorrhage secondary to alveolar damage. Renal involvement often appears several weeks after respiratory symptoms and is characterized by the deterioration of renal function over a period of hours or days (acute renal failure) leading to *uraemia* (the retention of waste products, including urea). Although *oliguria* (reduced urine output) or *anuria* (absence of urine production) are frequently seen in acute renal failure this is not always so. *Haematuria* (blood in the urine) may be seen in many other urinary tract diseases and is therefore not specific. *Hyperkalaemia* (raised blood potassium), due to inadequate renal excretion of potassium, may produce life-threatening cardiac dysrhythmias early in the course of acute renal failure.

Oedema, often seen in acute renal failure, is the accumulation of excess fluid in the interstitial space, presenting in this case as swollen ankles. In acute renal failure, oedema is usually the result of inappropriate sodium and water retention which increases extracellular fluid volume. Rarely, if urinary protein losses are great, there may be a significant decrease in plasma protein concentration. This may contribute to the oedema via the resultant passage of water out of capillaries and into the interstitial space.

Treatment and prognosis

Treatment is usually by a combination of plasmapheresis (plasma exchange), which eliminates both circulating autoantibodies and secondary inflammatory mediators, and drug therapy with glucocorticosteroids and cyclophosphamide. Dialysis support may be required for patients in renal failure.

The prognosis for patients with Goodpasture's syndrome is favourable if an early diagnosis is made, and with aggressive treatment renal function is maintained in more than 50% of patients. Extensive crescent formation within glomeruli is a poor prognostic sign.

Questions

1 What do you think are the likely causes of anaemia in this patient?
2 The patient was hypertensive. How do you account for this?

Answers on p. 304.

CASE STUDY 9

Breathlessness in a young man

Clinical features

A 23-year-old schoolteacher presented to his GP complaining of a 3-week history of 'shortness of breath', which was particularly troublesome after exercise. He was an occasional smoker and had a history of mild eczema and hay fever since childhood but had never suffered any serious illnesses. On examination his doctor noticed mild conjunctivitis and small areas of chronic eczema on the backs of his hands. Examination of his chest was unremarkable except for a few scattered inspiratory rhonchi (wheezes) heard throughout his lung fields.

Given these findings, his GP diagnosed asthma and prescribed a salbutamol inhaler with the advice that the teacher should take two puffs whenever he felt short of breath.

Two weeks later, after playing in a school cricket match, the teacher became breathless despite taking puffs of his inhaler. He became increasingly wheezy and his chest 'felt tight', a concerned colleague drove him to hospital.

On admission to the accident and emergency department he was barely able to speak because of his breathlessness. His pulse rate was 120 b.p.m. and on examination of his chest the doctor commented that it sounded almost 'silent'.

He was given nebulized salbutamol and ipratopium bromide and an intravenous dose of corticosteroids. He was admitted for observation and prescribed a 5-day course of oral steroids.

Investigations

Laboratory investigations included those shown in Table CS9.1.

A chest radiograph revealed hyperinflated lung fields but no areas of consolidation.

Table CS9.1 Laboratory investigations carried out.

Analyte	Value	Reference range
Blood		
Haemoglobin	15 g/dL	13.0–18.0
White blood cell count	8×10^9/L	4.0–11.0
Urea	6 mmol/L	2.5–6.7
Sodium	144 mmol/L	135–146
Potassium	3.2 mmol/L	3.5–5.0

Diagnosis

The patient had presented with acute severe asthma, which is a life-threatening condition. He required emergency treatment and admission to hospital where he remained for several days. The important questions are why did this happen to a previously healthy individual and could it have been prevented?

Diagnosis: acute severe asthma.

Discussion

Although this patient suggested to his doctor that his breathlessness was a new symptom, it should have been tied in with the background history and clinical features of conjunctivitis which clearly define an atopic tendency. The association with exercise was noted but a more detailed history would have elicited that exercise in winter months was not associated with symptoms and therefore this was more likely to be associated with the patient's recognized pollen allergy (hay fever). Had the seasonal nature of the symptoms been recognized, a more appropriate therapeutic strategy might have been instituted which would have prevented the need for hospital admission.

Adequate history taking is the key to identifying likely allergens in the atopic individual. In addition, the appropriate use of further investigations can be helpful. In this case the patient was followed up at an immunology clinic and had some further investigations. Total serum immunoglobulin E (IgE) was raised at 544 U/L (normal reference range: 1.5–120 U/L) and pulmonary function testing showed a moderate obstructive pattern which reversed with β_2-agonists. The consultant who saw him performed skin prick testing which demonstrated strong reactions to grass and tree pollens. Testing for allergen-specific IgE was not performed as it was not felt that this would add any useful information. Blood tests for allergen-specific IgE are only indicated where skin testing is not possible due to the risk of an anaphylactic response, the presence of severe eczema, the need for antihistamine therapy which cannot be withdrawn, or occasionally in young children.

Treatment and prognosis

Preventative therapy was instituted in this case. Inhaled disodium cromoglycate was prescribed as a mast cell stabilizer. This drug must be taken on a regular, daily, basis and acts by preventing the immediate release of mast cell mediators in response to allergen. In addition, the patient continued to carry his salbutamol inhaler and take it prior to participating in any outdoor activities.

This simple approach was adequate in controlling the teacher's symptoms, but in more refractory cases regular β_2-agonists would be required with the possible addition of inhaled corticosteroids.

Questions

1 Why were the other investigations listed in the table performed?
2 Why were corticosteroids administered and what is the mechanism of their action?

Answers on p. 304.

Diarrhoea, jaundice and rash

Clinical Features

A 27-year-old woman presented three weeks after her successful allogeneic bone marrow transplantation (BMT) with 1.2 L liquid stool per day, yellow colour of eye sclerae and skin rash. On examination, she was dehydrated and had a maculo papular rash over 40% of her body surface. The patient was febrile (temperature: 38°C). The heart rate was regular, 96 beats per minute, and her blood pressure was normal.

Investigations

The results of laboratory investigations are shown in Table CS10.1.

The total and differential white blood cell counts are normal and confirm a successful haematological recovery after the allogeneic BMT. The haemoglobin, red blood cell and platelet counts also indicate a sustained haematological recovery. The serum bilirubin was above the reference range.

Table CS10.1 Results of laboratory investigations.

Analyte	Value	Reference
Blood		
Total white cell count	4×10^9/L	4.0–11.0
Red cell count	3.1×10^{12}/L	3.8–5.8
Haemoglobin	10 g/dL	11.5–16.5
Haematocrit	0.37	0.37–0.47
Mean cell volume	85 fl	82–92
Mean cell haemoglobin	28 pg	27–32
Platelets	150×10^9/L	150–400
Urea	5.0 mmol/L	2.5–6.7
Urate	0.3 mmol/L	0.18–0.42
Serum bilirubin	45 µmol/L	< 17
Blood Film		
White cell differential		
Neutrophils	75%	
Lymphocytes	14%	
Monocyes	4%	
Eosinophils	5%	
Basophils	2%	

Diagnosis

The patient was severely dehydrated due to the large amount of body fluid lost in her diarrhoea. The patient also had jaundice and a typical maculopapular rash over 40% of her body surface. The clinical picture is consistent with a diagnosis of acute graft versus host disease (GvHD). The volume of liquid stools per day, degree of jaundice and extent of the maculopapular skin rash indicate Grade II acute GvHD.

Diagnosis: acute graft versus host disease.

Table CS10.2 Risk factors for acute graft versus host disease (GvHD).

Recipient
- Over 30 years old
- Cytomegalovirus infection
- Other viral infections

Donor
- Previous transfusions
- Previous pregnancies

Donor–recipient matching
- Sex mismatch
- HLA-A, -B, -DR mismatch
- Unrelated donor

Discussion

Acute graft versus host disease (GvHD) occurs in about 40% of allogeneic BMT recipients within the first 100 days after transplantation. The main reason for GvHD is the reaction of immunologically competent T-lymphocytes derived from the donor against antigens expressed on recipient tissues.

The main risk factors for acute GvHD are listed in Table CS10.2.

Treatment and prognosis

A combination of immunosuppressive drugs, methylprednisolone plus cyclosporine, is administered and once symptoms and signs abate, the dose is gradually reduced over several weeks. In severe cases, additional second-line agents such as antithymocyte globulin (ATG) should be administered.

The prognosis of acute GvHD is highly dependent on the clinical grade as summarized in Table CS10.3. Patients with grade I or II usually respond well to

Table CS10.3 Clinical grading of acute graft versus host disease.

Clinical grade	Skin rash	Jaundice	Diarrhoea
I	Rash < 25% of body	2–3 mg/dL	0.5–1 litres/day
II	Rash 25–50%	> 3–6 mg/dL	1–1.5 litres/day
III	Generalized erythroderma	> 6–15 mg/dL	> 1.5 litres/day
IV	G. erythroderma + bullae	> 15 mg/dL	+ abdominal pain

traditional immunosuppression therapy. On the other hand, the mortality is almost 100% in cases with grade IV acute GvHD, despite aggressive immuno-suppression, and often results from the complication of super-infections rather than direct organ failure from acute GvHD. Also, patients with severe acute GvHD are more likely to develop chronic GvHD. In this case the patient responded to treatment and made a successful recovery.

Questions

1 What is the effect of acute GvHD on immune reconstitution?
2 What are the possible late complications of allogeneic BMT?

Answers on p. 304.

CASE STUDY 11

Protein in the urine and high blood pressure

Clinical features

A 45-year-old man was found to have protein in his urine on dipstick testing at an employment medical. He was also hypertensive (blood pressure: 180/100). On questioning he admitted to having had some swelling of his ankles at the end of the day for the last 6 months, but otherwise had no symptoms.

Investigations

Laboratory investigations included those shown in Table CS11.1.

Antinuclear antibodies were not detectable. Renal ultrasound showed normal size and appearance of kidneys.

A renal biopsy was performed. Histological analysis of the renal biopsy showed glomer-ulonephritis (inflammation of the renal glomeruli) of membranous type, characterized by thickening of the glomerular basement membrane and sclerosis (scarring) of individual glomeruli. Immunofluores-cent analysis showed granular deposition of immu-noglobulin G (IgG) within the glomerular basement membranes. On electron microscopy there were

Table CS11.1 Investigations performed.

Analyte	Value	Reference range
Blood		
Albumin	27 g/L	34–48
Sodium	138 mmol/L	135–146
Potassium	3.8 mmol/L	3.5–5.0
Urea	11.2 mmol/L	2.5–6.7
Creatinine	155 µmol/L	60–120
Creatinine clearance	64 mL/min	75–140
Fasting glucose	4.6 mmol/L	4.5–5.6
Cholesterol	9.2 mmol/L	3.5–6.5
Urine		
24-h urinary protein	6.3 g/24 h	< 0.15

electron-dense deposits within glomerular base-ment membranes.

Diagnosis

The moderately large amount of protein in the urine (proteinuria) is consistent with chronic glomer-ulonephritis. Other forms of renal disease such as chronic pyelonephritis and chronic interstitial nephritis produce much less severe proteinuria. The absence of antinuclear antibodies would tend to rule out systemic lupus erythematosus (see Chapter 11) as a cause of the renal disease. Other forms of glomerulonephritis, e.g. proliferative glomerulonephritis, are excluded as are other causes of heavy proteinuria such as diabetic nephropathy (fasting blood glucose levels were within the reference range).

Diagnosis: membranous glomerulonephritis.

Discussion

Membranous glomerulonephritis is due to the deposition of antigen–antibody complexes (immune complexes) within the glomerular basement membranes. These immune complexes can be detected by immunofluorescence analysis or as electron-dense deposits on electron microscopy.

The precise stimulus for the formation of these immune complexes cannot always be clearly identified. Rarely, in some cases exogenous antigens (e.g. hepatitis B virus, *Treponema pallidum* antigens) and endogenous antigens (e.g. thyroglobulin) have been implicated. The deposition of immune complexes within glomeruli leads to glomerular inflammation, glomerular damage, including the deposition of collagen within glomeruli (glomerular sclerosis), and subsequent impairment of renal function. In membranous glomerulonephritis the changes in the basement membrane are manifested as the leakage of protein through the damaged basement membrane and into the urine. This patient has moderately severe proteinuria sufficient to reduce the blood albumin levels below normal (hypoalbuminaemia). The hypoalbuminaemia has in turn caused a reduction in the oncotic pressure of the blood, with leakage of fluid into the tissues resulting in the accumulation of fluid (oedema) in the legs. The triad of proteinuria, hypoalbuminaemia and oedema is termed *nephrotic syndrome*. The patient shows evidence of impaired renal function with a slight elevation of blood urea and creatinine and

reduction in creatinine clearance. The history of oedema for 6 months suggests the condition is not of recent origin. Hypertension has developed secondary to renal disease. Most cases of hypertension are of unknown cause and are termed 'essential hypertension' or 'idiopathic hypertension'. Approximately 5% of hypertension is due to other medical conditions, and the majority of 'secondary hypertension' is the result of renal disease.

Treatment and prognosis

Diuretics, either orally or intravenously, can be used to increase water excretion and reduce oedema. Where oedema is resistant then intravenous albumin infusions can be used to raise plasma oncotic pressure and facilitate diuresis. In some forms of glomerulonephritis corticosteroids can be used to suppress the glomerular inflammation. There are two possible outcomes of patients with membranous glomerulonephritis. In some patients there will be a partial resolution of proteinuria with stabilization of renal function. Alternatively, renal function may decline progressively over the course of between 5 and 20 years, eventually requiring dialysis. In the latter group of patients, corticosteroids have been shown to have no effect. Hypertension will accelerate the decline of renal function and treatment of hypertension is therefore indicated.

Questions

1 Hypercholesterolaemia (raised blood cholesterol level) is frequently encountered in patients with the nephrotic syndrome. Why is it important to administer lipid-lowering drugs to this group of patients?
2 Why is plasma creatinine a useful marker of renal function? Are there more accurate methods for the measurement of renal function?

Answers on p. 304.

CASE STUDY 12

Fever and cervical lymph node enlargement

Clinical features

A 23-year-old woman with a history of renal transplantation for chronic renal failure secondary to thrombotic thrombocytopenic purpura, was admitted to the hospital with new onset *cervical lymphadenopathy* (enlarged neck lymph nodes) and renal failure. At the time of transplantation, the patient had been started on prednisone and azothioprine immunosuppression to prevent rejection of the allograft. However, 3 weeks later the serum creatinine rose and a percutaneous renal biopsy yielded a diagnosis of acute rejection. This was treated by increasing the immunosuppression with an intravenous infusion of OKT3 (a mouse monoclonal anti-T-lymphocyte antibody). Eleven days after the monoclonal antibody infusion, the patient developed pharyngitis, cervical and submandibular lymphadenopathy and fever.

On examination the patient was mildly hypertensive (blood pressure: 170/95) and febrile (temperature: 38.5°C). The tonsils were enlarged and there was pharyngeal erythema (redness). There was bilateral submandibular and cervical lymphadenopathy, and hepatosplenomegaly (enlarged liver and spleen).

Investigations

Laboratory investigations included those shown in Table CS12.1.

The clinical features and laboratory results suggest a systemic infection. Systemic infection is supported by pharyngitis, fever, lymphadenopathy and hepatosplenomegaly. This syndrome is suggestive of Epstein–Barr virus (EBV)—associated infectious mononucleosis (glandular fever) typically characterized by: pharyngitis; fever; cervical lymphadenopathy; hepatosplenomegaly; and a

Table CS12.1 Investigations performed.

Analyte	Value	Reference range
Blood		
Urea	17 mmol/L	2.5–6.7
Creatinine	1112 μmol/L	60–120
White blood cell count	1.8×10^9/L	4.0–11.0
VCA-IgM titre	1 : 128	–

leucocytosis (increased white cell count) with atypical lymphocytes. Other infections, including cytomegalovirus, herpesvirus 6, human immunodeficiency virus infections and toxoplasmosis can produce similar or overlapping syndromes with lymphadenopathy and systemic symptoms. However, pharyngitis is not part of the constellation of symptoms in these diseases and is typical of EBV-associated infectious mononucleosis. The depressed white blood cell count and absence of atypical lymphocytes in this patient is unusual in infectious mononucleosis but may reflect treatment with the *myelosuppressive* (bone marrow suppressing) and lympholytic agents employed (azothioprine, prednisone and OKT3). Detection of an immunoglobulin M (IgM) antibody titre to the EBV viral capsid antigen (VCA) is diagnostic of a recent EBV infection and is consistent with this interpretation.

In addition to infectious mononucleosis, a second diagnosis must be considered: post-transplant lymphoproliferative disease. Patients who are immunosuppressed, particularly with respect to T-cell function are at risk for developing uncontrolled proliferation of EBV-infected B lymphocytes. This disease process may occur with or without an infectious mononucleosis-like syndrome. Lymphadenopathy in the post-transplant setting must always raise this concern.

A submandibular lymph node was biopsied and a proliferation of large activated B lymphocytes (B immunoblasts) was diagnosed. Nephrectomy of the transplanted kidney was performed and showed focal proliferation of B immunoblasts as well as acute rejection. *In situ* hybridization showed the presence of EBV within the immunoblasts in both tissues. Southern blot hybridization using an immunoglobulin heavy chain probe showed a clonal population of cells in the submandibular lymph node and a distinct clonal population in the kidney. No chromosome translocations were detected by conventional cytogenetics.

Diagnosis

The diagnosis of post-transplant lymphoproliferative disease is confirmed by study of the biopsied lymph node and the nephrectomy specimen showing proliferation of B immunoblasts. This syndrome is virtually always associated with EBV. Any potential confusion with the benign lymphoid hyperplasia that may accompany infectious mononucleosis is eliminated by the demonstration of monoclonal populations of cells and the identification of the EBV within virtually all of the B immunoblasts. The presence of one or more distinct clonal B-cell populations and the absence of chromosomal translocations is characteristic of post-transplant lymphoproliferative disease.

Diagnosis: B-cell lymphoproliferative disease in an organ transplant recipient.

Discussion

EBV-associated B-cell lymphoproliferative disease is recognized in patients with congenital immunodeficiencies (such as the X-linked lymphoproliferative syndrome), HIV infection and in organ transplant recipients. In organ transplant recipients, the incidence of the disease seems to be a function of the particular immunosuppressive regimen used to prevent organ rejection. Patients receiving cyclosporin A or anti-T-cell antibodies are at highest risk. The pathogenesis of the disease is thought to be related to the ability of EBV to immortalize human B lymphocytes. EBV-immortalized B lymphocytes will proliferate indefinitely *in vitro* and will grow as tumours in mice with *severe combined immunodeficiency* (SCID mice). However, in the presence of memory T cells, *in vitro* or *in vivo*, the EBV-induced lymphoproliferation is suppressed. In immunosuppressed patients, the inadequate T-cell response allows the outgrowth of EBV-infected B cells. Histologically, these tumours may have features of benign hyperplasia or frank malignancy.

A tendency to involve extranodal sites is characteristic of these opportunistic lymphoproliferative diseases and involvement of the allograft itself is particularly common. Although the disease may mimic a viral illness or be entirely asymptomatic at presentation, and may appear to be histologically benign, the lymphoproliferation will result in the death of the patient in most instances unless appropriate interventions are undertaken.

Treatment and prognosis

When immunosuppressive agents are discontinued, tumours will resolve in approximately half of cases. When the graft is involved by tumour and can be sacrificed without endangering the patient, as is the case with renal transplants, the graft is generally removed. If these measures fail, other interventions including antiviral agents to inhibit further spread of viral infection, interferon, anti-B-cell antibodies, such as the anti-CD20 monoclonal antibody, Rituximab, or combination chemotherapy have all been reported to be of benefit in some patients.

Questions

1 This patient's lymphoma was associated with EBV. Are other viral infections associated with lymphomas?
2 This patient was deliberately immunosuppressed in order to prevent graft rejection. This immunosuppression allowed the development of EBV-associated lymphoma. Is immunosuppression associated with a global increase in risk for all kinds of malignancy?

Answers on p. 305.

CASE STUDY 13

Neutropenia and recurrent infection in a patient with rheumatoid arthritis

Clinical features

A 67-year-old lady was admitted to hospital with a severe chest infection having presented with breathlessness, a productive cough and mild confusion. She had had rheumatoid arthritis (RA) for the past 25 years and was under the care of a hospital rheumatology department. Despite her condition she led an active life and was normally mentally alert. Six months previously she also had a chest infection, although this episode did not require hospital admission. However, at that time she was noted to be neutropenic.

Investigations

The results of laboratory investigations are shown in Table CS13.1. Although the total blood cell white count is within the normal range, the differential is clearly abnormal. There is a profound reduction in the neutrophil count. The absolute lymphocyte count, at 5.1×10^9/L, although not dramatically increased, is above the upper limit of normal, and on the blood film has a large granular lymphocyte morphology. She is slightly anaemic and her mean corpuscular volume (MCV) is low.

In addition to the laboratory investigations,

Table CS13.1 Investigations performed.

Analyte	Value	Reference range
Blood		
Total white cell count	6×10^9/L	4.0–11.0
Red cell count	4.27×10^{12}/L	3.8–5.8
Haemoglobin	10.6 g/dL	11.5–16.5
MCV	74.4 fl	82–92
Mean cell haemoglobin	24.8 pg	27–32
Platelets	343×10^9/L	150–400
Vitamin B$_{12}$	260 pg/mL	160–760
Serum folate	4.1 ng/L	3.0–20.0
Blood film		
White blood cell differential		
Neutrophils	9%	40–75%
Total lymphocytes	85%*	20–45%
Monocytes	3%	1–10%
Eosinophils	2%	1–6%
Basophils	1%	0–1%

* Large granular lymphocytes comprise 70–80% of total lymphocytes; reference range 0–15%

Note: mean corpuscular volume; if iron deficient, the average size of the red blood cell decreases.

peripheral blood lymphocytes were also analysed on a fluorescent-activated cell sorter (FACS) machine. The results showed that they were predominantly CD8 lymphocytes and carried the CD57 marker (expressed on large granular lymphocytes) on about 85% of the cells. There was also an inverted CD4 : CD8 ratio.

Diagnosis

The anaemia in this case is described as microcytic, i.e. the red blood cells are reduced in size (low mean cell volume), which could indicate iron deficiency. Patients on non-steroidal anti-inflammatory tablets are at risk of losing iron through the gastrointestinal tract due to peptic ulceration. Alternatively, microcytosis is typical in anaemia associated with chronic inflammatory diseases such as RA, in which the anaemia does not respond to treatment with iron (see Chapter 14).

In the context of RA a low neutrophil count in the absence of any other specific cause is likely to be Felty's syndrome. This describes the association of unexplained neutropenia and RA. The patient is usually sero-positive for rheumatoid factor (see later) and in the severe end of the spectrum (although this is not always the case) the arthritis is often quiescent by the time Felty's syndrome develops. The original description also included splenomegaly, but this is not now felt to be obligatory. Some patients with Felty's syndrome, also have an expansion of large granular lymphocytes. These are easily identified on the blood film by an experienced haematologist.

Felty's syndrome occurs in about 1% of patients with RA. The diagnostic finding is that of neutropenia. If this is mild, i.e. above 1×10^9/L, the risk of infections is relatively low but as the neutrophil count drops further, patients are at greater risk of infections, and if untreated there is a high mortality rate. Some patients will also have a thrombocytopenia and/or lymphopenia, but anaemia is not usually a feature of Felty's syndrome alone. About a third of patients with Felty's syndrome will also have an expansion of large granule lymphocytes; ranging from a very subtle to a substantial increase in lymphocyte counts with virtually all being clonal

CD3+ CD8+ and CD57+. Interestingly, T cells with similar immunophenotype are found in patients with human immunodeficiency virus (HIV) infection which might suggest the possibility of a retroviral aetiology in this subgroup of patients. In patients with RA this phenomenon occurs as a benign condition and often resolves spontaneously over a number of years. Interestingly, another form of large granular lymphocyte syndrome affects natural killer (NK) cells rather than lymphocytes. NK cell leukaemia is often a disease with a poor prognosis but is not usually found in the patients with Felty's syndrome.

RA is a complex systemic autoimmune disease, of unknown aetiology, characterized by chronic inflammation of the joints which in some cases may lead to severe disability. The disease may start in the small joints, e.g. metacarpophalangeal (knuckle) joints of the hand and progress to the wrists and large joints such as knees and elbows. Typically, the inflammation of the joints is manifested by erythema and swelling which progressively gets worse; the patients suffering with pain, stiffness and restricted movement. For the clinician, diagnosis is dependent on the patient presenting with certain clinical signs and symptoms as defined by the American Rheumatism Association (Table CS13.2). It should be pointed out that about 75% of RA patients are rheumatoid factor (RF) positive. Intriguingly, the presence of RF is associated with a poorer prognosis and extra-articular manifestations

Table CS13.2 Revised diagnostic criteria for the classification of rheumatoid arthritis (RA) (1987 American Rheumatism Association).

1 Morning stiffness in and around joints lasting at least 1 h before maximal improvement
2 Soft tissue swelling (arthritis) of three or more joint areas observed by a physician
3 Swelling (arthritis) of the proximal interphalangeal, metacarpophalangeal, or wrist joints
4 Symmetric swelling (arthritis)
5 Rheumatoid nodules
6 Rheumatoid factor positivity
7 Radiographic erosions and/or periarticular osteopenia in hand and/or wrist joints

Criteria 1–4 must have been present for at least 6 weeks.
RA is defined by the presence of four or more criteria.

which may include subcutaneous nodules, cardiac involvement, vasculitis and Felty's syndrome: in the latter case patients tend to have high titres of RF. RFs are autoantibodies largely of the IgM isotype (but may also include IgG and IgA isotypes) which bind to the Fc region of IgG and are associated with immune complex formation.

Treatment and prognosis

If the neutrophil count is not dramatically suppressed (i.e. above $1 \times 10^9/L$) and the patient is not suffering from infection then there is no absolute requirement for treatment. However, if there is a profoundly low neutrophil count and/or recurring infections, then it is sensible to treat in order to prevent a life-threatening infection. It is usually helpful to perform a bone marrow aspirate: in the majority of patients this will be an active marrow and provides reassurance that it is safe to treat with immunosuppressive drugs. Occasionally, patients will have bone marrow that is infiltrated with large granular lymphocytes or possess high levels of antineutrophil antibodies causing a hypocellular marrow.

Drugs that are most effective in treating patients with Felty's syndrome include methotrexate and cyclosporin. Indeed, a few reports in the literature highlight a dramatic improvement when using cyclosporin. If the patient is profoundly neutropenic, it may be worthwhile and as a precaution, to cover the introduction of methotrexate or cyclosporin with granulocyte–macrophage colony-stimulating factor (GM-CSF) which can be given twice weekly, weekly or even monthly depending on the level of response. There is little evidence that corticosteroids *per se* are beneficial. Corticosteroids can increase the peripheral neutrophil count, although this may be due to a redistribution of existing neutrophils and consequently may not have a positive affect on the disease. If the patient is carefully monitored and the neutrophil count maintained above $1 \times 10^9/L$ (and preferably $2 \times 10^9/L$), then the outcome should be similar to that of any other patient with RA.

Questions

1 What is the cause of the neutropenia?
2 What links Felty's syndrome, large granular lymphocyte syndrome and neutropenia?

Answers on p. 305.

Fever and leg ulcer

Clinical features

A 54-year-old man presented to an accident and emergency department with fever and a large ulcer on the sole of his right foot. This had been present and gradually enlarging over 2 weeks. Earlier action had not been taken because the ulcer was painless. He claimed to be otherwise fit and well, although on direct questioning he had noticed increased thirst and urination over 18 months, a 10-kg weight loss over 2 years and non-specific lethargy of longer duration which had been attributed to 'old age'. On examination he was thin, somewhat dehydrated and febrile (temperature 39°C). Examination of his retina revealed capillary haemorrhages. He was unable to detect vibration sensation below his knees

Table CS14.1 Investigations performed.

Analyte	Value	Reference range
Blood		
Random glucose	24.7 mmol/L	3.5–8.9
Urea	19.4 mmol/L	2.5–6.7
Creatinine	157 µmol/L	60–120
Bicarbonate	23 mmol/L	22–30

and had lost soft touch sensation below his ankles. There was a large deep malodorous ulcer under his great toe that was surrounded by spreading skin infection. Exploration of this ulcer revealed a cavity full of pus tracking deep along the sole of his foot. His dipstick urine analysis showed 3⁺ glucose, 2⁺ protein and 3⁺ ketones.

Investigations

The results of laboratory investigations are shown in Table CS14.1.

No islet cell or insulin autoantibodies were detected.

A radiograph of the patient's right foot showed destruction of the bone in the great toe.

Microbiological analysis of the pus from the ulcer showed the presence of both aerobic (including *Staphylococcus aureus*) and anaerobic bacteria.

Diagnosis

The patient has *hyperglycaemia* (raised blood glucose levels) confirming diabetes mellitus. The raised blood urea and creatinine indicate poor renal function, almost certainly due to diabetic renal disease (diabetic nephropathy). This is further supported by the proteinuria (protein in the urine) which is the result of protein leaking through a damaged renal glomerular capillary basement membrane. The dehydration is the result of the osmotic loss of water induced by glycosuria (glucose in the urine) resulting in increased urination and stimulation of thirst. His bicarbonate levels were normal so the blood accumulation of ketone bodies (i.e. acetoacetate and 3-hydroxybutyrate which are the breakdown prod-

ucts of non-esterified fatty acid metabolism) was not sufficient to cause acidosis (lowered blood pH).

The failure to detect islet and insulin autoantibodies is against a diagnosis to type 1 diabetes mellitus which usually has an autoimmune basis (see Chapter 11). Clearly he has had diabetes for a long time. Microvascular complications involving the eyes (diabetic retinopathy, manifested by the presence of retinal capillary haemorrhages) and kidneys and peripheral nerve damage (diabetic neuropathy) relate to a long exposure to high blood glucose levels. His onset of diabetes was insidious, possibly developing 10 years or so before presentation, and so this is probably type 2 diabetes mellitus. The mean prediagnosis duration of unrecognized hyperglycaemia is estimated at 4 years. Ten per cent of patients with type 2 diabetes have complications at diagnosis.

Diagnosis: type 2 diabetes mellitus with diabetic nephropathy, diabetic neuropathy and infected neuropathic foot ulcer.

Discussion

Diabetes mellitus is a metabolic disorder in which blood glucose concentrations are elevated. Conventionally, two major forms of diabetes mellitus are recognized. Type 1 diabetes (juvenile onset, insulin-dependent diabetes mellitus) usually presents acutely in young patients and is the result of an autoimmune attack on the insulin-producing pancreatic β-cells. This leads to destruction of the β-cells with consequent lack of secretion of insulin. There is a genetic predisposition to type 1 diabetes which is explained in part by association with specific human leucocyte antigen (HLA) types (see Chapter 6); however, it is likely that a triggering environmental factor such as a viral infection is involved in initiating the disease process. This hypothesis is supported by the finding that the rate of concordance for type 1 diabetes in identical twins is found to be under 50% in most studies.

Insulin is a potent anabolic hormone which promotes synthesis and storage of triacylglycerol (fat) primarily in adipocytes and of glycogen (glucose polysaccharide) in skeletal muscle and liver. Its major role, acting on these insulin-sensitive tissues is to lower blood glucose levels by stimulating glucose uptake and storage. It also increases protein synthesis and inhibits lipolysis (fat breakdown), including inhibition of the release of fatty acids from adipose cells. In the absence of insulin these fatty acids are released from adipose cells and converted to ketones in the liver resulting in the accumulation of ketones in the blood and their excretion in the urine (ketonuria). The excess ketoacids in the blood require buffering by the bicarbonate ion; this leads to a marked decrease in serum bicarbonate concentrations and thus acidosis. Patients with type 1 diabetes mellitus therefore have a mandatory requirement for insulin injection therapy to prevent acidosis-induced coma and inevitable death.

In contrast, patients with type 2 diabetes (maturity onset, non-insulin-dependent diabetes mellitus) are usually older, often obese, and there is usually an insidious or gradual onset of symptoms. Type 2 diabetes is far more common than type 1, affecting some 90% of diabetes patients. Genetic factors are even more important than in type 1 diabetes and among identical twins there is a concordance rate of about 90%. However, type 2 diabetes is not linked to any HLA haplotype and there is no evidence that autoimmune mechanisms are involved in its pathogenesis. Postmortem examination of sections of pancreas from type 2 diabetics often reveals evidence of the accumulation of amyloid plaques around the β-cells. The plaque has been shown to be composed of fibrils of β-pleated stacks of islet-amyloid polypeptide (IAPP or amylin) which is able to destroy β-cells and which may have a pathogenic role in type 2 diabetes.

The following two metabolic defects characterize type 2 diabetes.

A relative but not absolute *insulin deficiency*. The cause of this insulin deficiency is not known but may be related to a progressive loss of β-cell function and β-cell mass.

An inability of peripheral tissues to respond to insulin, termed *insulin resistance*, due to a number of abnormalities of postreceptor stimulation of glucose transport. Insulin resistance alone is not sufficient to cause type 2 diabetes: many obese individuals exhibit severe insulin resistance without any accompanying diabetes since they are sufficiently hyperinsulinaemic to compensate for the decreased insulin sensitivity. Susceptible individuals, presumably with a genetic predisposition, are not able to sustain sufficient insulin secretion and once the loss of β-cell mass (possibly due to amyloid accumulation) is extensive enough diabetes becomes apparent.

In clinical practice, the distinction between type 1 and 2 diabetes mellitus is not always clear cut and an appreciation of the underlying biochemical abnormalities often aids therapeutic decision making.

Treatment and prognosis

Insulin resistance can be reduced by weight loss and exercise, but insulin deficiency is of greater significance. Altering the diet by reducing the content of simple, refined carbohydrates and increasing complex carbohydrates and fibre reduces the rate of entry of glucose into the circulation. This may be to a sufficiently low level such that the diminished insulin secretion in type 2 diabetes may more easily cope.

If still insufficient to achieve good glucose control, then oral hypoglycaemic drugs (e.g. sulphonylureas) can be used. These act by stimulating insulin secretion from the β-cell and by enhancing the effect of insulin at the postreceptor level in peripheral tissues. However, if insulin deficiency and β-cell loss are marked then these drugs become ineffective in the treatment of type 2 diabetes. Obviously these drugs are not used in type 1 diabetes where insulin deficiency is absolute. On average, because of the slow progression of type 2 diabetes, a patient responding initially to diet alone will require oral hypoglycaemic agents after a period of approximately 3 years and insulin treatment some 7 years later.

This patient was started on twice daily insulin injection therapy with rapid disappearance of urinary ketones and correction of blood glucose. Despite antibiotic therapy he required surgical removal of the infected tissue losing his first two toes and part of his forefoot. With healing his mobility remained impaired and he never returned to employment. His retinopathy was stabilized using retinal laser photocoagulation to prevent blindness. Normal kidney function was not restored. Slow but progressive decline of renal function would be expected and he will eventually require dialysis. Six months after commencing therapy he was given a trial of oral hypoglycaemic tablets, but had a brisk recurrence of symptomatic hyperglycaemia and ketonuria and was restarted on insulin therapy for life.

Questions

1 Given that a number of patients with type 2 diabetes respond well to dietary restriction and/or oral hypoglycaemic agents, why was the patient started on insulin therapy?
2 How can you explain the leg ulcer in this patient?

Answers on p. 305.

CASE STUDY 15

Chest pain radiating to the left arm

Clinical features

A 53-year-old Asian man was admitted to hospital with severe crushing central chest pain, coming on at rest, which radiated to the left arm. This was associated with sweating, nausea, vomiting and breathlessness. On questioning, he had experienced similar but less severe pain for the previous month whilst walking. He had not seen a doctor for many years. He smoked 20 cigarettes a day. His father was diabetic and died from 'heart trouble' aged 48 years.

On examination he was obese, pale and sweaty. His heart rate was 100 b.p.m. and irregular. He was hypertensive (blood pressure: 170/100 mmHg).

Investigations

Investigations included those shown in Table CS15.1.

Clinical investigations included an electrocardiogram (ECG) and a chest radiograph. The ECG showed atrial fibrillation, left ventricular hypertrophy and raised ST segments in anterior chest leads. The chest radiograph showed evidence of slight cardiac enlargement and mild pulmonary oedema.

Diagnosis

The clinical history and features are suggestive of myocardial infarction (MI) preceded by a short history of angina pectoris (see Chapter 17). The diagnosis is supported by the ECG ST segment

Table CS15.1 Initial investigations performed.

Analyte	Value	Reference range
Blood		
Sodium	148 mmol/L	135–146
Potassium	4.3 mmol/L	3.5–5.0
Urea	5.7 mmol/L	2.5–6.7
Creatinine	98 µmol/L	60–120
Cholesterol	8.2 mmol/L	3.6–6.7
Fasting glucose	13.6 mmol/L	4.5–5.6
Aspartate transaminase	235 U/L	10–40
Lactate dehydrogenase	2263 U/L	240–460
Urine (dipstick tests)		
Glucose	2+*	0–trace
Protein	0	0–trace

* A 2+ glucose reading approximates to a urinary glucose of at least 28 mmol/L.

elevation in the anterior region of the heart (i.e. the left ventricle) and the raised levels of the cardiac enzymes, aspartate transaminase (AST) and lactate dehydrogenase (LDH).

Diagnosis: acute MI.

Discussion

MI defines death of myocardial tissue. It is the result of inadequate blood flow to the myocardium (myocardial ischaemia) sufficient to produce lethal cell injury. Myocardial ischaemia is most often due to thrombosis in a coronary artery, usually at a site of a previous atheromatous plaque (see Chapter 17).

Following MI, some parts of the damaged heart are unable to conduct impulses. These changes in impulse conduction can be detected on the ECG and are one basis for determining whether an infarct has occurred and its likely location. This can result in the development of abnormal heart rhythms (dysrhythmias) some of which may be life threatening.

Myocardial cell death also results in the release of intracellular enzymes into the extracellular fluid. Monitoring the serum levels of these enzymes can be useful indicators of the presence and extent of an MI. The substantial rise in the levels of the cardiac isoenzymes, LDH and AST, observed in this patient suggests significant myocardial damage. Myocardial creatinine kinase (CKMB) and troponin levels can also be measured.

The previous history of angina pectoris, due to transient myocardial ischaemia, suggests that blood flow to the myocardium may have been compromised for some time in this patient. This has produced an overall reduction in cardiac function resulting in mild cardiac failure. This is supported by enlargement of the heart and the accumulation of fluid in lungs (*pulmonary oedema*).

Treatment and prognosis

The management of a patient with an MI is in three stages. Firstly, the patient is treated with bed rest, analgesia using diamorphine and oxygen to try to reduce the myocardial ischaemia. Thrombolytic therapy (e.g. using intravenous streptokinase or

tissue plasminogen activator (tPA) to promote fibrinolysis) is also given and can reduce the size of the infarction if given early enough. In this patient the myocardial ischaemia produced an irregular rhythm and atrial fibrillation. Digoxin can revert the heart to its normal rhythm and will also improve cardiac contractility. After 48 h in bed the patient should commence mobilization and provided there are no further complications, may be discharged after 5–7 days. Rehabilitation continues over the following 6 weeks.

Secondly, it is important to identify any risk factors for MI. The patient is a smoker, has *hypercholesterolaemia* (raised blood cholesterol levels) and left ventricular hypertrophy suggesting long-standing previously undiagnosed hypertension. The elevated blood glucose level suggests mild, maturity onset diabetes mellitus (non-insulin-dependent diabetes mellitus, type 2 diabetes). Mild diabetes is frequently asymptomatic and may be present for a number of years before it is detected. The normal blood urea, sodium and potassium and absence of proteinuria (protein in the urine) suggests that the patient has not yet developed diabetic renal disease. The early death of his father from heart disease suggests an inherited risk of MI which may be the result of genetically determined hypercholesterolaemia, hypertension or diabetes. There is increasing interest in the role of high insulin levels as a risk factor for MI. In the UK Asian patients, in particular, have an increased risk of death from MI which is 40% above that of the British Caucasian population. They also have a four times greater risk of developing diabetes.

Finally, additional investigations and treatment may be necessary to prevent further MI. Most importantly, the patient must stop smoking as this is an important risk factor. An exercise test on a treadmill is also generally performed 6 weeks after MI. If further ischaemic changes develop on ECG then coronary angiography needs to be performed. If there is significant stenosis or occlusion of the coronary arteries then coronary artery bypass–graft or percutaneous coronary artery angioplasty should be considered.

The progress of most patients is monitored in an outpatient clinic. In this case, the patient had

Table CS15.2 Blood lipid profile.

Analyte	Value	Optimal value
Triglyceride	1.4 mmol/L	< 2.1
Cholesterol	7.7 mmol/L	< 5.2
High density lipoprotein cholesterol	1.2 mmol/L	> 1.0
Lipoprotein A	811 mmol/L	< 300

been clearly overweight at the time of his MI. Since then, he had seen a dietitian who had given him advice on healthy eating and suggested a reduction of his fat intake to less than 30% of his total energy intake. The patient was noted to have *corneal arcus* (deposition of lipids in the periphery of the cornea), which is often, though not always, indicative of hyperlipidaemia. A full profile of his blood lipids was performed, the results are shown in Table CS15.2.

In order to prevent further accumulation of cholesterol in his arteries the patient was prescribed a drug to lower his cholesterol levels. This drug acts as an inhibitor of a key enzyme involved in the synthesis of cholesterol by the liver. The patient was again advised to stop smoking and to take more exercise. His diabetes was successfully controlled by the administration of oral hypoglycaemic agents (sulphonylureas, see case study 14). Low dose aspirin as an antiplatelet agent (see Chapter 14) and β-blockers were also prescribed. Both of these agents have been shown to reduce the incidence of reinfarction.

Questions

1 What is the physiological basis of left ventricular hypertrophy in long-standing hypertension?
2 How do you account for the pulmonary oedema observed in this patient?

Answers on p. 306.

CASE STUDY 16

Unexpected death in a young man

Clinical features

A 32-year-old man attended his local hospital following a referral from his GP. He was complaining of a retrosternal pain that appeared suddenly at 2 a.m. while he was attending a party. He had never been seriously ill and was active in sports. He worked as a representative of an industrial company and had no other significant medical history.

Investigations

Physical examination including examination of the chest was normal. Blood pressure was 130/80 mmHg, pulse rate 70/min and regular, respiratory rate 12/min. The electrocardiogram (ECG) was normal on admission. Laboratory investigations were normal.

The patient was further suffering from some chest discomfort and was kept on observation for suspicion of a myocardial ischaemia or pericarditis, in spite of normal laboratory values. Later in the evening on the day of admission he reported a sudden increase of pain, became short of breath and was severely hypotensive. ECG showed ventricular fibrillation and flutter. Defibrillation was unsuccessful and the patient was pronounced dead at 11.35 p.m.

A postmortem examination showed the left ventricle of the heart to be thicker than normal. The pericardial sac was filled with blood. In addition, there was a tear in the wall of the ascending aorta measuring 2.5 cm in length. The rest of the aorta was normal except for some atherosclerotic plaques and fatty streaks located in both the ascending and the descending aorta. There were no other abnormal findings. Histological examination of the aortic tissues showed focal disappearance of elastic fibres and accumulation of glycosaminoglycans characteristic of cystic medial necrosis.

Diagnosis

Cystic medial necrosis of the aorta with aortic dissection and intrapericardial aortic rupture and cardiac tamponade.

Discussion

Aortic dissection is caused by a tear in the tunica intima (inner layer) of the aorta which exposes the tunica media (middle layer) to blood from the lumen of the aorta. This blood is at high pressure and the medial layer splits into two (dissection) causing a false lumen along which blood can travel. The dissection may cause obstruction to branches of the aorta as it spreads along its length, which may in turn lead to cerebral or renal ischaemia, for example. The false lumen may go on to rupture externally into the left pleural space or pericardium (as in the case patient) or internally into the true lumen of the aorta. The sudden increase in pressure on the heart as a result of the presence of blood in the pericardial sac often leads to heart failure (this type of heart failure is often referred to as cardiac tamponade).

Aortic dissection develops mostly in 40–60-year-old patients with hypertension where it apparently results from the damaging effect of high blood pressure on the aortic wall. In younger patients aortic rupture sometimes develops as a complication of Marfan's syndrome. This autosomal dominant condition is characterized by skeletal, ocular and cardiovascular manifestations and is caused by a defect in *fibrillin*, a connective tissue protein that participates in formation of elastic fibres.

In the case patient, the histology of the aortic tissues was characteristic of a degeneration of the tunica media of the aorta known as cystic medial necrosis. Cystic medial necrosis has been found in some cases of aortic rupture and aortic dissection but its role in the pathogenesis of the lesion remains uncertain, since it can be sometimes seen in elderly patients as an incidental finding without aortic rupture.

The patient also had an enlarged left ventricle, which is considered a sign of arterial hypertension.

Treatment and prognosis

Aortic dissection and aortic rupture are serious conditions that frequently lead to sudden death due to massive bleeding. Lesions in the descending aorta can be corrected by surgery. Intrapericardial rupture of the ascending aorta is almost invariably lethal due to cardiac tamponade.

Questions

1 What is the definition of 'sudden death'?
2 What are the main causes of sudden death?

Answers on p. 306.

CASE STUDY 17

Easy bruising and recurrent nose bleeds

Clinical features

A 5-year-old boy presented with a 12-month history of easy bruising and recurrent nosebleeds. He was otherwise extremely well. In his past history he had had prolonged bleeding following a tonsillectomy at the age of 3 years. On examination he looked well but had several large bruises on his upper and lower limbs. His mother had a history of life-long easy bruising and also suffered with menorrhagia (excessive menstrual bleeding). The child's 10-year-old sister was well with no history of bleeding problems.

Investigations

The results of the laboratory investigations are shown in Table CS17.1. The platelet count and the prothrombin time (PT) are normal, but the activated partial thromboplastin time (APTT) is prolonged. Factor VIII and von Willebrand factor (vWF) antigen levels are both reduced to 30%, and vWF activity levels are reduced to 2%. Other investigations included the following.

Table CS17.1 Investigations performed.

Analyte	Value	Reference range
Total white cell count	8×10^9/L	5.0–15.0
Haemoglobin	12 g/dL	12.0–14.0
Platelet count	210×10^9/L	150–400
PT	11 s	11–15
APTT	50 s	26–35
APTT 50 : 50 mix	35 s	26–35
Factor VIII	0.3 U/mL	0.5–1.5
vWF antigen	0.3 U/mL	0.5–1.5
vWF activity	0.02 U/mL	0.5–1.5

- Platelet aggregation studies—these showed absent aggregation with ristocetin.
- vWF multimer analysis—this showed loss of large molecular weight multimers (Fig. CS17.1).

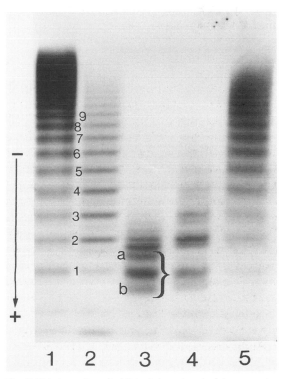

Fig. CS17.1 Autoradiograph of SDS gel electrophoresis of plasma samples on 1.2% agarose gel. Lane 1: normal plasma. Lane 2: type 2A (phenotype IID) von Willebrand disease. Lane 3: type 2A (phenotype IIA)—patient in this case study. Lane 4: type 2B (phenotype IIB). Lane 5: type 1. Note the absence of high and intermediate molecular weight bands in type 2A (phenotype IIA) together with abnormal triplet banding. Type 2A (phenotype IID) also shows aberrant multimer banding. In type 2B there is loss of the highest molecular weight multimers only. Lighter staining reflects the low levels of vWF in type 1. The bands are visualized by staining with ^{125}I-labelled monoclonal anti-vWF antibody. The direction of electrophoresis ($- \rightarrow +$) is from top to bottom.

Diagnosis

Both factor VIII and vWF antigen levels are reduced consistent with a diagnosis of von Willebrand disease. The vWF activity levels are lower than vWF antigen levels and there is absent aggregation of platelets with ristocetin. These findings together with the absence of high molecular weight multimers confirm the diagnosis of type 2A von Willebrand disease.

Differential diagnosis:
• Haemophilia A (prolonged APTT, reduced factor VIII levels, normal vWF antigen, activity and multimers, normal platelet aggregation).
• Other types of von Willebrand disease (see later for laboratory features).

Discussion

Background

Von Willebrand disease is the commonest inherited bleeding disorder and is characterized by either a quantitative or a qualitative abnormality of vWF.

vWF is a large multimeric glycoprotein synthesized in megakaryocytes in the bone marrow and in endothelial cells. It is stored in specific cellular storage granules in endothelial cells (Weibel–Palade bodies) and in platelets (α-granules), and is also present circulating in the plasma as a series of multimers of variable molecular weight. It may be measured immunologically as von Willebrand antigen, or using a biological assay to determine its functional activity.

vWF is involved in haemostasis and has several functions.
• Mediation of *platelet adhesion* to the subendothelium at sites of vascular injury, resulting in the formation of platelet thrombi (Fig. CS17.2a).
• Mediation of platelet–platelet interaction by activation of bound platelets resulting in *platelet aggregation* (Fig. CS17.2b).
• Serves as a *carrier protein* for the coagulation factor VIII preventing its degradation.

Von Willebrand disease is a heterogeneous disorder that results from a variety of genetic defects. It is often a mild disease and its true incidence is therefore not well defined. However, it is probably present in approximately 1% of the population although most affected individuals will have minimal symptoms. Males and females are equally affected, and von Willebrand disease occurs in all racial groups. It usually shows autosomal dominant inheritance, although occasional patients with autosomal recessive inheritance and severe disease are seen. It is important to note that sporadic cases can also occur.

Clinical features

Von Willebrand disease shows a mild to moderate bleeding tendency with mucocutaneous bleeding (i.e. bleeding from mucous membranes and the skin) including epistaxis, easy bruising and menorrhagia. The clinical expression, however, is extremely variable. Females with von Willebrand disease may develop iron deficiency anaemia due to menorrhagia. Rare patients with severe disease may have a clinical picture similar to haemophilia A or B with large haematoma formation and haemarthroses (joint bleeds), in addition to mucocutaneous bleeding.

A careful clinical history is important and may reveal previous episodes of bleeding, especially following minor surgery such as dental extraction that was previously overlooked. A family history must be taken and may identify symptoms in parents or siblings as in this case.

The diagnosis of von Willebrand disease is frequently missed until later in life when excessive bleeding occurs following minor surgery or dental extraction.

Classification

There are several types of von Willebrand disease and a standard classification was published in 1997.

Primary classification

• Type 1—partial quantitative deficiency of vWF. This is the commonest type and is characterized by a parallel reduction of vWF antigen and activity (~80% of cases).

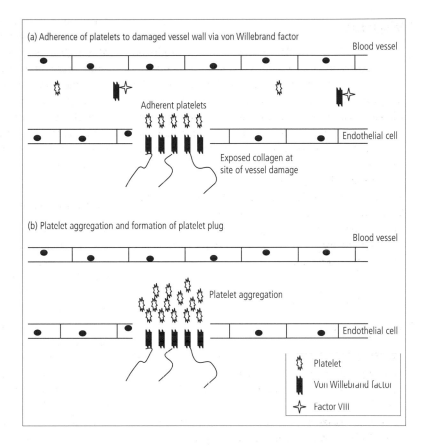

Fig. CS17.2 (a) Adherence of platelets to damaged vessel wall via vWF. (b) Platelet aggregation and formation of platelet plug.

Table CS17.2 Pattern of results in von Willebrand disease.

	Type 1	Type 2A	Type 2B	Type 3
Factor VIII	Low	Low/normal	Low/normal	Low
vWF antigen	Low	Low	Low/normal	Very low
vWF activity	Low	Very low	Low	Very low
Platelet aggregation with ristocetin	Absent	Absent	Increased	Absent
Bleeding time	Normal/prolonged	Prolonged	Prolonged	Prolonged

- Type 2—qualitative deficiency of vWF (15–20% of cases). See below and Table CS17.2.
- Type 3—virtual complete deficiency of vWF with antigen and activity levels of < 5% (rare).

Secondary classification (von Willebrand disease type 2)

- Type 2A—absence of high molecular weight multimers, with a more marked reduction in vWF activity levels than antigen levels (several subtypes).
- Type 2B—loss of high molecular weight multimers with increased binding of platelets which may lead to thrombocytopenia.
- Type 2M—qualitative deficiency as 2A but with a normal multimer pattern.
- Type 2N—decreased affinity for factor VIII resulting in accelerated clearance of unbound factor VIII

and markedly reduced factor VIII levels. This subtype is often misdiagnosed as mild haemophilia A.

Laboratory investigations

The laboratory findings in von Willebrand disease are highly variable. A routine full blood count should be performed in order to check the platelet count and to look for iron deficiency anaemia from chronic blood loss.

Coagulation screening tests (PT, APTT) may be normal especially in type 1, and therefore a normal PT and APTT should not exclude the diagnosis. If the plasma vWF level is significantly reduced however, the associated low factor VIII level may result in a prolonged APTT.

A bleeding time is not essential for diagnosis and it is especially difficult to perform in young children. It is usually prolonged but as with the screening coagulation tests may be normal.

Investigations required to diagnose von Willebrand disease and its type include the following.
• vWF antigen.
• vWF activity.
• Factor VIII coagulant levels.
• Platelet aggregation studies with ristocetin.
• Multimeric analysis.
• Factor VIII binding assay (for type 2N).

Table CS17.2 shows the pattern of results in the four main types of von Willebrand disease.

It is important to note that levels of vWF may be altered by various genetic and environmental influences. Patients with blood group O have lower levels than those with other blood groups, infection may increase levels, as does stress including that following difficulty in obtaining a blood sample. Levels also increase during pregnancy and in patients receiving oestrogen therapy. It is important that these influences are kept in mind when interpreting results. Investigations may need to be repeated if results are normal but clinical suspicion for von Willebrand disease is high.

Treatment

Some patients may not need any specific treatment.

If treatment is required, however, it is important to consider the type of von Willebrand disease, the nature of the haemostatic challenge and the patient's bleeding history.

Products available

Desmopressin/DDAVP
This synthetic vasopressin analogue stimulates release of endogenous vWF from endothelial cell stores resulting in a two- to fourfold increase in plasma levels of both vWF and factor VIII within ~30 min of an intravenous injection. It can also be given subcutaneously or intranasally.

It is usually used in patients with type 1 disease, although there will be occasional patients (< 10%) who do not respond. It is therefore usual, once the diagnosis of von Willebrand disease has been made, to conduct a therapeutic trial of DDAVP to determine an individual patient's responsiveness. Patients with type 3 disease do not usually respond and require alternative treatment. For those with type 2 disease the role of DDAVP is unclear. Some may respond and a therapeutic trial may be worthwhile. It may, however, result in worsening of thrombocytopenia in type 2B patients and generally should be avoided.

DDAVP is generally used prophylactically or therapeutically for minor bleeding and minor surgical procedures. Major surgery and life-threatening bleeds should be treated with coagulation factor concentrates.

Coagulation factor concentrates
In those patients in whom DDAVP is ineffective or contraindicated the alternative is to provide exogenous vWF from coagulation factor concentrates. These patients should be counselled about the low risk of viral transmission from blood products, and should be vaccinated against hepatitis A and B. The products available containing vWF are intermediate purity factor VIII concentrates and purified vWF concentrate, which have had virucidal treatment. These are effective in all types of von Willebrand disease, but should only be used when there are clear indications.

Tranexamic acid

This antifibrinolytic agent can be used orally, intravenously or topically for mucocutaneous bleeding, either alone or together with DDAVP or coagulation factor concentrates depending on the severity of bleeding.

Oestrogens

These may be of use in reducing menstrual bleeding.

Miscellaneous

Patients with von Willebrand disease should never use aspirin or other non-steroidal anti-inflammatory drugs that interfere with platelet function.

As von Willebrand disease is an inherited disorder all affected families should receive genetic counselling.

Questions

1 What is the significance of the correction of the APTT with normal plasma?
2 What happens during pregnancy?
3 Can von Willebrand disease be acquired?

Answers on p. 306.

CASE STUDY 18

Diarrhoea and abdominal distension

Clinical features

A 50-year-old woman presented with diarrhoea. She gave a 10-year history of intermittent diarrhoea and tiredness but symptoms had worsened considerably in the last 2 weeks. The diarrhoea was up to five times daily, described as creamy-white and associated with wind and abdominal distension. She was not on any medication.

On examination the patient was pale and her abdomen was distended. There was marked ankle swelling.

Investigations

Laboratory investigations included those shown in Table CS18.1.

Colonoscopy, gastroscopy and small bowel barium meal X-ray were all normal. A jejunal biopsy

was performed. This showed a flat mucosal surface with a total loss of villi (subtotal villous atrophy). A chronic inflammatory infiltrate was present within the lamina propria.

Table CS18.1 Investigations performed.

Analyte	Value	Reference range
Blood		
Haemoglobin	10.1 g/dL	11.5–16.5
Serum folate	0.6 µg/L	3.0–20.0
Red cell folate	84 µg/L	160–640
Vitamin B$_{12}$	255 ng/L	160–760
Ferritin	6 µg/L	15–300
Albumin	18 g/L	34–48
Thyroid-stimulating hormone	40.8 mU/L	0.4–4.0
Free thyroxine	9.8 pmol/L	9.0–24.0

Diagnosis

The histological appearance of the jejunal biopsy showed subtotal villous atrophy consistent with coeliac disease. The laboratory findings are also consistent with a malabsorption syndrome. Low serum albumin, anaemia with low folate and ferritin levels but a normal vitamin B_{12} concentration all suggest malabsorption.

Diagnosis: coeliac disease.

Discussion

Adult coeliac disease can be defined as a condition in which there is an abnormal jejunal mucosa which improves when treated with a gluten-free diet and relapses when gluten is reintroduced. The highest incidence of coeliac disease in the world is found in the west of Ireland where 1 in 300 of the population are affected. In the UK, the incidence is around 1 in 2000. There is a familial tendency which may be explained in part by the association of coeliac disease with HLA DQw2.

Coeliac disease is the result of a sensitivity to gluten which is a constituent of wheat, rye and barley. More specifically, the responsible protein is contained in the alcohol-soluble fraction of gluten, known as gliadin. The precise mechanisms of the damage to the small intestine are unknown but are thought to be due to a local immunological reaction to gliadin.

Recently, it has been proposed that there are two stages in the development of the disease. Firstly, a genetically determined state of inappropriate immunity (hypersensitivity) to gliadin is induced in local intraepithelial T lymphocytes. This does not produce overt disease until exposure to a second factor occurs. The nature of the second factor is unknown but may be sudden exposure to gliadin or to an infectious agent. Exposure to the second factor activates the damaging immunological mechanisms and disease results.

Coeliac disease primarily affects the proximal small bowel. Loss of normal villi results in a mucosa which appears flat with elongated intestinal crypts. There is often an infiltrate of inflammatory cells present within adjacent connective tissue (the *lamina propria*) and numbers of intraepithelial lymphocytes are increased.

The clinical features of coeliac disease are common to all types of malabsorption and include weight loss, weakness and diarrhoea due to fat malabsorption. The stools are pale, bulky and offensive. In addition to deficiencies of iron and folate, there may also be *hypocalcaemia* (low serum calcium concentration), due to vitamin D malabsorption which, if long standing, may result in *osteomalacia* (a decrease in calcified bone due to poor mineralization).

A number of other diseases are associated with coeliac disease including chronic liver diseases and certain endocrine abnormalities. The high thyroid-stimulating hormone (TSH) concentration in this patient is indicative of *hypothyroidism*. The thyroid deficiency was rapidly corrected by replacement therapy with thyroxine.

Recently, a serum test of antiendomysial antibodies has shown promise as a sensitive blood test for coeliac disease.

Treatment and prognosis

A gluten-free diet combined with oral folic acid and iron supplementation produced a remarkable clinical response in this patient. Within 4 months all the laboratory indices, including the serum albumin had returned to normal. Life-long dietary gluten exclusion is recommended for adult patients. Rarely, coeliac disease can be complicated by the development of intestinal lymphoma.

Questions

1 Explain the typical finding of folate and iron deficiency in coeliac disease.
2 Explain the significance of the increased concentration of TSH in hypothyroidism.

Answers on p. 306.

CASE STUDY 19

Abdominal pain and diarrhoea

Clinical features

A 46-year-old woman complained of right-sided colicky abdominal pain and diarrhoea for 6 weeks. She had lost 2 stone in weight but passed no blood in the stools. On examination, she was pale and had mouth ulceration. A tender mobile mass was felt in the lower abdomen.

Investigations

Laboratory investigations included those shown in Table CS19.1.

Examination of the colon by sigmoidoscopy and abdominal ultrasound tests were normal. A

Table CS19.1 Blood investigations.

Analyte	Value	Reference range
Total white cell count	11.9×10^9/L	4.0–11.0
Haemoglobin	9.3 g/dL	11.5–16.5
Haematocrit	0.302	0.37–0.47
Mean cell volume	73.0 fl	82–92
Mean cell haemoglobin	22.46 pg	27.0–32.0
Platelet count	400×10^9/L	150–400
Erythrocyte sedimentation rate	103 mm/h	0–12
Blood film		
White blood cell differential		
Neutrophils	76%	
Lymphocytes	17%	
Monocytes	5%	
Eosinophils	2%	
Basophils	0%	

The total leucocyte (white cell) count is slightly high, with a mild neutrophilia.
Erythrocyte morphology: microcytic (cells reduced in size) and hypochromic (staining intensity reduced). Normal erythrocytes would appear normocytic and normochromic (see Chapter 14). The erythrocyte sedimentation rate (ESR) is very high, reflecting active inflammatory disease.

small bowel barium meal X-ray showed narrowing and thickening of the distal ileum consistent with Crohn's disease.

Diagnosis

The combination of weight loss and diarrhoea over a short period of time suggests significant bowel pathology. This is supported by the iron deficiency anaemia (indicated by the low mean cell volume or MCV) and raised ESR (erythrocyte sedimentation rate). Active inflammation or malignant disease are most likely to produce these results while the normal sigmoidoscopy makes colitis unlikely. Typical Crohn's disease was shown by the small bowel barium meal X-ray. The distal ileum is the most common site of presentation.

Diagnosis: Crohn's disease.

Discussion

Each year, in most developed countries, Crohn's disease is diagnosed in approximately five people in every 100 000. The disease affects more women than men, often presents before the age of 30, and tends to occur more frequently in certain families, suggesting genetic susceptibility in some people. Typical symptoms of Crohn's disease and other inflammatory bowel disorders (notably ulcerative colitis), include colicky abdominal pain, diarrhoea, fever, weight loss and anorexia. Fistula formation is relatively common in Crohn's disease and may require surgical intervention. Changes associated with Crohn's disease may extend beyond the affected area indicated by radiography or laparotomy (exploratory abdominal surgery). Abnormalities in proximal small intestinal permeability to folic acid and sugars have been demonstrated in patients in whom disease was apparently confined to the distal ileum and colon.

It can be difficult to make a precise diagnosis in inflammatory bowel disease because the clinical features of Crohn's disease and ulcerative colitis can be similar. In both conditions, there may also be systemic complications, including iritis (inflammation of the iris), arthritis and in some long-standing cases, sclerosing cholangitis (inflammation and fibrosis of the bile ducts).

The causes of Crohn's disease (and ulcerative colitis) are as yet unknown. Recently, it has been suggested that patients born during measles epidemics are more likely to develop Crohn's disease than those who were not. There was no such association with ulcerative colitis. The significance of this finding remains to be established.

Treatment and prognosis

The patient was commenced on high dose corticosteroids. Initially there was a good response to treatment. However, 3 months later the patient returned with fever and right-sided pain. An abscess obstructing the right kidney was diagnosed and surgical resection was performed.

As with many other chronic inflammatory diseases, Crohn's disease is characterized by periods of remission and relapse. Remission is induced by high dose steroids which are then gradually reduced. Aminosalicylates are beneficial in ulcerative colitis and may be combined with corticosteroids in Crohn's disease with colonic involvement.

Inflammatory bowel disease affecting the colon is associated with an increased risk of colorectal cancer.

Questions

1 Can you explain the haematological findings?
2 How does Crohn's disease differ from ulcerative colitis?

Answers on p. 306.

Recurrent epigastric pain with abnormal liver function tests

Clinical features

A 52-year-old publican was admitted to hospital with severe epigastric pain (pain in the upper central region of the abdomen) radiating to the back. The pain had developed with increasing intensity over six to eight hours and the patient had also experienced retching and vomiting.

This patient had been seen in the Outpatient Department three months previously for investigation of recurrent epigastric pain and steatorrhoea (the passage of bulky greasy stools due to fat malabsorption). Typically the abdominal pain lasted for three to four days, was accompanied by nausea, and could be eased slightly by sitting forward. An abdominal radiograph had revealed pancreatic calcification and after further investigations a diagnosis of chronic pancreatitis had been made.

On admission to hospital the patient's blood pressure was a little high at 175 mm systolic, 95 mm diastolic. A full blood count, ESR and blood biochemistry were requested. The results are shown in Table CS20.1.

Diagnosis

The most likely cause of the acute onset of epigastric pain in this case is acute exacerbation (sudden

Table CS20.1

Analyte	Value	Reference range
Total white cell count	12.6×10^9/L	4.0–11.0
Haemoglobin (Hb)	14.2 g/dL	13.0–18.0
Haematocrit (Hct)	0.42	0.40–0.54
Mean cell volume (MCV)	100 fl	82–92
Platelet count	180×10^9/L	150–400
Erythrocyte sedimentation rate	20 mm	0–14
Blood film		
WBC differential		
Neutrophils	79%	
Lymphocytes	16%	
Monocytes	4%	
Eosinophils	1%	
Basophils	0%	
Biochemistry		
Random blood glucose	3.6 mmol/L	3.5–8.9
Total bilirubin	30 µmol/L	< 17
Aspartate aminotransferase (ASAT)	68 µ/L	10–40
Alanine aminotransferase (ALAT)	115 µ/L	5–40
Gamma glutamyltransferase (gammaGT)	190 µ/L	11–50
Serum amylase	1600 units/L	< 220

increased severity) of chronic relapsing pancreatitis. However, it is important to exclude other, unrelated, conditions for which surgery might be indicated. Damage to the exocrine pancreas results in the release of pancreatic enzymes into body fluids, so the very high serum amylase is indicative of acute pancreatitis. However, serum amylase levels also rise in perforated peptic ulcer, acute intestinal obstruction and acute biliary obstruction, but peak levels are usually less than five times the upper range of normal. In acute pancreatitis serum amylase usually increases to at least five times the upper reference range within 24 hours. Other pancreatic enzymes such as trypsin and lipase also increase in acute pancreatitis. In this case the serum amylase was approximately eight times the upper reference range.

The most common cause of pancreatitis is chronic alcohol abuse but other possible causes include hyperparathyroidism, protein calorie malnutrition and trauma. High levels of bilirubin and transaminase enzymes together with red cell macrocytosis

(see Chapter 14) indicate liver damage, again possibly due to alcohol abuse. In some cases of pancreatitis there is cholestatic jaundice, due to pressure from the swollen head of pancreas on the common bile duct, but jaundice may also be due to hepatocellular damage. Pancreatitis can also affect the endocrine pancreas, causing diabetes mellitus. In this case blood glucose was normal, indicating that diabetes mellitus had not developed.

Diagnosis: Chronic relapsing pancreatitis, with liver damage due to alcohol abuse.

Treatment and prognosis

The patient was treated conservatively with bed rest and a low fat diet and the acute condition resolved. On further direct questioning, the patient admitted to excess alcohol intake, and he was counselled to abstain. He was discharged from hospital and was eventually referred to a psychiatric clinic and to self help groups when it became apparent that he was continuing to drink heavily.

Clinical outcome and discussion

The patient continued to drink heavily, began to neglect himself and eventually lost his job. He attended his general practitioner's surgery every three months to collect a prescription for vitamins and on each occasion he would claim to be in control of his drinking. One day, the patient collapsed at home, vomited material resembling coffee grounds and an emergency admission to hospital was arranged. On admission to hospital haematemesis due to upper gastrointestinal bleeding was confirmed, and gross abdominal ascites were noted. An endoscopic examination revealed oesophageal varices. Laboratory results on this occasion are shown in Table CS20.2.

The white cell differential count revealed an absolute neutrophilia. The haemoglobin concentration and red cell count were low due to acute blood loss.

Bleeding persisted and the patient was transfused. Despite this, the haemoglobin remained low indicating continued bleeding, so blood coagulation tests were requested.

The prothrombin time was prolonged (17 seconds, normal control 13 seconds). The activated partial thromboplastin time was also prolonged (60 seconds, normal control 41 seconds). Because most coagulation factors are synthesized in the liver, these abnormalities reflect hepatocellular damage. Vitamin K and fresh frozen plasma were administered in an attempt to correct the coagulation defect and the bleeding was eventually controlled.

The patient was discharged from hospital, but he died at home 6 weeks later. At *post mortem* examination the liver was found to be enlarged to a weight

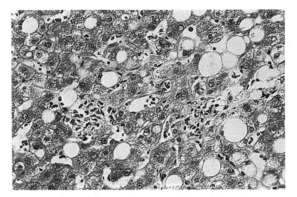

Fig. CS20.1 Typical histological appearance of alcoholic liver disease showing the 'ground glass' appearance of hepatocytes, which also contain fatty vacuoles, together with neutrophil infiltration.

of 2165 g. On slicing the liver was rather yellow coloured and greasy in texture. Histological examination showed that many of the hepatocytes were swollen and that large vacuoles were present in their cytoplasm (Fig. CS20.1). A frozen section was taken, and when stained appropriately showed that the vacuoles were full of lipid.

The liver in this patient showed the appearances of so-called 'fatty change' or steatosis. This is not a feature specifically related to alcohol abuse and can occur under the influence of numerous other agents.

Alcohol abuse accounts for substantial worldwide morbidity, causing a range of medical, psychological and sociological problems. In addition the consequences of alcohol abuse include substantial mortality from disease or trauma. Although most attention focuses on the effects of alcohol on the liver and gastrointestinal tract, there are also wide-ranging adverse effects on the central nervous and cardiovascular systems and on mental health.

Table CS20.2 Blood investigations.

Analyte	Value	Reference range (female)
Total white cell count	11.5×10^9/L	4.0–11.0
Red cell count	3.90×10^{12}/L	3.8–5.8
Haemoglobin (Hb)	9.6 g per d/L	13.0–18.0
Mean cell volume (MCV)	108 fl	82–92
Platelet count	120×10^9/L	150–400

Questions

1 What is the cause of red cell macrocytosis in liver disease?
2 Why was the prothrombin time prolonged in this patient?
3 What are the likely causes of gastrointestinal bleeding in alcoholic liver disease?

Answers on p. 307.

CASE STUDY 21

Sudden onset of severe pain in the leg

Clinical features

A 20-year-old Afro-Caribbean man with known sickle cell disease attended casualty with sudden onset of pain in his right thigh of 6 h duration. He had initially tried to control the pain with oral paracetamol but this had had little effect.

On examination, the patient was in obvious discomfort and reluctant to move his right leg. The pain was localized to the right thigh but there was nothing to see on examination. He was febrile (temperature 37.8°C) and the sclerae were yellow, indicating mild jaundice.

Investigations

Laboratory investigations included those shown in Table CS21.1.

The patient is anaemic with a high reticulocyte count indicating haemolysis (reduced red blood cell

Table CS21.1 Investigations performed.

Analyte	Value	Reference range
Blood		
Total white cell count	20.0×10^9/L	4.0–11.0
Red cell count	2.2×10^{12}/L	4.5–6.5
Haemoglobin	7.1 g/dL	13.0–18.0
Haematocrit	21.6	0.40–0.54
Mean cell volume	98.7 fl	82–92
Mean cell haemoglobin	32.3 pg	27–32
Platelets	460×10^9/L	150–400
Absolute reticulocyte count	279×10^9/L	50–100
Bilirubin	42 μmol	< 17
Alanine aminotransferase	25 IU/L	5–40
Alkaline phosphatase	70 IU/L	25–115
Urea	2.0 mmol/L	2.5–6.7
Creatinine	70 μmol/L	60–120
C-reactive protein (CRP)	20 mg/L	< 10
Blood culture	No growth	
Blood film		
White blood cell differential		
Neutrophils	86%	
Lymphocytes	4%	
Monocytes	8%	
Eosinophils	2%	
Red blood cell morphology	Sickled red cells +	
Radiology		
X-ray lumbar spine, right femur	–	No abnormality seen

survival). The blood film shows sickled red blood cells consistent with sickle cell anaemia.

There is a neutrophilia and mild thrombocytosis which can represent a response to either acute infection or inflammation. The observation that the C-reactive protein (CRP) concentration is not dramatically raised indicates that an infective cause of bone pain, such as osteomyelitis, is unlikely. The elevated bilirubin, in the absence of abnormal liver enzymes, is a typical feature of *haemolytic disorder*, due to the increased breakdown of red blood cells and consequent increased turnover of haemoglobin (see Chapter 14).

Diagnosis

The patient was known to have sickle cell disease from childhood, confirmed by haemoglobin electrophoresis showing 98% haemoglobin S (HbS) and 2% haemoglobin F (HbF). He had been relatively well during childhood apart from dactylitis (swelling and inflammation of the hands) at the age of 5 and an episode of pneumonia at the age of 16.

He presented with sudden onset of a deep-seated bony pain in his right thigh with no history of trauma. The CRP is raised but not to levels that would indicate infection. The acute onset of pain and splinting (holding the limb rigid) with no evidence of bony abnormality on X-ray is typical of an acute sickle cell crisis.

Diagnosis: acute sickle cell crisis involving the right femur.

Discussion

Sickle cell disease is one of a group of disorders classified as the haemoglobinopathies (see Chapter 14). Haemoglobin is present in solution in the red cell as a tetramer composed of two α-chains and two non-α-chains. The majority of adult haemoglobin is composed of two α- and two β-chains (HbA) with small quantities of two α- with two δ-chains (HbA$_2$) and two α- with two γ-chains (HbF). Haemoglobinopathies are of two types: (a) quantitative disorders, the thalassaemias, where there is deficient production of normal haemoglobin chains, usually due to gene deletion; and (b) qualitative disorders

such as sickle cell disease where there is production of an abnormal haemoglobin. This is usually due to a substitution in one of the codons of the genetic code giving rise to the translation of a wrong amino acid within the amino acid sequence of the haemoglobin protein. In sickle cell disease the codon for the sixth amino acid in the β-chain is changed from GAG to GUG, leading to the substitution of glutamic acid by valine (see also Chapter 19).

HbS, under conditions of reduced oxygenation, precipitates into elongated rigid polymers forming characteristic sickle cells that do not flow well through small vessels and are more adherent than normal to vascular endothelium, leading to vascular occlusion and sickle cell crises as well as chronic red cell haemolysis. This process occurs if the percentage of HbS is high in the red cells as in homozygous sickle cell anaemia (HbSS) where the patient has inherited HbS from both parents or sickle cell β-thalassaemia where the patient has inherited HbS from one parent and a non-producing haemoglobin gene from the other. Patients who have inherited only one HbS gene, and the other is normal, have sickle cell trait (the carrier state) and are totally asymptomatic with normal blood parameters.

The sickle β-haemoglobin gene is spread throughout equatorial Africa with pockets in the Mediterranean countries, the Middle East and India, and has been carried by migration to the Caribbean, America and Europe. The frequency of the carrier state is up to 20% in West Africa and 10% in Afro-Caribbeans.

Treatment and prognosis

As the vaso-occlusive event cannot be reversed, treatment of the crisis in sickle cell disease is purely symptomatic. This is centred on pain relief, usually requiring opiate analgesia, such as morphine, diamorphine or pethidine. As sickle cell patients can get easily dehydrated due to poor renal concentrating ability, intravenous fluid replacement is also given. Sickle cell crises can occur spontaneously or may be precipitated by dehydration, cold, infection and possibly stress. It is therefore important to exclude a treatable infection as the cause. Though the white blood cell count and temperature are raised, this can occur in response to tissue damage resulting from vaso-occlusion and subsequent infarction rather than to infection. The CRP result is against an infection but a chest X-ray, blood and urine culture are usually taken and the patient started on a penicillin antibiotic, such as amoxycillin. The painful crisis subsides over 4–6 days though the time course can be quite variable.

Sickle cell disease is a chronic debilitating condition with an average life expectancy in the mid-40s, though the clinical variability of the condition means that some individuals may never experience any symptoms. Usually it presents in early childhood with vaso-occlusion within the bones of the hands and feet, causing pain and swelling (dactylitis). Patients are also prone to acute splenic sequestration causing a sudden severe anaemia as their blood volume pools and sequesters within a rapidly enlarging spleen. The spleen eventually infarcts leading to hyposplenism. Repeated infections are

also common in childhood. In adulthood painful crises in long bones predominate. Other complications are vaso-occlusion of cerebral vessels leading to cerebrovascular accident (stroke), while sickling within the lung (chest syndrome) causes increasing hypoxia with a poor prognosis if not dealt with urgently. Later, repeated bone infarctions result in joint destruction while chronic organ damage occurs to lung and kidneys.

Questions

1 Why has the sickle gene predominated in equatorial Africa?
2 Why is the blood urea concentration low?
3 Why may the patient not have the severity of symptoms which would be typical for the degree of anaemia?

Answers on p. 307.

CASE STUDY 22

Rectal bleeding with diarrhoea

Clinical features

A 17-year-old girl was referred to the gastroenterology department with a 6-month history of rectal bleeding and diarrhoea. When asked about the delay in seeing a doctor she replied that her father had died when she was 6 years old from what her mother called 'bowel problems' and that she had been afraid she might have the same problem.

Details of her father's medical history showed that he had died from a metastatic colonic adenocarcinoma when only 35 years old. The postmortem report revealed that he also had multiple polypoid adenomas situated throughout the entire length of his colon.

Previous family history revealed that the patient's brother had died from a rare form of liver cell cancer, known as *hepatoblastoma*, when only 5 years old.

Investigations

The results of laboratory investigations performed are shown in Table CS22.1.

The total white cell count is towards the upper limit of normal. The differential white cell count is normal.

Erythrocyte morphology showed microcytic (cells reduced in size) and hypochromic (staining intensity reduced) red blood cells. Normal erythrocytes

Table CS22.1 Laboratory investigations.

Analyte	Value	Reference range (female)
Total white cell count	10.6×10^9/L	4.0–11.0
Red cell count	3.46×10^{12}/L	3.8–5.8
Haemoglobin	7.6 g/dL	11.5–16.5
Haematocrit	0.244	0.37–0.47
Mean cell volume	70.5 fl	82–92
Mean cell haemoglobin	21.96 pg	27.0–32.0
Platelet count	460×10^9/L	150–400
Blood film		
White blood cell differential		
Neutrophils	70%	
Lymphocytes	22%	
Monocytes	6%	
Eosinophils	2%	
Basophils	0%	

would appear normocytic and normochromic (see Chapter 14).

The blood count results indicate iron deficiency anaemia. Iron deficiency can arise due to dietary deficiency, malabsorption or chronic blood loss (see Chapter 14). In this case, in view of the clinical history and presentation, the most likely cause is chronic rectal blood loss.

Chronic rectal bleeding and diarrhoea may be due to a number of inflammatory conditions of the colon, including ulcerative colitis and Crohn's disease (see case study 19), or may have an infective cause. Examination of the colon and rectum by sigmoidoscopy is therefore indicated. On sigmoidoscopy, multiple polyps were observed throughout the patient's colon and rectum, some of which were biopsied. Histological examination of these polyps revealed that these were benign tumours of colonic epithelial cells (*adenomas*). Microbiological culture of the stools was negative.

Diagnosis

The presence of multiple polypoid adenomas in the colon indicates a diagnosis of *familial adenomatous polyposis* (FAP). This is consistent with the early

onset of colonic adenocarcinoma in the patient's father which had presumably arisen in at least one of the multiple adenomas situated throughout his colon (see also case study 34).

Diagnosis: FAP.

Discussion

FAP is an autosomal dominant condition, therefore any offspring of an affected parent have a 50% risk of developing the disease. FAP can now be traced to germline mutations of the *APC* gene. Hepatoblastoma is a relatively rare childhood tumour but is often found in association with FAP. A diagnosis of FAP in the deceased boy is therefore highly likely. The genetic basis of FAP is discussed in detail in Chapter 19.

Screening of children in FAP families begins at the age when polyps start to develop (i.e. usually in the mid-teens). The three ways in which screening can be carried out are as follows.

• Annual clinical investigations from mid-teens until mid-40s. This involves inspection of the colon by sigmoidoscopy and eye examination. Approximately 90% of FAP patients have lesions in their eye known as *congenital hypertrophy of the retinal pigment epithelium* (CHRPE). These lesions, if present in affected members of a family, are good markers of gene carriers. Patients generally accept eye examination better than sigmoidoscopy (although sigmoidoscopy is still necessary once a patient is identified by eye examination).

• Linkage analysis using microsatellite markers, e.g. dinucleotide repeats around the FAP gene locus can be carried out in suitable families. This can be used to identify those at highest risk, who can then be screened annually as above. Those individuals identified to be at low risk by RFLP analysis (see Chapter 19) may still need to be screened occasionally by sigmoidoscopy as the technique can produce false negative results.

• Finally, it may be possible and more preferable to identify the specific mutation in an affected family member. At-risk family members can then be screened for the presence of this mutation. The detection of mutations in this way is more accurate than microsatellite analysis.

A mutation in exon 15 of the *FAP* gene at codon 1309 was identified in the patient described above. This mutation is the most common in FAP families, occurring in about 10% of families worldwide and would be the first to be tested for in any new family.

A full pedigree of the case family revealed that there were two younger male siblings, aged 14 and 11, both of whom are at a 50% risk of developing the disease. The mutation was not found in the 14-year-old sibling so further screening was not necessary in his case. The 11-year-old brother was too young to be screened since there was no evidence of a particularly early onset of the disease in this family. Testing would be offered to the younger boy in 2–3 years time unless requested earlier by the family, or if symptoms appeared.

Treatment and prognosis

Since it is certain that one of the adenomas in affected individuals will become malignant, treatment is by removal of the colon. The prognosis for patients who have had this type of surgery at an early stage is relatively good. However, regular investigations to check for the presence of any further polyps developing in the remains of the rectal tissue or in the upper gastrointestinal tract are essential.

Questions

1 What is the likely diagnosis in a family showing a history of colonic cancer in which affected members develop right-sided tumours at around 40–50 years of age without any prior evidence of adenomas?
2 Can you explain the basis of the iron deficiency anaemia observed in this patient?

Answers on p. 308.

CASE STUDY 23

Heart murmur and cleft palate

Clinical features

A 10-day-old baby boy with cleft palate and a cardiac murmur required assisted ventilation. Several hours later he developed twitching, neuromuscular irritability and convulsions.

Investigations

Laboratory investigations revealed a plasma calcium level of 1.6 mmol/L (reference range: 2.2–2.6). Values for all other analytes measured were within normal reference ranges.

Investigation at a regional paediatric cardio-thoracic centre by echocardiography revealed obstructive lesions of the left (pulmonary) outflow tract together with a ventral septal defect (VSD).

A clinical geneticist reviewing the case noted that the facial features were slightly *dysmorphic* (mis-shapen). Inner canthi were slightly displaced and the palpebral fissures were short. The root and bridge of the nose were noted to be wide and prominent. The mouth was relatively small. The ears were low set and posteriorly rotated. Deficient upper helices together with an increase in anteroposterior diameter gave a relatively circular shape to the ear. Previous family history revealed that a half-sibling from the father's previous marriage had died from cardiac failure within 5 weeks of birth. A postmortem examination had revealed the presence of congenital heart defects together with *hypoplastic* (underdeveloped) thymus and parathyroid glands. Further questioning of the family also revealed that the patient's father had

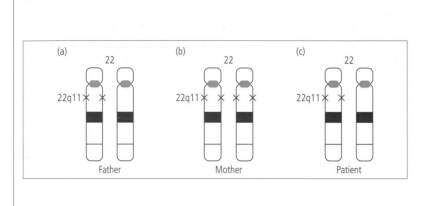

Fig. CS23.1 Fluorescence *in situ* hybridization (FISH) analysis of chromosomes from the case family. (a) Father's chromosome 22 pair. Fluorescent dye-labelled probe to a region within the DiGeorge commonly deleted region (DGCR) hybridizes (shown as star) to one chromosome 22 only. (b) Mother's chromosome 22 pair. Hybridization of probe to both chromosomes. (c) Patient's chromosome 22 pair. The probe only hybridizes to one chromosome 22. These results suggest that the patient and his father have a deletion of the DGCR on one copy of chromosome 22. The mother is deletion negative.

learning problems at school and a repaired cleft palate.

Blood samples were taken from the patient and his parents for chromosome analysis. No abnormalities were detected on conventional cytogenetic analysis using banding techniques (see Chapter 20).

Fluorescence *in situ* hybridization (FISH) analysis of the patient's chromosomes using a probe specific to certain regions of chromosome 22 (Fig. CS23.1 and Plate CS23.1, facing p. 276) revealed a submicroscopic deletion on one copy of chromosome 22 at band q11. This region encompasses the so-called *DiGeorge commonly deleted region (DGCR)* (Fig. CS23.2). The same abnormality was also present in the father's case, but the mother's chromosomes were normal.

Further laboratory investigations revealed reduced numbers of circulating T lymphocytes. A chest radiograph failed to show any conclusive evidence of thymus gland hypoplasia.

Diagnosis

The association of congenital cardiac defect, dysmorphic facies, thymus gland hypoplasia, cleft palate and *hypocalcaemia* (reduced serum calcium levels), together with a microdeletion of chromosome 22 at q11 suggests a diagnosis of DiGeorge syndrome. The FISH results show that the patient has inherited the chromosome abnormality from his father (Fig. CS23.3).

Diagnosis: DiGeorge syndrome.

Discussion

DiGeorge syndrome comprises thymus and parathyroid gland hypoplasia, hypocalcaemia, cardiac

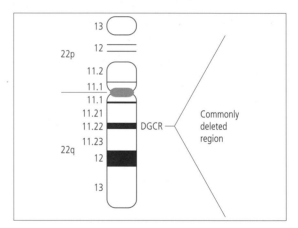

Fig. CS23.2 DiGeorge syndrome is characterized by deletions of chromosome 22 within subband 22q11. The DiGeorge commonly deleted region (DGCR) spans approximately 2 megabases of DNA.

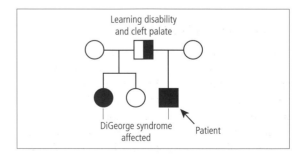

Fig. CS23.3 Family pedigree of case family.

outflow tract defects, and dysmorphic facies. It is almost invariably associated with an interstitial microdeletion of chromosome 22 encompassing the DGCR which comprises about 2 megabases of DNA. The hypocalcaemia seen in DiGeorge syndrome is due to an underdeveloped parathyroid gland which produces less than normal levels of parathyroid hormone (parathyroid hormone increases serum calcium levels). Clinically, hypocalcaemia manifests as neuromuscular irritability and convulsions.

DiGeorge syndrome is now thought to be at the severe end of a spectrum of overlapping clinical disorders associated with the same deletion. *Conotruncal anomaly face syndrome* (dysmorphic facial appearance and cardiac outflow defects) and *velocardiofacial syndrome* (VCFS) (cleft palate, cardiac anomalies and characteristic facial appearance) show a deletion within 22q11 in most cases. All three syndromes show considerable phenotypic overlap and variability even within a single family. The acronym CATCH-22 (cardiac defects; abnormal facies; thymic hypoplasia; cleft palate; hypocalcaemia) has been coined as an umbrella term for this overlapping group of syndromes.

Some surveys have suggested that as many as 25% of DiGeorge/VCFS deletions may be familial —that is, the deletion is present in one or other parent. Anecdotal evidence now suggests a more conservative estimate of 5–10%.

A great deal of effort is currently being expended to unravel the molecular basis of these conditions and to identify the relevant gene or genes. A better understanding of the molecular basis of the disease will allow more accurate diagnosis and prognosis and ultimately pave the way for gene therapy.

Treatment and prognosis

Convulsions are controlled by administering 2.5% calcium gluconate in a 5% glucose solution which is given intravenously until the convulsions cease. It is important to monitor heart rate during treatment since *bradycardia* (a decreased heart rate, usually defined as less than 60 b.p.m.) may develop. From then on, calcium gluconate is added to feeds until the serum calcium concentration rises to normal.

Any congenital heart defects will require surgery in an appropriate unit.

In one recent study, 24 children with DiGeorge syndrome were assessed during the first few weeks after diagnosis. All the patients studied had a cardiac defect. Thirteen of the 24 children died during the period of study, 11 as a consequence of their cardiac defect and two as a result of infection secondary to severe immunodeficiency. It should be noted that thymus gland hypoplasia in DiGeorge syndrome, whilst resulting in underproduction of T lymphocytes, does not normally produce a life-threatening immunodeficiency (see also Chapter 12). However, common infections may occur frequently up to 2–3 years of age which is then often followed by a spontaneous improvement.

Moderate to severe developmental delay may be expected to occur in approximately half of all patients with DiGeorge syndrome who survive beyond infancy. Symptoms of deafness may be present in older children and this should be confirmed by formal testing.

Genetic counselling of parents of children with DiGeorge syndrome depends on whether a parent has the deletion. When one parent has the deletion the risk of any offspring being affected is 50%.

The value of FISH in the diagnosis of chromosome abnormalities is well illustrated in this case. FISH may also be useful in the prenatal diagnosis of DiGeorge syndrome. Screening for microdeletions of 22q11 using FISH has been successfully accomplished on cells from chorionic villus samples at 11–12 weeks of pregnancy. Counselling for this approach may still present clinical and ethical dilemmas because of the phenotypic variability that is seen in affected individuals.

Questions

1 Why do you think the patient is more severely affected than his father?
2 Does the risk of having affected offspring increase or decrease in a man or woman who is a known deletion carrier who has two 'normal' (i.e. deletion-negative) offspring?

Answers on p. 308.

Seizures, aggressive behaviour; Rett syndrome—affected sister

Clinical features

The index patient was an 8-year-old girl with non-specific mental retardation, seizures and aggressive behaviour. She was small for her age. She was referred for cytogenetic analysis coincidentally as part of a study of Rett syndrome patients. Rett syndrome is a progressive neurological disorder, limited to females, characterized by psychomotor deterioration and specific behavioural traits notably stereotypical hand movements, e.g. hand-wringing. The molecular basis for the disorder is not yet known.

Her older sister had been diagnosed with Rett syndrome and a cytogenetic survey was being conducted on all such patients and their first-degree relatives (parents and siblings).

Investigations

Examination of the index patient revealed an apparent subtle deletion of the tip of the short arm of one copy of chromosome 1. This deletion is shown diagrammatically in Fig. CS24.1. Although the loss of material appeared to be consistent, the small size of the deletion, at the limit resolution of the light microscope, did not allow the possibility that the patient had a balanced rearrangement involving this region to be excluded. Fluorescence *in situ* hybridization (FISH) studies were performed with the probe p1.79 (D1Z2), which maps to the tip of the short arm of chromosome 1 at 1p36.3 together with a control probe, puc 1.77 (D1Z1), which hybridizes to the heterochromatic variable region just below the centromere of chromosome 1 (Fig. CS24.1). This probe was cohybridized to metaphase spreads to allow unequivocal identification of chromosome 1 and to allow short arm/long arm identification. The FISH results in the index patient and her mother are shown in Plates CS24.1 and CS24.2 (facing p. 276). Identical results to those seen in the mother were seen in the father and the Rett syndrome affected sister. Both parents and the sister had apparently normal chromosomes as judged by G-banded analysis.

Diagnosis

The index patient had a terminal deletion of the tip of the short arm of chromosome 1. Her karyotype may be written as 46,XX, del(1) (p36.3) *de novo*. There are now reports in the literature of more than 20 cases with simple deletions of 1p. Careful comparison of their phenotypes reveals that they tend to share common clinical features. This deletion therefore appears to be syndromic, i.e. the individuals with the deletion tend to share certain features (see Chapter 20). Clinical features associated with this particular deletion include (percentage of patients affected in brackets): large anterior fontanelle

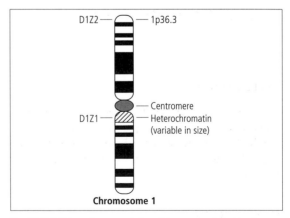

Fig. CS24.1 Schematic representation of chromosome 1 showing the position of the heterochromatic variable region just below the centromere, and the regions recognized by the FISH probes used in this case (see text).

(100%), *moderate to severe mental retardation* (92%), *growth delay* (85%), eye/vision problems (75%), hearing deficits (56%), *abusive/aggressive behaviour* (56%) and deep-set eyes (50%). The features in italic are known to be present in the index patient.

Discussion

This case study illustrates the power of FISH to detect the presence of a subtle chromosome abnormality and to distinguish between this patient from her chromosomally normal sister diagnosed with Rett syndrome.

FISH confirmed the presence of a suspected deletion but more importantly:

• Excluded the possibility that the deleted material had been translocated elsewhere in the karyotype, thus confirming that there was chromosomal imbalance.

• Confirmed that the abnormality was not present in either parent or her sister in balanced or unbalanced form.

These two observations clearly have clinical consequences. The most important of which is that the clinician can assign some if not all of the child's clinical problems to the presence of the deletion. Many parents in such a situation find it helpful to have a reason for the problem. The case may represent an example of a new contiguous gene disorder with a number of genes in close proximity within the deleted region. Variability in the size of the deletion may account for some of the differences in phenotype seen in this group of patients. Support for this idea is provided by recent studies at the molecular level, which show that size of deletions is variable.

Questions

1 If the deleted 1p had been found in apparently unbalanced form in one or other parent, what further tests might have been performed?
2 From which parent was the *de novo* deleted chromosome 1 most likely to have been inherited? What tests could be performed to try to confirm your answer?

Answers on p. 308.

CASE STUDY 25

Recurrent miscarriage

Clinical features

A 36-year-old woman and her 28-year-old husband had been attempting to conceive for 5 years. She had experienced four miscarriages, three were first trimester and the longest gestational period was 14 weeks.

Investigations

The cause of recurrent miscarriage can be very difficult to determine. The first step in investigation is a detailed personal and family history. Exclusion of anatomical disorders, such as uterine malformation, is important. Endocrine factors such as inadequate luteal function and polycystic ovary disease should be considered. Immunological causes are autoimmune disease and antiphospholipid syndrome. There are a variety of other factors, such as cervical incompetence and fibroids, which may or may not be associated with the problem.

A range of obstetric investigations at local hospitals had revealed no problems in this couple; a visit to a specialist infertility centre resulted in blood

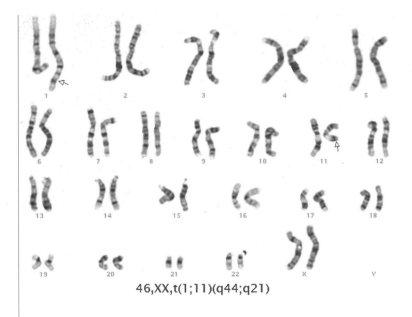

46,XX,t(1;11)(q44;q21)

Fig. CS25.1 Karyotype of the 36-year-old female showing a balanced translocation involving chromosomes 1 and 11.

samples being sent for chromosome analysis. The male partner's karyotype was normal but the female was shown to be carrying an apparently balanced reciprocal translocation of material between the long arm of chromosome 1 and the long arm of chromosome 11.

Diagnosis

Cytogenetic analysis revealed the karyotype: 46,XX t(1;11)(q44;q21). This indicated a female karyotype with an apparently balanced reciprocal translocation between the distal long arm of chromosome 1 and the long arm of chromosome 11 (Figs CS25.1 and CS25.2). This is consistent with recurrent miscarriage due to formation of unbalanced products of the translocation.

Although it is likely that the unbalanced products will lead to fetal loss, there is an associated risk of an abnormal live born child with mental or physical abnormality coming to term. An empirical estimate of this risk is between 1 in 20 and 1 in 100; a family study may help to define the figure more accurately and to identify other family members who may carry the translocation.

However, if the translocation is the only factor affecting the fetal loss, then this couple does have

the potential to establish a successful pregnancy with a normal or balanced chromosome complement. Any established pregnancy could be monitored by prenatal diagnosis. The patients would benefit from referral for genetic counselling, where the comparative risks associated with this translocation could be discussed and a family study instigated.

Diagnosis: balanced translocation involving chromosomes 1 and 11.

Discussion

Chromosome abnormality is a very common reason for fetal loss; it is thought that 50–60% of early miscarriage is due to this cause. However, these are normally sporadic events associated with errors in gametogenesis and do not recur. For a small number of couples who have had two or more miscarriages, a balanced chromosome rearrangement leads to a high frequency of pregnancy loss. These rearrangements, which include translocation of material between two or more chromosomes or inversion of material within a chromosome, do not affect the health or phenotype of the carrier in any way other than their reproductive fitness, since the number of genes present is not affected. When the

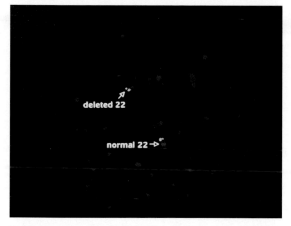

Plate CS23.1 Metaphase spread demonstrating the use of fluorescence *in situ* hybridization (FISH) for the detection of a microdeletion within 22q11.

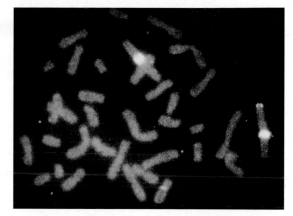

Plate CS24.1 Metaphase spread of the index patient demonstrating the FISH detection of a microdeletion within 1p36. The control probe DIZ1 hybridizes to the region just below the centromere on both copies of chromosome 1. However, the DIZ2 probe (which identifies 1p36 at the tip of chromosome 1) does not hybridize to one copy.

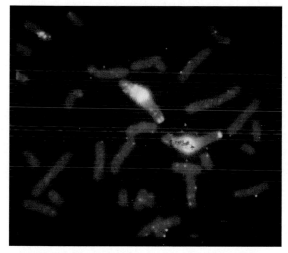

Plate CS24.2 Metaphase spread of the mother of the index patient using the same probes as in Plate CS24.1. Again, the DIZ1 probe recognises both copies of chromosome 1. However, the DIZ2 probe hybridizes to the tips of both copies, indicating that no deletion is present.

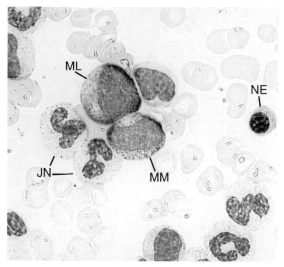

Plate CS29.1 Photomicrograph of a blood film from a patient with chronic myeloid leukaemia. The majority of cells are normal non-nucleated red blood cells with some platelets scattered in between. The large nucleated cells are myelocytes (ML), metamyelocytes (MM) and juvenile neutrophils (JN). A nucleated erythrocyte precursor (NE) is also present.

[Facing p. 276]

46,XX,t(1;11)(q44;q21)

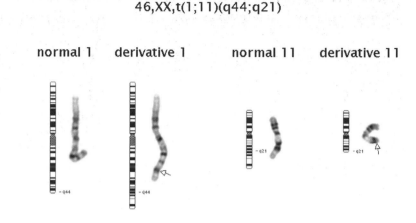

normal 1   derivative 1   normal 11   derivative 11

Fig. CS25.2 Karyotype of the 36-year-old female showing normal copies of chromosome 1 and 11 and the two derivative chromosomes 1 and 11 (derived from the translocation).

meiotic reduction division occurs to produce sperm or ova with a haploid karyotype in a translocation carrier, some gametes will inherit only one of the translocated chromosomes without its reciprocal partner, so resulting in chromosome imbalance in those gametes. Depending on the type and degree of imbalance, the resulting conception may abort or develop into a live born child with physical and mental abnormalities More rarely, a balanced familial translocation is detected by the birth of an abnormal child rather than by recurrent miscarriage.

Treatment and prognosis

To some extent, the likelihood of lethality of the imbalance or the expected prognosis for a live born child can be predicted by knowledge of the chromosomal regions involved and by a family study of carriers. This is why a referral for genetic counselling is important following diagnosis; pre-natal fetal chromosome analysis should only be

considered if there is a significant risk of a live born abnormal child as no established pregnancy should be put at risk by that test unnecessarily. For most couples, an explanation for their recurrent mis-carriages is a positive event, particularly if the diagnosis does not exclude the possibility of a successful pregnancy. Identification of carrier status can also help a couple to decide on whether assisted reproduction techniques, such as sperm or ovum donation, might be appropriate.

Questions

1 Fertility problems affect around 1 in 10 couples attempting to conceive. At what stage should chromosome analysis be considered?

2 How would we know for certain that carrier status of a balanced reciprocal translocation in a patient experiencing recurrent miscarriage was not a coincidental finding?

Answers on p. 308.

Neonate with dysmorphic features and high-pitched cry

Clinical features

A female baby was observed at birth to have dysmorphic (misshapen) features comprising downward slanting palpebral fissures, wide and depressed nasal bridge, hypertelorism (wide-set eyes), slight micrognathia (receding chin), low-set ears, short neck and high-arched palate. The birth was normal and American Pediatric Gross Assessment Record (APGAR) scores were 8 and 10 at 1 and 5 min. The only other physical features were mild jaundice and anteriorly placed anus, but the child also had a very distinctive high-pitched, piercing cry, reminiscent of a mewling kitten.

The baby was discharged and at a review appointment 3 weeks later was feeding well and thriving. The jaundice had resolved and she could fix objects and follow movement. The high-pitched cry was still pronounced; her head circumference was noted to be small, lying on the 25th centile against her weight and length, which were on the 91st centile. Cardiovascular, respiratory and abdominal examinations were unremarkable. There was a patent soft fontanelle and normal Moro and palmar grasp reflexes.

Investigations

In view of the dysmorphic features and unusual cry, blood samples were taken for chromosomes, electrolytes and calcium investigations. The two latter investigations were within normal ranges (Table CS26.1) but the chromosome analysis showed a deletion of part of the short arm of chromosome 5 (Fig. CS26.1).

Diagnosis

The cytogenetic analysis showed the karyotype:

Table CS26.1 Blood biochemistry.

Analyte	Value	Reference range
Sodium	137 mmol/L	135–146
Potassium	4.7 mmol/L	3.5–5.0
Bicarbonate	23 mmol/L	22–30
Calcium	2.53 mmol/L	2.20–2.67

46,XX,del(5)(p14). This indicates a female karyotype with a deletion of the distal region of the short arm of chromosome 5, between band p14 and the telomere. *In situ* hybridization with a gene probe specific for the locus D5S23, critical for the cri-du-chat syndrome, showed deletion of the p15.2 region, confirming a diagnosis of cri-du-chat syndrome. Parental karyotypes should be investigated at some stage to exclude a balanced familial situation. The family may benefit from referral for genetic counselling. The karyotype is illustrated in Figs CS26.1 and CS26.2.

Diagnosis: cri-du-chat syndrome.

Discussion

As the name implies, cri-du-chat syndrome is characterized by a high-pitched, shrill cry in infancy, caused by hypertrophy of the larynx. The cry is monotone and almost an octave higher than normal; its resemblance to the mewing of a kitten is striking and in itself can suggest the diagnosis. The syndrome was first described in 1963 and was one of the earliest clinical syndromes to be associated with a structural chromosome abnormality. It is one of the more common chromosome deletion syndromes with an estimated incidence of 1 in 50 000 births. As well as the cat-like cry, the infantile craniofacial dysmorphism is also very suggestive of the

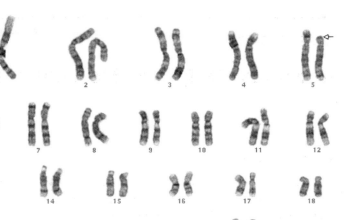

46,XX,del(5)(p14)

Fig. CS26.1 Karyotype of the patient showing deletion of part of one copy of chromosome 5.

46,XX,del(5)(p14)

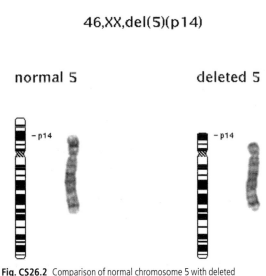

normal 5

deleted 5

Fig. CS26.2 Comparison of normal chromosome 5 with deleted chromosome 5 showing the location of the deleted region.

syndrome. The small head circumference, the wide apart and deep-set eyes, broad flat nasal bridge and slightly receding chin give a characteristic moon-like face.

It has been known for many years that not all deletions of the short arm of chromosome 5 give rise to cri-du-chat syndrome. Deletions in this region have been associated with varying clinical phenotypes, from severe mental retardation and dysmor-phism to clinically normal phenotypes, suggesting a critical region specific for the syndrome. Molecular and phenotypic mapping of short arm 5 deletions has allowed delineation of this critical region to within band 5p15.2. The size of this region is around 2 megabases of DNA, which could code for between two and 40 genes. A gene probe for the D5S23 locus can be used with the *in situ* hybridization technique to assess likely prognosis in short arm 5 deletion cases.

Treatment and prognosis

Malformations are relatively rare in this syndrome and life expectancy is generally not reduced. However, the prognosis for affected individuals is poor, as mental deficiency is mostly severe, with some patients having an IQ less than 25 and not attaining language or motor skills. The characteristic dys-morphism of infancy is lost with age and the face becomes thin. The cat cry disappears quite rapidly, sometimes within weeks of birth. Parental chromosomes should be investigated as a small proportion of cases are due to unbalanced forms of balanced inherited rearrangements; in these cases, there is an approximately 10% risk of recurrence for future pregnancies compared to the negligible risk of recurrence associated with the *de novo* cases. The families are usually offered genetic counselling as the diagnosis can be a traumatic event and they have many questions to be answered. Affected children are monitored closely and regularly by paediatricians for developmental assessment.

Questions

1 When would it be particularly useful to apply the D5S23 locus probe to a detected case of short arm 5 deletion?
2 Would the expected prognosis be the same for all cases of cri-du-chat syndrome?

Answers on p. 309.

CASE STUDY 27

Meconium ileus in a newborn

Clinical features

A newborn female baby had meconium ileus, indicated by distended abdomen and detected by X-ray. The meconium was passed naturally after 34 h.

Investigations

A sweat sample was tested in the biochemistry laboratory for sodium and chloride electrolytes. Any value below 50 mmol/L for both these ions is considered to fall within the normal range. If concentrations of approximately 50 mmol/L are detected this is an equivocal result and the test is repeated. For this patient, tests detected concentrations of 110 mmol/L of these ions. These elevated values required further investigations.

A blood sample was sent to the molecular genetics laboratory where DNA was extracted from the sample, which was then tested for the presence of 12 common cystic fibrosis (CF) mutations. Molecular analysis showed that the child was a compound heterozygote for the $^\Delta$F508 and 621 + 1 G > T mutations.

Diagnosis

Following birth, a delay in passage of meconium of between 24 and 36 h, is one of the earliest clinical symptoms of CF and is observed in around 10% of CF patients. Elevated values of sodium and chloride ions in sweat are diagnostic of CF, however, a false negative result can be obtained from this test for some genotypes.

In this case the diagnosis of CF is confirmed by the detection of two known CF mutations.

Discussion

CF is one of the most common autosomal recessive conditions, with an average carrier frequency of approximately 1 in 20 and incidence of 1 in 2500 for North European Caucasian populations. The disease is much less common in some ethnic populations. Confirmation of the condition can be provided by genetic tests. Currently there are over 800 known mutations in the CF transmembrane conductance regulator (*CFTR*) gene that are linked with CF. Many of these mutations are specific (known as 'private' mutations) to one family, however, others are much more common. The $^\Delta$F508 CF mutation accounts for 75% of all CF mutations seen in the UK. Genetics laboratories routinely test for the presence of the most common mutations. One such test directly detects the presence of 12 common mutations, these together account for 85% of mutations found in North European Caucasians.

This child's parents were tested to confirm their CF carrier status. The mother was found to be heterozygous for the ^ΔF508 CF mutation, the father was confirmed as the carrier of the 621 + 1 G > T mutation. Referral of the family to the clinical genetics unit for counselling and appropriate family studies followed. This couple was advised that prenatal testing is an option to consider in any future pregnancy. The genetics unit also counselled appropriate family members about the availability and implications of CF carrier status testing in a cascade screening programme.

In this case (see pedigree of this family; Fig. CS27.1) the father of the case patient has a brother (shown as individual number 4) who is a possible carrier of the familial 621 + 1 G > T CF mutation. The brother's partner (5) has no family history of CF, but was found to be 9 weeks pregnant. Hence, the couple (individuals 4 and 5) were referred to the molecular genetics laboratory for urgent screening of CF mutations. Individual number 4 was found not to carry the familial mutation, or any of the other 11 most common mutations. This reduces his risk of being a carrier of CF to approximately 0.4%. However, individual number 5 was found to be a carrier of the ^ΔF508 mutation, despite having no family history of the condition. The risk of the unborn child being affected is therefore very low, but the risk of its being a carrier is approximately 50%. In view of these results the relevant family

members of individual number 5 can also be screened for CF mutations if required.

Cascade screening enables identification of at-risk couples and if appropriate prenatal diagnosis can be offered. Future preimplantation technology will almost certainly be able to offer at-risk couples access to tests that will allow them to have an unaffected fetus without having to contemplate termination, which to some couples is ethically or culturally unacceptable.

Treatment and prognosis

Pancreatic ducts that deliver digestive enzymes to the intestine become occluded in CF and this causes malabsorption of fats and fat-soluble vitamins, and also occasionally results in diabetes. This can be treated by oral ingestion of supplementary digestive enzymes taken with food. Due to the pancreatic insufficiency associated with CF, a high calorie diet and extra vitamins must be used actively to maintain growth of the patient.

CF is characterized by abnormally thick mucus on epithelia lining the respiratory tract. Bronchioles and bronchial tubes often become obstructed. Patients are prone to recurring bacterial infections and hence long-term damage. Management of lung involvement is by chest percussion and postural drainage which aid mucus clearance. Antibiotics can be used to control bacterial infection. Oral steroids can be taken for severe symptoms, but are associated with side-effects. Inhaled steroids have been shown to have anti-inflammatory effects but with fewer side-effects. Trials of non-steroidal anti-inflammatory drugs (NSAIDs) are ongoing but are not currently used routinely as dosage and safety information is being compiled. Patients with end-stage lung disease may be considered for a heart–lung transplant.

Infertility is observed in approximately 95% of males due to blockage of the vas deferens and subfertility is often seen in females. Fertility treatment is available, but counselling prior to this should be considered. Some males with CF may be only mildly affected and their only physical symptom is congenital bilateral absence of the vas deferens (CBAVD). This mild phenotype is associated with rare mutations in the *CFTR* gene.

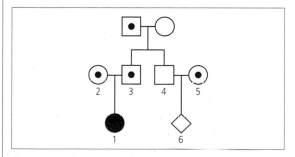

Fig. CS27.1 Pedigree analysis of the CF patient and her family. The affected female is represented as a closed circle (1). The child's mother (2) was a carrier of the ^ΔF508 mutation, and the child's father (3) was a carrier of the 621 + 1 G > T mutation. Screening of the father's brother (4) and his female partner (5) revealed that only the female partner was a carrier. Their unborn child (6) has a 50% risk of being a carrier.

A very small percentage of patients have liver involvement since plugging of small bile ducts can occur. Such patients will need to attend liver clinics for appropriate monitoring and treatment.

The prognosis for individuals born with CF has improved greatly over the last 30 years. Early diagnosis and a better understanding of the condition result in less lung tissue damage. Currently, patients born in the 1990s have a median life expectancy of 40 years. The prognosis for individuals will almost certainly continue to improve, as the underlying cause of the condition becomes better understood.

Clinical trials underway include gene therapy that involves delivery of intact wild-type *CFTR* gene to the affected tissues. As yet these trials have failed to fulfil their potential. Despite this, gene therapy remains a promising tool for the future treatment of CF.

Deoxyribonuclease has been shown to reduce the viscosity of sputum successfully. However, it is not presently available to those under 5 years of age.

Questions

1 Why are elevated levels of the electrolytes, sodium and chloride, diagnostic of CF?
2 What screening strategies other than the cascade model have been proposed for the detection of carriers of CF mutations?

Answers on p. 309.

Back pain, lethargy and weight loss

Clinical features

A 56-year-old woman attended her routine clinic appointment at the breast unit of her local hospital. Three years ago, following a mammogram performed as part of the national screening programme, she had undergone surgery to remove a primary breast cancer. On this occasion, she complained of increasing lower back pain associated with general lethargy. The doctor examining her found an enlarged lymph gland in the axilla on the same side as her previous breast surgery and tenderness over the lumbar spine.

Investigations

The results of the laboratory investigations performed are shown in Table CS28.1. They show a mild normocytic normochromic anaemia. The

Table CS28.1 Laboratory investigations.

Analyte	Value	Reference range
Blood		
Haemoglobin	10.0 g/dL	11.5–16.5
Haematocrit	0.31	0.37–0.47
Mean cell volume	88.4 fl	82–92
Mean cell haemoglobin	27.2 pg	27.0–32.0
Total white cell count	7.3×10^9/L	4.0–11.0
Platelet count	163×10^9/L	150–400
Albumin	32 g/L	34–48
Calcium (total)	2.74 mmol/L	2.20–2.67
Phosphate	1.25 mmol/L	0.8–1.5
Alkaline phosphatase	182 U/L	25–115
Serum bilirubin	15.4 mmol/L	< 17
Alanine aminotransferase	48 U/L	5–40
Total protein	62 g/L	62–80

elevated alkaline phosphatase and calcium reflect significant bone resorption. The abnormal liver blood tests raised the suspicion of liver metastases.

A fine-needle aspirate of the axillary lymph gland was undertaken immediately in clinic and cytological examination confirmed the presence of a moderately differentiated adenocarcinoma. X-ray of the lumbar spine showed a crush fracture of the fourth lumbar vertebra.

An isotope bone scan was requested and revealed multiple 'hot' spots scattered throughout the skeleton. A chest X-ray was clear, but the liver ultrasound showed several small hypoechoic lesions suspicious of metastases.

Diagnosis

The presenting symptoms and clinical features were suggestive of breast cancer recurrence. The laboratory data are in keeping with a chronic illness and specifically indicate hypercalcaemia (raised serum calcium levels) as a consequence of bone infiltration by metastatic tumour. The fine-needle aspiration cytology confirmed local lymph node spread from the previously resected primary cancer.

Diagnosis: recurrent breast cancer with local and distant metastases.

Discussion

Breast screening by mammography is routinely offered to women between the ages of 50 and 65 in the UK on a 3-yearly basis. Although it is a nationally agreed programme, the true benefits either to the individual or the population as a whole remain uncertain and controversial. Mammography is sensitive enough to detect early breast cancers less than 1 cm in size, which are difficult to detect on palpation. The theoretical advantages of early detection are to enable more conservative management of the primary tumour and to prevent disseminated disease. In the last few years, mortality rates from breast cancer have begun to decrease. However, this is attributed to the introduction of systemic therapies as adjuvants to primary surgery rather than to earlier detection by breast screening.

Unfortunately, even with optimal detection and treatment of early disease, many women will develop cancer recurrence. Breast cancer spreads locally via lymphatic vessels and more widely to distant sites via the blood stream. The prognosis of patients with advanced disease is variable and is dictated primarily by the extent and site of metastases. Local recurrence and skeletal involvement are common and are not immediately life threatening but spread to the liver and the lungs carries a much poorer prognosis. Systemic therapy currently impacts little on chance of survival and so treatment is offered primarily to palliate symptoms of disease.

Treatment and prognosis

At the time of diagnosis of the primary cancer, this patient underwent a wide local excision of a 1.5-cm moderately differentiated carcinoma. The tumour also strongly expressed oestrogen receptors, suggesting that the tumour would respond to antioestrogen drugs, such as tamoxifen. No axillary lymph nodes were involved. These features suggested a good prognosis with an 80% chance of being disease-free 5 years postsurgery. Patients routinely receive local radiotherapy to the affected side after breast-conserving surgery, primarily to reduce the risk of local recurrence. She was also commenced on adjuvant hormone therapy with tamoxifen, which has been shown significantly to reduce mortality from breast cancer.

Despite optimal treatment, the patient developed recurrent disease. Her main symptom was back pain associated with a vertebral crush fracture. The diagnosis was explained to her by the clinician, in the presence of the specialist nurse, offering additional support for the patient. She was immediately commenced on a non-steroidal analgesic and a single fraction of radiotherapy to the fractured vertebra was arranged for the following day.

The patient was commenced on an oral bisphosphonate to reduce the risk of further skeletal damage. Since at this stage, the patient's disease did not appear life threatening, and there was evidence of endocrine responsiveness, the tamoxifen was stopped and replaced by an aromatase inhibitor, as a second-line hormonal agent.

In fact, a repeat ultrasound scan 3 months later

confirmed changes in the liver consistent with meta-static spread. She was offered palliative chemotherapy as a means of controlling the cancer in the short term. The centre she was being treated at were taking part in a national clinical trial evaluating a novel chemotherapy regimen for efficacy, side-effects and impact on quality of life compared with the more standard treatment regimen. The study was explained to the patient, who was also given some written information to take home. A decision regarding choice of treatment would not be made until her next clinic visit.

Questions

1 What other complications of this lady's bone metastases should the clinician be alert to?
2 The patient attended her next appointment with her daughter, aged 30. Is the daughter's risk of developing breast cancer affected by her mother's illness?

Answers on p. 309.

Addendum: Approaches to cancer therapy

This case study and others later in this section testify to the complex nature of cancer therapies. This short section is intended to give an overview of such approaches and should promote easier appreciation of the discussion of treatment in each of the case studies.

Surgery

Most patients present with a lump, which is surgically biopsied or removed and diagnosed as cancer. With careful clinical, biochemical and radiological assessment of the patient, it is possible to identify the extent of disease at presentation and so determine whether surgical intervention has the potential to cure. Unfortunately, many patients undergoing surgery for cancer with curative intent will develop recurrent disease. Clearly, microscopic tumour cells must have disseminated beyond the surgical excision margins giving rise to metastases at a later date. Currently, while strategies to detect minimal residual disease are not yet available, the goal is

to include active therapies as adjuncts to surgery to reduce risk of recurrence: so-called adjuvant therapy is administered after surgery, neoadjuvant therapy is administered before surgery.

Chemotherapy

Most cytotoxic chemotherapy drugs exert their effect by inhibiting cell proliferation or by inducing apoptosis (see Chapter 4). In fact the mechanisms responsible for inducing apoptosis in this setting are increasingly well understood. Thus, many cytotoxic agents act by inducing cytochrome C release from mitochondria, which is followed by activation of caspase 9 and the initiation of apoptosis (see Chapter 4).

The DNA synthetic processes are essentially identical in normal and cancer cells. However, there is some selective cytotoxicity against cancer cells, since some tumours are generally more proliferative relative to normal cells (e.g. high grade lymphomas) or are defective in their ability to repair the DNA damage induced by cytotoxic agents. Even so, damage to normal tissues, especially the bone marrow, is the dose-limiting factor for most chemotherapy drugs. For some cytotoxic agents, a linear drug dose–tumour response effect has been demonstrated. However, it is unlikely that increasing the amount of drug one could safely administer would lead to the elimination of all cancer cells. Therefore, most chemotherapy drugs are given in low doses over a period of time (so-called 'fractional kill hypothesis'; Fig CS28.1). High dose chemotherapy with bone marrow supportive measures (e.g. bone marrow transplantation, see Chapter 14) is a concept being evaluated in the context of some cancers.

Acquired mutations during tumourigenesis may protect cancer cells against chemotherapy and drug resistance is the most common reason for treatment failure. Tumours may be intrinsically resistant and so fail to respond to therapy from the outset. Alternatively, tumours may acquire resistance after a period of successful treatment, due to an outgrowth of drug-resistant subclones. One strategy to overcome resistance is to combine drugs with differing mechanisms of action and side-effect profiles, to avoid cross-resistance and maximize the chances of killing the different tumour cell populations. This

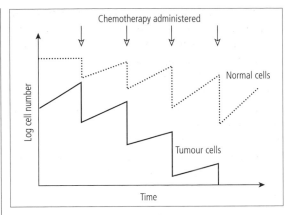

Fig. CS28.1 The fractional cell kill hypothesis.

is known as *combination chemotherapy*. Combination chemotherapy regimens are standard clinical practice in the treatment of most common cancers. In high grade lymphomas and testicular teratomas, combination regimens offer a significantly higher chance of cure compared with single agent therapy.

Radiotherapy

Various sources of ionizing radiation—both electromagnetic and particulate—are used to treat malignant disease and radiation-induced DNA damage is thought to be the critical target leading to cell death. Similarly to chemotherapy, the major drawback of treatment is the concomitant damage to normal tissue. Radiotherapy is therefore confined to the treatment of localized disease in tumour types found to be empirically radiosensitive, either alone or as an adjunct to surgery or chemotherapy. In patients with disseminated disease, radiotherapy plays an important role in symptom control, particularly with regard to pain relief, spinal cord compression and superior vena cava obstruction.

Biological approaches

Tamoxifen is the best example of a mechanistically targeted cancer therapy routinely used in clinical practice. Oestrogen is a key growth factor for breast cancer and tamoxifen induces cytostasis by combining with the cytosolic oestrogen receptor to block oestrogen-mediated stimulation of DNA synthesis.

In a meta-analysis of all clinical trials of adjuvant therapy in breast cancer, tamoxifen alone was shown to be almost as effective as combination chemotherapy in reducing mortality, and certainly far better tolerated by patients.

A greater understanding of the host immune system has led to development of a variety of immunotherapy approaches for cancer. Proteins naturally synthesized and secreted by lymphoid cells usually in tiny amounts have been shown either directly or indirectly to possess antitumour activity. Thus, recombinant interferon and interleukin 2 are nonspecific active immunotherapeutic agents that may have a role in treating certain haematological malignancies, melanoma and renal cancer. These drugs, however, are associated with significant systemic toxicity. Alternatively, tumours often overexpress certain antigens, which afford potential to target cancer therapy safely. Passive immunotherapy strategies include injection of monoclonal antibodies reacting with a specific tumour-associated antigen which can be conjugated with a toxin or radioisotope. Examples here include Rituximab, an anti-CD20 monoclonal antibody that is effective in the treatment of B-cell lymphomas and Herceptin, a monoclonal antibody directed against the *HER2/neu* oncogene that is overexpressed in some breast cancers. Another example of a related approach is the targeting of virus-associated cancer using cytotoxic T cells (CTLs) that are specific for a virus product. This approach has been been used successfully to treat Epstein–Barr virus (EBV)-associated post-transplant lymphoma (see case study 12). Active immunization strategies include tumour cells or tumour cell extracts prepared as vaccines, often conjugated with an immune stimulant such as bacillus Calmette–Guérin (BCG).

A growing understanding of the mechanisms of carcinogenesis at the cellular and molecular level is now yielding a variety of novel approaches to cancer treatment. Gene-directed therapy, drugs designed to inhibit proteases required for tumour invasion and angiogenesis inhibitors are just some of the new classes of agents now being tested in cancer clinical trials.

CASE STUDY 29

Easy bruising, weight loss and abdominal discomfort

Clinical features

A 57-year-old woman presented to her family doctor with shortness of breath, weight loss, and abdominal discomfort of 2 months duration. She had also noticed bruising after minor trauma. On examination she was pale and had marked *splenomegaly* (enlargement of the spleen), which was the cause of her abdominal discomfort. The heart rate was regular, 96 b.p.m., and the patient was *normotensive* (blood pressure was normal).

Investigations

The results of laboratory investigations are shown in Table CS29.1.

The total and differential white cell counts are clearly abnormal. There is an absolute increase in all cells of the granulocyte and monocyte series. Immature cells of the myeloid series (blast cells, myelocytes and metamyelocytes) are present (Plate CS29.1, facing p. 276). These immature haemopoietic cells are normally found in bone marrow, but are not usually seen in peripheral blood. This blood picture is consistent with a diagnosis of either leukaemia or leukaemoid reaction (see later).

Other investigations included the following two tests.
• Neutrophil alkaline phosphatase (NAP) score: 6 (reference range 20–100).
• Cytogenetic studies showed a reciprocal translocation involving chromosomes 9 and 22: t(9;22) (q34;q11).

Diagnosis

The patient is mildly anaemic with a very high white cell count, far in excess of that usually encountered as a result of infection or tissue damage. The differential leucocyte count, showing a range of

Table CS29.1 Investigations performed.

Analyte	Value	Reference range
Blood		
Total white cell count	98.6×10^9/L	4.0–11.0
Red cell count	3.40×10^{12}/L	3.8–5.8
Haemoglobin	11.0 g/dL	11.5–16.5
Haematocrit	0.335	0.37–0.47
Mean cell volume	98.5 fl	82–92
Mean cell haemoglobin	32.35 pg	27.0–32.0
Platelets	110×10^9/L	150–400
Vitamin B_{12}	1150 ng/L	160–760
Serum folate	3.0 µg/L	3.0–20.0
Urea	6.5 mmol/L	2.5–6.7
Urate	0.52 mmol/L	0.18–0.42
Blood film		
White blood cell differential		
Neutrophils	50%	
Lymphocytes	5%	
Monocytes	4%	
Eosinophils	4%	
Basophils	3%	
Metamyelocytes	10%	
Myelocytes	21%	
Blast cells	3%	

cells from immature blast cells to relatively mature myelocytes and metamyelocytes, is consistent with a diagnosis of chronic myeloid leukaemia (CML) and this is supported by the reduced NAP score. CML is confirmed by cytogenetic investigations showing the characteristic translocation involving chromosomes 9 and 22.

Diagnosis: CML (also referred to as chronic granulocytic leukaemia or CGL).

Discussion

The leukaemias are a group of neoplastic disorders

affecting haemopoietic tissue. Typical features of all leukaemias include: anaemia, *neutropenia* (low neutrophil count), often leading to secondary infection and *thrombocytopenia* (low platelet count) due to bone marrow infiltration by leukaemic cells. Infiltration of other organs and tissues with leukaemic white blood cells is another typical finding. Sweating and weight loss also occur, due to an increase in the basal metabolic rate.

Leukaemia is classified on the basis of the following two factors.
• The maturity of the proliferating cells, which determines whether the disease is termed acute or chronic. In acute leukaemias, large numbers of immature (blast) cells proliferate in the bone marrow and also appear in the peripheral blood. In chronic leukaemias the majority of cells in the peripheral blood have differentiated to form relatively mature cells.
• The cell type involved, which determines whether the disease is classified as myeloid or lymphoid in origin. Myeloid leukaemias are those in which the proliferating cells are derived from myeloid progenitor cells, and lymphatic leukaemias are those in which the predominant cells are derived from lymphoid progenitor cells (see Chapter 14).

Thus, there are four major classes of leukaemia.
• Acute myeloid (or myeloblastic) leukaemia (AML).
• Acute lymphatic (or lymphoblastic) leukaemia (ALL).
• Chronic myeloid (or granulocytic) leukaemia (CML or CGL).
• Chronic lymphatic (or lymphocytic) leukaemia (CLL).

There are further subdivisions of leukaemia, particularly the acute forms.

There are also a number of conditions which have many of the features of the leukaemias, but which are not themselves regarded as true leukaemias. These include the *myeloproliferative disorders* and *leukaemoid reactions*. Leukaemoid reactions are unrelated conditions which produce a blood picture resembling that of leukaemia. It is essential to differentiate these disorders from true leukaemias because treatment and prognosis differ.

Differentiation of leukaemia from myeloproli-

ferative disorders and from leukaemoid reactions depends on further clinical and laboratory investigations. The estimation of NAP activity within granulocytes by cytochemical methods is particularly useful in the diagnosis of CML. In leukaemoid reaction and myeloproliferative disorders, enzyme activity is normal or increased, whereas in CML it is invariably low.

The incidence of CML is approximately 1 per 100 000 of the population per year in the UK. CML is characterized by proliferation of large numbers of relatively mature cells of myeloid origin. The excessive *myelopoiesis* (white blood cell formation) which is a feature of CML usually causes a reduction in the rate of erythropoiesis and thrombopoiesis resulting in low numbers of circulating erythrocytes and platelets, respectively. However, this is not always the case and red cell count and platelet counts may be normal or raised in some patients with CML.

CML is a neoplasm derived from myeloid stem cells (see Chapter 14) and is characterized by a chromosomal abnormality which is present in all neoplastic myeloid cell lines (myelomonocytic, megakaryocytic and erythroid). This chromosomal abnormality is a translocation involving chromosomes 9 and 22 t(9; 22) (q34; q11) giving rise to a small chromosome 22 (22q–) called the *Philadelphia chromosome*. As a result of this translocation, the *ABL* oncogene becomes transferred from chromosome 9 to combine with the *BCR* gene on chromosome 22. The result is the production of a fusion gene (*BCR-ABL*). The precise function of normal ABL protein is not clear although recent evidence suggests it is a nuclear kinase that is activated by DNA damaging agents and mediates growth arrest in a p53-dependent manner. However, the ABL-BCR hybrid protein has a cytoplasmic location and acts as a tyrosine kinase protein, interacts with RAS and is able to activate MYC and cyclin D1 resulting in cell proliferation.

This translocation may also be seen in ALL where it is associated with poor prognosis.

Transformation of CML to 'blast crisis' is associated with the development of other chromosomal abnormalities and defects in oncogenes, notably those involving the *p53* gene (see Chapter 22).

Treatment and prognosis

Treatment of CML aims to reduce the leucocyte count to normal and to prevent progression to its more aggressive terminal stage (blast crisis). This is usually achieved using alkylating agents or other cytotoxic drugs. Allopurinol is also useful if the plasma urate concentration is high. Some patients remain in a stable chronic phase of the disorder for many months or years (median survival is 3–4 years), but most patients with CML eventually undergo 'blast transformation', in which a distinct change in the population of leukaemia cells occurs. In the chronic phase most of the proliferating cells are relatively mature whereas after transformation the majority of the cells in the peripheral blood are myeloblasts or other primitive cells. At this stage the disease has many more features of acute leuk-

aemia and is much more resistant to treatment than when in the chronic phase. Survival after blast transformation is typically 1–3 months. For this reason some patients are considered for potential cure by bone marrow transplantation at an early stage after diagnosis of CML while the disease is still in the chronic phase.

Questions

1 What is the significance of the raised concentration of plasma urate?

2 Why are serum vitamin B_{12} concentrations typically very high in CML?

3 What is the relationship between myeloproliferative disorders and CML?

Answers on p. 309.

Bleeding from the nose and gums with fever

Clinical features

A 57-year-old man presented to his family doctor with bleeding from the nose and gums, red urine and faintness of 1-week duration. On examination, he was very pale and had a petechial rash on his arms and thighs. The patient was febrile (temperature: 39°C). The heart rate was regular at 100 b.p.m., his blood pressure was normal.

Laboratory investigations

The results of laboratory investigations are shown in Table CS30.1.

The total and differential white blood cell counts are clearly abnormal. There is a significant increase in the white blood cell count due to the presence of

promyelocytes (large cells with numerous primary granules that coalesce into eosinophilic needle-like aggregates called *Auer rods*).

The promyelocytes are normally without Auer rods and are usually present only in the bone marrow and not in the peripheral blood. The Auer rods are seen only in *acute myeloid leukaemia* (AML).

Cytogenetic studies showed a reciprocal translocation between chromosomes 15 and 17 t(15;17) (q22;q12). This translocation involves two oncogenes; the retinoic acid receptor (*RAR*) gene and the *PML* gene.

Diagnosis

The patient is severely anaemic with a very high white cell count, far in excess of that usually encoun-

Table CS30.1 Results of laboratory investigations.

Analyte	Value	Normal reference
Blood		
Total white cell count	48×10^9/L	4.0–11.0
Red cell count	1.1×10^{12}/L	4.5–6.5
Haemoglobin concentration	6 g/dL	13.0–18.0
Haemotocrit	0.26	0.40–0.54
Mean cell volume	85 fl	82–92
Mean cell haemoglobin	28 pg	27–32
Platelet count	8×10^9/L	150–400
Urea	7.0 mmol/L	2.5–6.7
Urate	0.6 mmol/L	0.18–0.42
Blood film		
White cell differential		
Neutrophils	10%	
Lymphocytes	4%	
Monocytes	1%	
Eosinophils	0%	
Basophils	0%	
Promyelocytes*	85%	

* Most have Auer rods.

tered as a result of infection. The patient also has severe *thrombocytopenia* (very low platelet count) which causes the bleeding and petechial rash and neutropenia (low neutrophil count) is responsible for the fever. The blood picture is consistent with a diagnosis of AML of subtype M3, called acute promyelocytic leukaemia (APL). The diagnosis of APL is confirmed by the presence of the characteristic translocation between chromosomes 15 and 17, t(15;17) (q22;q12).

Discussion

The acute leukaemias are classified according to the nature of the cell type involved. AML is therefore neoplasia involving cells of the myeloid system.

AML is more common in adults than in children with a peak incidence in late adult life (65 or more years old). Sixty per cent of AML patients are over the age of 60 years. AML is diagnosed in more than 10 per 100 000 individuals over the age of 70 years each year. The main criteria for the widely used French–American–British (FAB) classification of AML are listed in Table CS30.2.

APL has a specific association with disseminated intravascular coagulation (DIC). Patients may present with severe bleeding and this may increase following treatment as the blast cells break down, leading to further consumption of clotting factors and platelets (see Chapter 16).

The translocation in APL links ligand and DNA binding sequences of the *RAR* gene on chromosome 17 to sequences of the *PML* gene on chromosome 15. The resultant fusion protein arrests differentiation in the promyelocyte stage. *All* transretinoic acid therapy is believed to work by inducing differentiation of these abnormal promyelocytes producing differentiated myeloid cells that have a limited lifespan in the circulation.

Table CS30.2 FAB classification of acute myeloid leukaemia (AML).

Type	Name	Cell type	Cytogenetic abnormality
M1	AML without differentiation	> 30% myeloblasts	Several abnormalities
M2	AML with differentiation	> 30% myeloblasts and > 10% granulocytes	t(8;21)
M3	Acute promyelocytic leukaemia	> 30% promyelocytes	t(15;17) (q22;q12)
M4	Acute myelomonocytic leukaemia	> 30% blasts, > 20% granulocytes and 20% monocytic cells	inv or del (16)
M5	Acute monocytic leukaemia	> 30% monoblasts and > 20% monocytic cells	t or del(11) (q23)
M6	Acute erythroleukaemia	> 30% myeblasts and > 50% erythroblasts	Several
M7	Acute megakaryocytic leukaemia	> 30% megakaryblasts	Several

Factor	Favourable	Unfavourable
Age	< 45 years	> 60 years
Diagnosis	*De novo*	Secondary (e.g. after chronic myeloid leukaemia)
WBC count	$< 25 \times 10^9$/L	$< 100 \times 10^9$/L
Cytogenetic picture	t(8;21)	−5, del(5q)
	t(15;17)	−7, del(7q)
	inv(16)	11q23 abnormalities
	del(16q)	3q21 abnormalities

Table CS30.3 Prognostic factors in acute myeloid leukaemia.

Treatment and prognosis

Therapy of all AML types except APL includes the use of an anthracycline (daunorubicin or idarubicin) intravenously for 2 days plus twice daily infusion of cytarabine for 7–10 days. Treatment with one or two cycles of this combined chemotherapy can achieve complete remission in 75–80% of young AML patients and in 50–60% of older AML patients. However, the relapse rate is the highest among all haematological malignancies and the 5-year survival is only 10–15%.

Treatment of APL is completely different to the other types and involves oral administration of *all*-transretinoic acid daily until complete remission is achieved.

Several prognostic factors have been identified in AML patients and these are summarized in Table CS30.3.

Questions

1 What is the effect of the age of the patient on the biology of AML?

2 What is the role of cytokines in the biology of AML?

Answers on p. 310.

Night sweats and cervical lymph node enlargement

Clinical features

A 20-year-old female presented with a 2-month history of drenching night sweats and pruritus (itching). Examination revealed a mobile firm enlarged 2.5-cm diameter lymph node on the left side of the neck. There was no evidence of other palpably enlarged nodes and the liver and spleen were not enlarged. An intermittent pyrexia (fever) of 39°C was noted.

Investigations

Investigations revealed a normal blood count and elevated serum levels of lactate dehydrogenase (LDH) and β_2-microglobulin. A cervical lymph node biopsy was undertaken and this showed loss of the normal lymph node architecture with cellular nodules of lymphocytes, eosinophils, histiocytes and Hodgkin–Reed–Sternberg cells (HRS cells) sur-

Table CS31.1 Staging system for Hodgkin's disease.

Stage I	Involvement of a single node region
Stage II	Involvement of two or more lymph node regions on the same side of the diaphragm
	A—without symptoms
	B—with symptoms (see below)
Stage III	Involvement of lymph node regions on both sides of the diaphragm
	A—without symptoms
	B—with symptoms (see below)
Stage IV	Extensive extralymphatic involvement and/or disseminated disease with involvement of liver, bone marrow, lung or skin
	A—without symptoms
	B—with symptoms

B symptoms
- Unexplained weight loss of more than 10% of the previous body weight during the past 6 months
- Unexplained persistent or recurrent fever with temperatures above 38°C during the previous month
- Recurrent drenching night sweats during the previous month

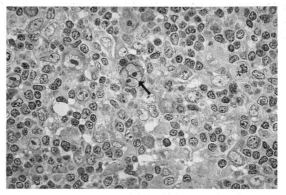

Fig. CS31.1 Histological appearance of Hodgkin's disease. This unusual malignancy is characterized by relatively few malignant Hodgkin–Reed–Sternberg (HRS) cells surrounded by numerous non-malignant cells. Shown here is a typical HRS cell (arrowed).

rounded by broad bands of fibrous tissue (collagenous connective tissue).

A chest radiograph showed widening of the mediastinum. A computed tomography (CT) scan showed gross enlargement of the mediastinal lymph nodes.

An iliac crest bone marrow trephine biopsy was taken for staging purposes and this was shown to be unaffected by Hodgkin's disease (HD). CT scans were performed on the abdomen and no other enlarged lymph nodes were found. The liver and spleen were normal.

Diagnosis

A diagnosis of nodular sclerosis Hodgkin's disease (NSHD) was made and the patient was found to have stage IIB disease (Table CS31.1).

Discussion

HD is a malignant lymphoma characterized by a minority of tumour cells, known as HRS cells surrounded by a mixture of non-malignant cells (Fig. CS31.1). HD is classified on the basis of the appearance of the HRS cells and on the nature of the non-malignant cell population.

The classification of HD in the REAL (Revised European–American Lymphoma) classification is similar to the Rye classification with several modifications. Lymphocyte predominance HD (LPHD) is considered an entity distinct from the other types of HD—nodular sclerosis, mixed cellularity and lymphocyte depletion. The latter have been grouped together under the heading of classic HD. In addition, a new provisional entity has been proposed, known as lymphocyte-rich classic HD (Tables CS31.2 and CS31.3).

The incidence of HD in the UK is about 2/100 000 with little regional variation. There is a male preponderance with a 3 : 2 male to female ratio. There is a bimodal age distribution with a distinct peak in the 15–34 years age group with the incidence increasing into the sixth decade. In the younger patients the male predominance is less marked and almost all cases are of the nodular sclerosis type.

Overall, NSHD is the most common type of HD in Europe and the USA, constituting approximately 70% of all cases. Patients commonly present with cervical or supraclavicular lymphadenopathy (enlarged lymph nodes). The mediastinum is frequently involved and most patients have stage I or II disease at presentation. The disease spreads contiguously to adjacent nodes with late involvement of bone marrow and extranodal sites.

Hodgkin's disease type	Features
Lymphocyte predominance (LPHD)	Few HRS cells, numerous non-malignant lymphocytes
Classic Hodgkin's disease (HD)	
Nodular sclerosis (NSHD)	Nodules of tumour separated by bands of fibrous tissue
Mixed cellularity (MCHD)	Moderate numbers of HRS cells with a mixture of different non-malignant cells
Lymphocyte depletion (LDHD)	Numerous HRS cells, few non-malignant cells
Lymphocyte-rich classic (provisional entity)	

Table CS31.2 Classification of Hodgkin's disease: Revised European–American Lymphoma (REAL) system.

Table CS31.3 General features of classic-type Hodgkin's disease.

Morphology	Classical or lacunar type HRS cells in a background of T and B lymphocytes, histiocytes and eosinophils. Nodular fibrosis in NSHD
Immunophenotype	CD15+, CD30+, CD45–, CD3–, EMA–. Rosettes of adherent T cells are often present
Cytogenetics	No specific abnormality
Pattern of disease	Contiguous nodal spread beginning in neck or mediastinum

It is essential that the pattern of disease at presentation is considered together with the biopsy features in making a firm diagnosis. The accurate diagnosis of HD involves demonstrating destruction of the normal nodal architecture by an infiltrate that includes HRS cells in the appropriate cellular background.

The proportion of HRS cells varies greatly from case to case and attempts have been made to subgrade NSHD to identify cases that would be expected to carry a better or worse prognosis. Cases without an excessive number of tumour cells have been designated NS1, those with prominent areas of lymphocyte depletion have been called NS2. Some earlier studies have shown that NS2 patients have a worse prognosis but this difference is less marked in more recent series where optimal or aggressive therapy has been used.

Phenotyping of the HRS cells by immunohistochemistry is essential for the accurate diagnosis of HD. In almost every case the HRS cells express CD30. CD30 is a growth factor receptor that has been shown to be a member of the tumour necrosis factor receptor (TNFR) family. A smaller percentage of cases will also express CD15. CD15 is a carbohydrate antigen expressed on myeloid cells and some epithelial cells. In a proportion (10–20%) of cases of classic HD the HRS cells may express the B-cell marker, CD20.

In most cases of classic HD the HRS cells are of B-cell origin. Since B lymphocytes rearrange their immunoglobulin genes early in their development (see Chapter 6), and each rearrangement is unique to an individual B lymphocyte, analysis of rearrangements can establish whether a clonal population of B cells is present. A clonal B-cell rearrangement can be detected in about 30% of cases of HD. More sensitive microdissection techniques have been used to isolate and study individual HRS cells and these data show that most HRS cells have rearranged immunoglobulin genes, although in a few cases the HRS cells sampled are not monoclonal. This suggests that monoclonal HRS cells may develop from polyclonal or oligoclonal populations of HRS cells during the course of the disease. A further interesting observation is the finding that the immunoglobulin genes show evidence that they have undergone somatic hypermutation indicating that they are derived from postgerminal centre B cells (see Chapter 6). This has led to the suggestion that a critical element in the pathogenesis of classic HD is the ability of the HRS cells to escape apoptosis, the usual fate of abnormal germinal centre cells.

Approximately 40% of cases of HD from Europe and the USA are associated with the Epstein–Barr virus (EBV) where the virus can be detected within the HRS cells. The most convincing evidence to suggest that EBV is important in the pathogenesis of HD is the detection of viral latent membrane protein (LMP-1) expression by the HRS cells. This protein is oncogenic and its characteristics are discussed more fully in Chapter 23.

Some of the pathological and clinical features of NSHD are not due to tumour invasion but are related to cytokine release by HRS cells. Thus, cytokines are believed to be responsible for fever, night sweats, weight loss and pruritus; collectively known as B symptoms (Table CS31.1).

Therefore, a key feature of HD may be dysregulation of cytokine production. As well as mediating systemic effects cytokine production may govern the interaction between the HRS cells and the non-malignant cell population that make up most of the mass of the node. Thus, the non-malignant cells may have a part to play in the growth of HRS cells—they express many growth-promoting ligands (such as CD40L, CD30L) for growth factor receptors (such as CD40, CD30) expressed on the HRS cells. Other cytokines produced by HRS cells may downregulate cytotoxic T cell (CTL) responses to the tumour cells (e.g. interleukin 10 or IL-10) or may produce the fibrosis characteristic of NSHD (e.g. transforming growth factor or TGF β, IL-1).

Most patients are staged using a combination of routine radiography and CT scanning. Stage of disease is one of the main prognostic factors in HD. The staging system for HD is shown in Table CS31.1 (based on Ann Abor classification). The case patient was stage IIB.

Treatment and prognosis

Patients with localized disease (stage I and stage IIA, non-bulky disease) can be treated by radiotherapy and have an excellent response.

Chemotherapy is the treatment of choice for stage III and IV disease and in all patients with B symptoms. This patient received combination chemotherapy and achieved sustained complete remission and has an excellent chance of cure.

A relatively small number of patients have disease refractory to standard treatment or relapse within 1 year of treatment. Some of these patients will respond to second-line chemotherapy. High dose chemotherapy used together with autologous haemopoietic stem cell transplant (see Chapter 13) may be useful in patients with relapsed or refractory disease.

Questions

1 What is the main differential diagnosis in this patient based on the appearances of the lymph node biopsy specimen?
2 What is the risk of a second malignancy in patients treated for HD?

Answers on p. 310.

CASE STUDY 32

Hoarseness and weight loss

Clinical features

A 71-year-old retired plumber attended his family doctor's surgery regularly for monitoring of his diabetes (which was controlled by dietary re-

striction) and his hypertension. On one visit, his doctor noticed that he had lost about 10 pounds in weight and was about to commend his efforts at dieting when she noticed how hoarse his voice sounded. The patient had noticed this symptom for approximately 6 weeks but since there was no pain in his throat had thought little of it. He put it down to the strain of smoker's cough. In fact he had brought up flecks of blood.

The patient had smoked at least 20 cigarettes daily since serving in the army. On questioning, he admitted to being rather short of breath for the last few months and to feeling rather wheezy at night.

On examination the patient was pale and was mildly breathless at rest. He was not blue (which would indicate hypoxia) but his fingers were club shaped, which is often a sign of heart or lung disease. There was a pronounced wheeze localized to the upper lung but no evidence of infection or fluid around the lung. There was no lymphadenopathy (enlargement of the lymph nodes) and the liver was not palpable. Urgent investigations were arranged.

Investigations

The laboratory investigations shown in Table CS32.1 were performed.

The results show a mild normocytic normochromic anaemia (see Chapter 14) and a raised erythrocyte sedimentation rate (ESR). The total leucocyte count is high, the majority of cells being neutrophils. A blood film showed the presence of immature leucocytes and nucleated red blood cells. This finding (known as a *leucoerythroblastic blood picture*) suggests bone marrow infiltration by tumour which replaces normal haemopoietic cells.

A chest radiograph showed a large opacity in the left lung. The patient was referred urgently to the chest clinic and bronchoscopy was performed. He was found to have a tumour in the left main bronchus. Histological analysis of a biopsy specimen taken at bronchoscopy showed a large cell carcinoma. Closer examination of his chest X-ray revealed the presence of several metastases in his ribs.

Diagnosis

The clinical features and laboratory data confirm the presence of a tumour in the left lung. Histology showed this to be a large cell carcinoma. The presence of metastases in the ribs and blood film results suggest significant involvement of bone marrow. The absence of any lymphadenopathy, hepatomegaly (enlargement of the liver) and the normal values for the enzymes alkaline phosphatase, alanine aminotransferase and aspartate aminotransferase suggest there was no metastatic spread to the lymph nodes or liver.

Diagnosis: large cell carcinoma of the left lung.

Discussion

From a clinical viewpoint lung cancer can be divided into two main groups. The first comprises squamous carcinomas, adenocarcinomas and large cell carcinomas, collectively referred to as non-small cell lung cancers (NSCLC). These are clinically different to small cell lung cancers (SCLC). NSCLCs account for approximately 75% of all lung cancers.

This patient's carcinoma was almost certainly a result of his cigarette smoking. This type of bronchial neoplasm is uncommon in non-smokers. Over the last 80 years the incidence of this disease has closely paralleled cigarette smoking patterns. In the mid-1970s it was estimated that cigarette smoking was responsible for 95% of all lung neoplasms in men.

Populations in which smoking has been reduced or low tar preparations favoured, have experienced a decline in the incidence of the disease. Women, who tended not to smoke before the 1940s, are increasingly victims of the disease. Other possible environmental carcinogens are asbestos, coal smoke, radon (in certain areas such as Cornwall) and other atmospheric pollutants. All the available evidence suggests that these account for only a small minority of cases.

Mutations in key oncogenes and tumour suppressor genes have been identified in lung cancer some of which are apparently induced by several tobacco carcinogens. Members of the *Ras* and *Myc* family are frequently mutated. Several tumour suppressor genes, including *p53* and the CdK inhibitor, *p16* (see Chapter 22) are also commonly inactivated in lung cancer.

The anaemia present in this case was almost certainly due to infiltration of the bone marrow by tumour which had displaced normal haemopoietic tissue (see Chapter 14).

Table CS32.1 Investigations performed.

Analyte	Value	Reference range
Haematology		
Haemoglobin concentration	10.7 g/dL	13.0–18.0
Red cell count	3.84×10^{12}/L	4.5–6.5
Haematocrit	0.325	0.40–0.54
Mean cell volume	84.6 fl	82–92
Mean cell haemoglobin	27.9 pg	27.0–32.0
Mean cell haemoglobin concentration	33.0 g/dL	30.0–35.0
Erythrocyte sedimentation rate	84 mm/h	0–14
White cells		
Total white cell count	13.6×10^9/L	4.0–11.0
Neutrophils	11.2×10^9/L (83%)	2.0–7.5
Lymphocytes	1.25×10^9/L (9%)	1.5–4.0
Monocytes	1.00×10^9/L (7%)	0.2 0.8
Eosinophils	0.10×10^9/L (1%)	Up to 0.4
Basophils	0.05×10^9/L (< 1%)	Up to 0.1
Platelet count	258×10^9/L	150–400
Blood picture	Neutrophilia with some toxic granulation; occasional nucleated red blood cells and myelocytes present	
Biochemistry		
Urea	8.4 mmol/l	2.5–6.7
Creatinine	134 µmol/L	60 120
Urate	0.3 mmol/L	0.18–0.42
Random glucose	8.0 mmol/L	3.5–8.9
Phosphate	1.25 mmol/L	0.8–1.5
Total bilirubin	15.2 µmol/L	< 17
Alkaline phosphatase	86 U/L	25–115
Alanine aminotransferase	7 U/L	5–40
Aspartate aminotransferase	18 U/L	10–40
Gamma glutamyltransferase	13 U/L	11–50
Total protein	77 g/L	62–80
Albumin	35 g/L	34–48
Globulin	42 g/L	16–37
Cholesterol	2.47 mmol/L	3.5–6.5
Triglycerides	0.85 mmol/L	0.7–2.1

Treatment and prognosis

For the NSCLC group early surgery is indicated where possible since metastases occur late. However, even for the limited stage of NSCLC, 5-year cure rates are only 50%. Conversely, SCLC is one of the most lethal forms of cancer known in humans with 5-year survival rates of only 5%.

Three weeks later his wife rang the doctor for advice. The patient was complaining of thirst and constantly going to pass urine. He was rather confused and was complaining of nausea, abdominal pain and constipation. The doctor suspected deterioration of his diabetes but analysis of his urine and blood glucose screen were normal. However, his serum calcium was found to be high at 3.3 mmol/L (reference range 2.2–2.6). He was admitted to hospital and treated with rehydration and cortico-steroids followed by calcitonin to control the hyper-calcaemia (raised blood calcium levels).

Questions

1 Was the patient's hoarseness caused by his tumour?
2 Can you explain the hypercalcaemia observed in this patient?

Answers on p. 310.

Burning sensation during urination, weight loss and skeletal pain

Clinical features

A 65-year-old man presented with both urgent and frequent urination and a urethral burning sensation during micturition which had developed gradually during the course of the last 5 years. The intensity of the symptoms had fluctuated during this time, but had become significantly worse in the last 2 weeks before presentation.

Investigations

Laboratory investigations were generally unre-markable with the exception of a significantly raised serum prostate-specific antigen (12.3 μg/L; reference value less than 4 μg/L). Microbiological investigation of the urine was negative.

Clinical investigation included palpation of the prostate gland per rectum. The examining physician found a tough textured prostate with a lumpy surface. Histological examination of a prostatic biopsy revealed the presence of a well-differentiated adenocarcinoma.

Diagnosis

The definitive diagnosis was established by biopsy and was supported by the high level of prostate-specific antigen in the serum.

Diagnosis: well-differentiated adenocarcinoma of the prostate gland.

Discussion

Prostatic adenocarcinoma is one of the most com-mon cancers affecting men. Its incidence increases dramatically in men over 40 years of age and this appears to be connected with changes in androgen levels at this age. Despite an 80% prevalence at autopsy by the age of 80 years, the clinical incidence is much lower. This means that many adenocarcin-omas will remain undiscovered during life and that their development is very slow, usually occurring over many years. Prostate cancer may have no specific presenting symptoms, and may often be clinically silent. Conversely, it may cause symptoms of the lower urinary tract mimicking benign nodu-lar hyperplasia of the prostate, which is itself very common in men of older age. In fact, most prostatic cancers arise in patients with concomitant benign hyperplasia. The enlargement of the prostate gland, which is a common symptom of benign prostatic hyperplasia, and prostate cancer both cause obstruction of urine flow through the prostatic urethrae. This obstruction causes the sensation of urgency and difficulty in initiating urination, diminished stream size and force, increased frequency, incomplete bladder emptying and nocturia (urination during the night). Other symptoms may arise secondary to the prostate cancer and are due to inflammation of the lower urinary tract (uretheral burning and the presence of leucocytes and bacteria in the urine).

Treatment and prognosis

The prognosis of prostate cancer depends on the clinical stage and on the hormone dependency (70–80% of prostatic neoplasms are androgen-sensitive tumours). The cancer sometimes manifests as metastasis in the lymph nodes or bone. Many prostate cancers are initially responsive to androgen withdrawal therapy. Unfortunately, in about 50% of cases, the cell clones that survive androgen ablation give rise to androgen-independent prostate carcin-

omas. Such subsequent tumours are clinically more aggressive and the prognosis after relapse is poor. So far there is no effective therapy for this hormone-refractory carcinoma.

In the present case the patient was treated with the antiandrogens, flutamide and Casodex. After 1 year of good response (disappearance of subjective symptoms, decrease of prostate-specific antigen level), the patient experienced the same symptoms as before together with additional symptoms which included an aversion to food, vomiting, weight loss and fever (38.5°C). Laboratory examinations suggested an infection of the lower urinary tract. Therefore, antiandrogen treatment was discontinued and the patient received antimicrobial therapy. After a short period of time he felt intense pain in the lumbar spine and in the pelvis. At this time the serum prostate-specific antigen was high (32 ng/mL) and the prostate was enlarged. Scintigraphy of the skeleton showed numerous metastases (Fig. CS33.1). At this time a new biopsy of the prostate revealed the presence of prostatic adenocarcinoma.

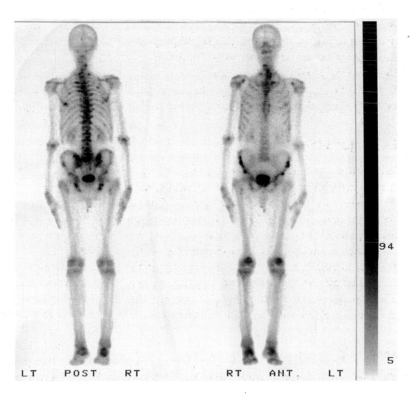

Fig. CS33.1 Scintigraphy reveals the presence of numerous metastatic deposits within the bones (shown as black areas).

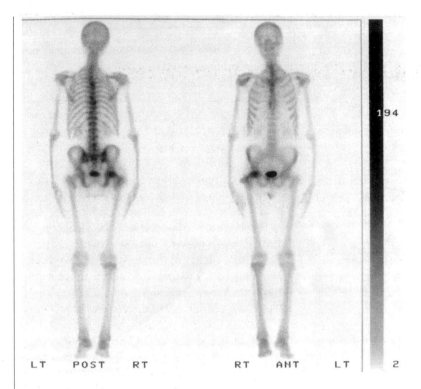

LT   POST   RT   RT   ANT   LT

Fig. CS33.2 Scintigraphy following antiandrogen therapy shows regression of the metastatic deposits.

Despite orchidectomy (surgical castration), testosterone levels were still high and the patient was commenced on Androcur (steroidal antiandrogen with central and peripheral effect). After this treatment a decrease in the levels of both testosterone and prostate-specific antigen was noted. The patient felt better and a further scintigraphy revealed the regression of the metastases (Fig. CS33.2). However, after 2 months there was a further relapse accompanied by a raised prostate-specific antigen (123 ng/mL), skeletal pain, fever and weight loss. The patient died soon after this. An autopsy revealed metastatic deposits in abdominal lymphatic nodes, liver, adrenal glands and bone. Hypertrophy and chronic inflammation of the bladder was also confirmed. The cause of death was pnuemonia.

The course of the disease in this patient is typical of refractory prostate cancer. After an initial very good response to treatment by antiandrogens there then followed a relapse of the disease and in spite of the subsequent total androgen ablation (including orchidectomy), the tumour cells revealed only limited sensitivity and the tumour progressed. Gradually, the tumour became unresponsive. The infectious complications due to metastases are very often the cause of death.

Questions

1 Is prostate cancer hereditary?
2 The BCL-2 protein is found more commonly in androgen-independent prostate cancer when compared to androgen-sensitive tumours. What is the significance of this?

Answers on p. 311.

Change of bowel habit and bleeding from the rectum

Clinical features

A 65-year-old man presented to his family doctor complaining of an alteration in his bowel habit over the past few months. This had taken the form of alternating constipation and diarrhoea, but in the last week he had also noticed fresh blood in his motions.

On examination he was slightly pale but there were no other external features of note. The doctor carried out a rectal examination and thought he could feel a mass in the rectum. The patient was therefore referred to a consultant surgeon for further investigation.

Investigations

The surgeon, on his examination, confirmed the presence of a lesion in the rectum at about 8 cm from the anal margin and therefore carried out a flexible sigmoidoscopy.

This enabled him to view the tumour mass in the rectum and to take a biopsy. No other lesion was found in the sigmoid colon or the rectum but the patient subsequently had a double-contrast barium enema performed in order to examine the entire length of the large bowel for other lesions. He also had a chest X-ray and a computed tomography (CT) scan of the liver in order to check for any distant tumour spread.

Diagnosis

The histopathology of the rectal biopsy confirmed the diagnosis of an adenocarcinoma of the rectum. No other lesion was detected in the colon or the rectum either on sigmoidoscopy or barium enema. No metastases were found in the lungs or the liver.

The surgeon assessed that the tumour had not spread into the surrounding pelvic tissues. The tumour and adjacent bowel were later removed by surgery.

Discussion

Adenocarcinoma of the colon and rectum is the second most common cancer, after lung cancer, in the UK. There are 28 000 new cases of this disease diagnosed each year and it is responsible for over 15 000 deaths (see p. 23). A change of bowel habit and bleeding from the rectum are the commonest presenting symptoms. The disease is more common in men than women and increases in frequency with advancing age, especially after 55 years. Predisposing conditions include ulcerative colitis, familial adenomatous polyposis (FAP), hereditary non-polyposis colorectal cancer and pre-existing polyps of the large bowel (see also case study 22).

The vast majority of colorectal cancers (70–90%) arise from these pre-existing benign polyps (also known as adenomas). A few tumours may arise *de novo* from non-polypoid colonic mucosa. Polyps which are greater than 2 cm in diameter, have a villous pattern or show dysplasia (premalignant histological changes) in the epithelium, are more likely to transform to a carcinoma than are other polyps.

Colorectal cancers, whether sporadic (non-inherited) or FAP associated, show multiple genetic alterations at the molecular level. The multistep theory of carcinogenesis in colorectal cancer is shown in Fig. CS34.1.

Colorectal cancer spreads in four ways and the extent of spread is of great importance in determining the outcome of the disease. Local spread involves the pelvic organs such as the bladder or the uterus. Lymphatic spread involves the local and regional lymph nodes and then the rest of the body. Blood spread results in tumour deposits

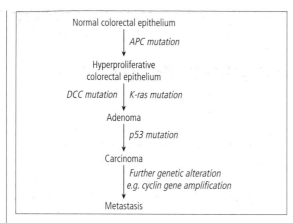

Normal colorectal epithelium

↓ *APC mutation*

Hyperproliferative
colorectal epithelium

DCC mutation | *K-ras mutation*

Adenoma

↓ *p53 mutation*

Carcinoma

*Further genetic alteration
e.g. cyclin gene amplification*

Metastasis

Fig. CS34.1 A genetic model for the development of colorectal cancer. The process of colorectal tumour evolution represents the acquisition of sequential mutations. Mutations in the *APC* gene, a putative tumour suppressor gene (see Chapter 22), are required to initiate the process. The normal *APC* gene produces a protein that seems to be able to induce apoptosis (physiological cell death, see Chapter 4). Therefore, inactivation of the *APC* gene may allow the development of clones of cells that are long lived. Eventually, one of these cells may acquire a mutation in the *ras* gene family (e.g. K-*ras*, see Chapter 22) and the *DCC* (deleted in colon cancer) gene (also a tumour suppressor gene with similarities to some adhesion molecules). Later, mutations, such as those involving *p53* (see Chapter 22), enable the development of full malignancy and metastatic spread. The whole process may take as long as 20–40 years.

(metastases) in the liver, lungs or other major organs and the tumour can also spread directly in the abdominal cavity, known as transcoelomic spread.

Accurate assessment of the tumour and surrounding bowel by the pathologist is essential to determine the extent of tumour spread. Depth of invasion, rather than the size of the tumour, is the best measure of the degree of local spread. In rectal cancer, in particular, it is very important to establish whether the peripheral or circumferential margin of

the specimen that is removed surgically is involved by tumour.

Lymph node involvement is assessed by examining all the lymph nodes from the mesorectal fat histologically for the presence of metastases. Blood vessels in the mesorectum are also examined for tumour involvement.

All these data are used to classify colorectal cancer using the Dukes' classification. Originally described in 1932, by Cuthbert Dukes this classification has been modified over the years but still remains the single most important measure of prognosis for any colorectal cancer patient.

The modified Dukes' classification in current use is as follows.
- Dukes A: tumour in the submucosa or muscularis propria, but not through it.
- Dukes B: tumour through the muscularis propria but not involving the lymph nodes.
- Dukes C1: tumour involvement of the lymph nodes, but not the highest node in the specimen.
- Dukes C2: tumour involvement of nodes, including the highest node in the specimen.
- Dukes D: presence of hepatic metastases.

Table CS34.1 shows the approximate frequency of these various stages and the 5-year survival in one study, which is representative of most series.

Treatment and prognosis

The patient in this case had a rectal carcinoma, shown in Fig. CS34.2, which had invaded through the full thickness of the muscle coats, but with a circumferential margin that was not involved by tumour. Four of the 15 lymph nodes recovered were involved by cancer but the highest node was free from tumour. There was no evidence of liver meta-

Table CS34.1 Colorectal cancer staging, stage distribution and survival.

Dukes' stage (modified)	Definition	Approximate frequency at diagnosis	5-year survival
A	Cancer localized within the bowel wall	11%	83%
B	Cancer which penetrates the bowel	35%	64%
C	Cancer spread to lymph nodes	26%	38%
D	Cancer with distant metastases (most often in the liver)	29%	3%

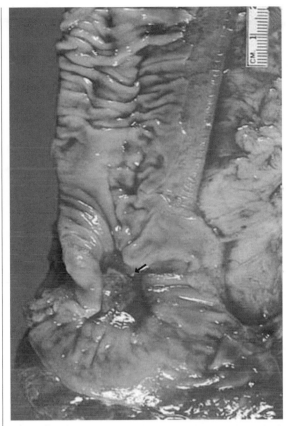

Fig. CS34.2 Specimen showing rectal cancer (here represented as a sunken lesion in the rectal mucosa and arrowed).

stases at operation. This was therefore a Dukes C1 tumour and 5-year survival would be expected in about 40% of such cases.

The patient had several forms of treatment. Firstly, because the tumour, on clinical assessment, was not thought to involve the surrounding tissues, the patient received short-term high dose radiotherapy to the tumour preoperatively. He then had an anterior resection of the rectum with total mesorectal excision and an end-to-end anastomosis of the proximal large bowel to the remaining rectal stump. Subsequently, following postoperative recovery, he was given a course of chemotherapy. The drugs used were 5-fluorouracil and levamisole since in Dukes C tumours, this approach has been shown to produce a 40% reduction in recurrence and a 33% reduction in mortality.

Questions

1 What methods are available to assess the prognosis of a patient with rectal carcinoma?
2 Does the size of a rectal carcinoma have any bearing on the outcome of the disease?
3 Would the systematic removal of adenomas reduce the incidence of colorectal cancer to zero?

Answers on p. 311.

Answers

Case Study 1

1 A routine full blood count and erythrocyte sedimentation rate are useful investigations to exclude physical causes of psychiatric symptoms. Thyroid function tests were performed because hyperthyroidism (overactivity of the thyroid gland) can produce agitation and anxiety (see also Chapter 2).

2 An increase in serum gamma-GT concentration is a sensitive marker of acute liver cell damage. Gamma-GT concentration is usually raised in alcohol abuse (see case study 20). Alcohol withdrawal could produce anxiety symptoms.

Case Study 2

1 Many drugs cross the placenta or may appear in breast milk. In the first trimester of pregnancy some are *teratogenic*, i.e. they may cause fetal malformation. Later in fetal development and in early life, drugs may cause serious physiological disturbance. Doxepin was chosen for this patient because it is the least able of all the tricyclic antidepressants to cross the placental barrier. However, it is secreted in breast milk and should be replaced during lactation by imipramine.

2 The value of ECT in the treatment of depressive illness has now been established in a number of double-blind trials in which the control group has been given muscle relaxant and anaesthetic but no ECT.

ECT is most effective in severe depressions in which there is marked retardation or agitation, or when some of the ideas are delusional. A *delusion* is a false belief, not amenable to reason and not shared by people with a similar educational and cultural background. *Retardation* is a slowing of the mind and a reduction in activity; when severe there is no speech and long periods of near immobility, a state referred to as *stupor*.

ECT may also be used to treat patients who are dangerously suicidal, who choose it, or for whom other measures such as drugs have failed. Depressive illness may relapse after a course of ECT, but the risk is reduced by treatment with an antidepressant drug in maintenance dose during the succeeding 6 months.

Case Study 3

1 Antibiotics destroy bacteria, resulting in the release of cell wall components (see above). This leads to the release of large amounts of pro-inflammatory cytokines and a particularly marked and potentially harmful inflammatory response.

2 *Haemophilus* vaccine is produced by conjugating the carbohydrate component of the bacterial cell wall to a protein 'carrier'. The infant's immune system sees the whole molecule as protein and produces antibodies to a variety of epitopes on it, including the carbohydrate portion. Similar vaccines are in preparation against the carbohydrate antigens of other clinically important bacteria.

Case Study 4

1 HIV infection is associated with a progressive increase in the frequency of certain tumours, including aggressive lymphomas of B lymphocytes, anal cancer (in HIV-positive homosexual men) and Kaposi's sarcoma. This suggests that the immune system may be important in preventing the development of some of these tumours in immunocompetent individuals (see also Chapters 21–23). Many tumours arising during immunosuppression are associated with viruses, e.g. lymphomas (EBV), Kaposi's sarcoma (KSHV) and more recently CIN (HPV). The

incidence of Kaposi's sarcoma and lymphomas has declined in the era of highly active antiretroviral therapy.

2 Patients with AIDS-associated tumours present a therapeutic dilemma because of the risk of further bone marrow suppression and hence immunosuppression that results from treatment with cytotoxic drugs.

Case Study 5

1 The main reason for the high virulence of *P. falciparum* parasites is their ability to sequester in blood vessels of the deep viscera like the brain. The parasites adhere to the vascular endothelium of different organs and also to surrounding uninfected red cells. Together these phenomena cause parasite accumulations in small blood vessels with mechanical obstruction and local induction of pathogenic levels of cytokines such as TNFα and IFNγ contributing to tissue damage that can lead to organ failure.

2 Persistence of parasites in blood, with or without clinical symptoms, in spite of antimalarial treatment or, more commonly, initial clinical and parasitological response to treatment that is followed by re-appearance of symptoms, and parasites within 28 days following initiation of treatment, are indicative of treatment failure. Symptoms that recur in these cases are commonly atypical and vague and repeated blood smears should be done for 28 days following treatment to ensure effective parasite elimination. Treatment failures with *P. falciparum* infections have been reported from most parts of the world where *P. falciparum* is endemic, being most severe in the South-east Asian countries of Vietnam, Laos, Cambodia and Myanmar where multi drug-resistant *P. falciparum* infections are common.

Case Study 6

1 It is not possible to differentiate reliably Gram-negative sepsis from bacteraemia caused by Gram-positive organisms, such as *Staphylococcus aureus* or *Streptococcus pyogenes*. However, with careful history taking and thorough clinical examination, it is often possible to identify a likely site of infection, and, on that basis, suggest the most probable causative organism.

2 *Pseudomonas aeruginosa* forms part of the normal faecal flora of only a minority of healthy subjects. However, it can also be found in food, particularly of vegetable origin, and in water. It is also intrinsically resistant to many commonly used antibiotic agents. In the immunocompromised patient, previous treatment with antimicrobial and chemotherapeutic drugs, coupled with the effects of their underlying illness, diminish the patient's resistance to colonization and the effectiveness of their mucosal and humoral defences against infection with this organism. The route of infection is often via the gastrointestinal tract, although there may be little or no evidence of gut damage.

3 Numerically, *E. coli* is the predominant aerobic Gram-negative bacillus in the faecal flora therefore, on a statistical basis, it is more likely to be involved in infections originating in the abdomen or after abdominal trauma or surgery. By virtue of its flagellae, fimbriae and protective capsular polysaccharide it is well equipped to colonize and infect the urinary tract, the most common focus of a septicaemic episode.

Case Study 7

1 Infection of the external auditory canal (otitis externa) is frequently seen in general practice. The delicate skin of this part of the ear is moist and, in its macerated condition may become infected by a variety of microorganisms, e.g. *Staphylococcus aureus*, *Pseudomonas aeruginosa*. However, a significant minority of infections is caused by *Aspergillus* species, the most dramatic being *Aspergillus niger* which produces powdery black spores.

2 Airborne spread of *Aspergillus* spores is the predominant route of infection, and hospital air may contain significant numbers. For the severely immunocompromised, the most effective protective measure is to provide their care in dedicated

rooms with high efficiency particulate air filters until such time as their immune function is recovering. Prophylactic administration of oral amphotericin B or itraconazole may also be of some benefit.

3 Aflatoxin is a poison produced by *Aspergillus* growth on foodstuffs, usually nuts, grains and seeds. Although the true extent to which aflatoxins affect man is not yet clear, aflatoxin B is a potent carcinogen and is also believed to cause direct liver damage (see Chapter 21). Storage of products under conditions of high temperature and humidity is closely related to toxin production.

Case Study 8

1 Anaemia is not a consistent feature of Goodpasture's syndrome but if blood losses are great an iron deficiency anaemia may result. In chronic renal failure, anaemia may be the result of decreased erythropoietin production by the damaged kidney and the retention of waste products which tend to shorten red cell lifespan and inhibit red cell production (see Chapter 14).

2 Two mechanisms are operative: (a) renal damage activates the renin–angiotensin–aldosterone system; (b) impaired renal excretion of sodium and water retention, an increase in blood volume and hence an increase in blood pressure.

Case Study 9

1 During his acute presentation in hospital the results of the emergency investigations were consistent with acute severe asthma. They were important in excluding other possible predisposing causes of his condition, including infection or spontaneous pneumothorax (defined as air in the pleural cavity, in spontaneous pneumothorax this is due to leakage of air from the lungs).

2 Corticosteroids were used to prevent a 'late phase' response which could have developed 4–6 h after his initial treatment. They are thought to act by blocking the synthesis of arachidonic acid meta-bolites and hence preventing the formation of the late phase/newly formed mediators (see Chapter 10).

Case Study 10

1 Early in the post-transplant period, evidence of donor cellular and humoral immunity can be demonstrated. This phenomenon is related to the transfer of mature donor T- and B-lymphocytes. As these mature cells disappear, they are replaced by naïve lymphocytes derived from transplanted haemopoietic stem cells. As naïve donor T-lymphocytes are re-educated in the presence of recipient antigens, tolerance develops. Reconstitution of humoral and cellular immunity in the transplant recipient is influenced by GvHD. In patients without evidence of GvHD, T-lymphocyte-dependent immunity is re-established 4–6 months after transplantation. Immune reconstitution is delayed or prevented by active GvHD and GvHD treatment with immunosuppressive drugs.

2 Most late complications after allogeneic BMT are related either to tissue damage from GvHD and/or immunosuppression by drugs or total body irradiation given as part of the conditioning regimen. Since most patients are under 40 years old and within the reproductive age group, fertility is a significant concern. Ovarian function returns to normal in 15% of postpubertal women and testicular function returns to normal in 25% of men. Late hypothyroidism and growth hormone deficiency can occur in children. Osteoporosis and cataracts may result from prolonged prednisolone therapy.

Case Study 11

1 Hypercholesterolaemia is associated with the development of atherosclerosis (see Chapter 17). In addition, the development of vascular damage associated with atherosclerosis is accelerated by hypertension.

2 Creatinine is released from skeletal muscle at a fairly constant rate and excreted in the urine. In renal disease, creatinine may accumulate in the blood as a result of impaired excretion. The rate of

creatinine clearance from the blood may therefore be a useful measure of renal function.

The relationship between plasma creatinine concentration and creatinine clearance rate is not linear. In some people, creatinine clearance may fall to 50 mL/min before plasma creatinine levels rise above the reference range. Glomerular filtration rate may be more accurately measured by intravenous injection of radioactive chromium-labelled EDTA (ethylenediamine tetra-acetic acid) followed by the measurement of its clearance over several hours. Alternatively, inulin clearance may be measured under certain experimental conditions.

Case Study 12

1 Human T-lymphotropic virus 1 (HTLV-1) infection is associated with adult T-cell leukaemia and lymphoma and is found within the tumour cells. HIV infection is associated with aggressive B-cell lymphomas but the viral genome is not found in the tumour cells and its role may be limited to bringing about immune dysfunction (see Chapters 9 and 22).

2 No, immunosuppression is associated with an increased risk of developing certain tumours but not others. For example, the increased risk of common solid tumours such as lung, breast or colon cancer is small or non-existent.

Case Study 13

1 One might expect that there would be a single pathophysiological mechanism underpinning this phenomenon. Since over 90% of the Felty's patients carry the HLA-DR4 subtype compared to about 70% of patients with rheumatoid arthritis alone and 25–30% of the healthy population, this would further support the idea of a single underlying mechanism. However the studies that have been carried out so far seem to show a variety of different processes occurring in different patients, and even combinations of mechanism in the same patient. These include reduced production of neutrophils by the bone marrow, failure of the neutrophils to get out of the bone marrow into the peripheral circulation, increased peripheral destruction and

splenic pooling. In some patients neutropenia is iatrogenic, linked to treatment with anti-inflammatory drugs.

2 This remains unclear. It is evident that there is a link between the large granular lymphocyte syndrome and neutropenia, in that patients who develop the LGL syndrome and who do not have rheumatoid arthritis often have neutropenia. It is even conceivable, that patients with Felty's syndrome who do not have overt large granular lymphocyte 'leukaemia' have a much more subtle version of the same process. Interestingly, large granular lymphocytes are often seen in viral infections such as HIV or CMV and it is therefore plausible that the two conditions (i.e. with and without LGL expansions) could have a viral aetiology. Whilst in some incidences the large granular lymphocytes can infiltrate the bone marrow, it appears that in most cases this is a benign condition (other than of course the necessity to treat the neutropenia).

Case Study 14

1 The patient was thin and losing weight, had marked hyperglycaemia and ketonuria. This pointed to severe insulin deficiency requiring insulin replacement therapy and predicted his subsequent failure to respond to oral hypoglycaemic agents. His diabetes was clearly well advanced at the time of diagnosis.

2 This man's foot had diminished sensation due to peripheral nerve damage (neuropathy) secondary to his diabetes. A further consequence of neurological damage is an abnormal gait leading to very high pressures in localized areas of the foot during walking. The consequent trauma very rapidly leads to ulcer formation which is often unrecognized by the patients. Once the skin is damaged, infection may ensue causing further inflammation and necrosis. The patient's ability to respond to infection is impaired because of circulatory disturbances due to microvascular disease together with other factors such as impaired leucocyte function which render patients with diabetes more susceptible to a number of forms of infection.

Case Study 15

1 The increased work of the heart in pumping against prolonged resistance in the form of high blood pressure causes thickening of the walls of the left ventricle (left ventricular hypertrophy).

2 A reduction in efficiency of the left side of the heart (left ventricular failure) increases the venous pressure in the pulmonary circulation. Hydrostatic pressure in the pulmonary capillary bed rises, forcing excess fluid into the interstitial spaces where it interferes with gaseous exchange. Eventually some fluid may pass into the alveoli causing marked *dyspnoea* (shortness of breath).

Case Study 16

1 The term 'sudden death' may be applied when an individual previously in good health falls ill and dies within minutes or at most a couple of hours after the onset of symptoms.

2 In most cases sudden death is the result of the complications of coronary artery disease and is usually due to a dysrhythmia (abnormal heart rhythm) caused by an acute myocardial infarction (see case study 15), myocardial ischaemia or scarring from an old myocardial infarct. Dysrhythmia also accounts for a percentage of sudden deaths from acute myocarditis (inflammation of the myocardium) and hypertrophic cardiomyopathy. Other non-cardiac causes of sudden death include cerebral haemorrhage.

Case Study 17

1 This indicates that the prolongation is due to deficiency of a coagulation factor in the patients' plasma, rather than due to the presence of an inhibitor of coagulation.

2 During pregnancy, levels of factor VIII and vWF generally increase and, in most patients with type 1 von Willebrand disease, levels become normal. Consequently most patients have few problems during pregnancy. In patients with type 3 disease levels do not increase and replacement with coagulation factor concentrates will be necessary to cover delivery. It is important to remember that the baby will need to be investigated for von Willebrand disease.

3 Acquired von Willebrand disease may occur in the setting of autoimmune or lymphoproliferative disorders, when an autoantibody is produced directed against vWF. The diagnosis should be considered in elderly patients who present with the characteristics of von Willebrand disease, but with no prior history of bleeding.

Case Study 18

1 Malabsorption of a wide range of nutrients occurs in coeliac disease and deficiencies of nutrients with relatively low body stores become apparent at an early stage. Iron and folate are absorbed mostly in the proximal small intestine, the area of the gut mainly affected by coeliac disease. Haemopoietic tissues have high demands for folate and iron, so anaemia soon follows the development of deficiency states. Anaemia may be predominantly due to iron deficiency (microcytic and hypochromic), to folate deficiency (macrocytic, normochromic) or may show features of both types of anaemia (see also Chapter 14).

2 TSH is secreted by the anterior pituitary gland in response to the action of thyrotropin-releasing hormone (TRH) from the hypothalamus. TSH stimulates the production of thyroid hormones and their release from the thyroid gland. Hypothyroidism (reduced activity of the thyroid gland) is characterized by reduced synthesis of the thyroid hormones, thyroxine (T_4) and tri-iodothyronine (T_3). The secretion of TSH is normally controlled by a negative feedback loop involving thyroxine, in which high levels of thyroxine depress TSH secretion. TSH levels increase in hypothyroidism in an attempt to stimulate the thyroid gland to secrete sufficient thyroxine for the maintenance of normal metabolic rate.

Case Study 19

1 The microcytic hypochromic anaemia could

indicate iron deficiency due either to chronic blood loss or malabsorption of iron. Alternatively, chronic inflammatory disorders can produce a similar haematological picture, with hypochromic and microcytic red blood cells. Iron deficiency is characterized by low serum iron, low serum ferritin and a raised serum transferrin concentration. The causes of anaemia due to chronic inflammation are complex, but the anaemia is probably due, at least in part, to a defect in the utilization of iron (see Chapter 14). In anaemia associated with chronic inflammation serum iron is also low, but serum ferritin is normal or high and serum transferrin is usually low. This patient's anaemia was probably due to a combination of chronic blood loss and inflammatory disease.

The ESR is a non-specific test which is raised in a wide variety of conditions, notably inflammatory and malignant disorders. Occasionally, especially in elderly patients, the ESR is raised and despite extensive investigations no cause is found. The measurement of plasma viscosity gives much the same information, and is subject to fewer variables, so is offered by some laboratories as an alternative to the ESR.

The raised leucocyte count, the majority of cells being neutrophils (neutrophilia), is consistent with an inflammatory disorder.

2 Clinically, Crohn's disease can be difficult to distinguish from ulcerative colitis since both diseases cause chronic inflammation and ulceration in the gut. However, whereas Crohn's disease can affect any area of the gut from the mouth to the anus, ulcerative colitis is confined to the colon. In addition, in Crohn's disease the inflammatory process typically extends through the gut wall, whereas, usually, in ulcerative colitis the mucosa and submucosa only are affected. Non-caseating granulomas (see Chapter 5) are a characteristic histological finding in Crohn's disease.

Case Study 20

1 Erythrocyte mean cell volume (MCV) is often high in alcoholic liver disease. This is sometimes due to folate deficiency resulting from poor diet,

but may also be due to liver damage. The precise mechanisms causing macrocytosis in alcoholic liver disease are not clear, but it has been suggested that acetaldehyde generated by oxidation of ethanol by bone marrow macrophages damages red cell precursors (see Chapter 14).

2 The liver synthesises most coagulation factors, so when there is hepatocellular (liver cell) damage synthesis of blood coagulation factors is often reduced. In addition, if there is cholestasis there is also malabsorption of fat, thus reducing absorption of fat soluble vitamins including vitamin K. Vitamin K is necessary for the synthesis of coagulation factors II, VII, IX and X, so in vitamin K deficiency their concentrations fall, thereby prolonging the prothrombin time and other coagulation tests (see Chapter 16).

3 Inflammation of the gastric mucosa and peptic ulceration are associated with alcohol abuse, and bleeding may occur in either condition. Furthermore, if the liver is damaged by cirrhosis (degenerative change resulting in fibrosis) pressure in the hepatic portal vein rises and a collateral circulation becomes established in other vessels to bypass the liver. One effect of this is that the veins of the lower oesophagus become dilated and distended (a condition known as oesophageal varices) and may bleed. Any bleeding is often exacerbated by reduced levels of blood coagulation factors, so the administration of vitamin K or the replacement of missing coagulation factors by transfusion of fresh frozen plasma may be indicated.

Case Study 21

1 The carrier state protects against malaria caused by *Plasmodium falciparum* (see also case study 5). The malarial parasite invades red cells where it replicates. In sickle cell trait the parasite produces such adverse conditions within the red cell that it sickles and is removed by the reticulo-endothelial system very early on. This has resulted in a benefit in carrying the gene, which has resulted in increased survival in those areas in which malaria is endemic.

2 As the kidneys lose their urine concentrating

ability, sickle patients pass large quantities of urine and hence drink increased amounts to prevent dehydration. The passage of large volumes of urine lowers the plasma urea.

3 HbS has a right-shifted oxygen dissociation curve which means that this haemoglobin variant more easily gives up its oxygen to the tissues than normal haemoglobin (HbA). The patient also has a chronic anaemia from childhood and the body can adapt by increasing cardiac output and reducing peripheral resistance thereby increasing blood flow to the tissues.

Case Study 22

1 FAP is only one of several inherited colon cancer syndromes. The later age of onset, in conjunction with tumours of the right side of the colon and a lack of adenomas suggests a diagnosis of *hereditary non-polyposis colon cancer* (HNPCC). This disease accounts for 10–15% of all colon cancer cases and is therefore more common than FAP. Five causative genes have so far been identified. These are DNA repair genes, one is situated on chromosome 2, and is responsible for approximately 60% of cases. The other, on chromosome 3, accounts for a further 30%. The other three genes account for the remainder of cases. Detection of mutations in HNPCC families is now possible.

2 The total iron content of the human body is typically 3–5 g, two-thirds of which is contained within erythrocytes. At the end of the erythrocyte lifespan, haemoglobin is catabolized and iron is released. The majority of this is conserved, being transported to iron stores or to the bone marrow for reincorporation into new erythrocytes. To compensate for the small amounts of iron which are lost normally, around 2 mg of iron are absorbed daily from dietary sources. Each millilitre of erythrocytes contains approximately 1 mg of iron, so in chronic blood loss there can be a substantial loss of iron from the iron pool, which must be replaced from other sources. Iron for haemopoiesis is drawn from iron stores and absorption increases to compensate for this. How-

ever, if blood loss is great, losses of iron invariably exceed iron available from iron stores and from dietary sources. Iron deficiency anaemia is the usual outcome. For this reason, patients presenting with unexplained iron deficiency anaemia must always be investigated for possible occult (hidden) blood loss. (See also Chapter 14.)

Case Study 23

1 Unlike some other inherited disorders (e.g. myotonic dystrophy) DiGeorge syndrome shows no evidence of increasing severity from one generation to the next. The most likely explanation in this case is that only mildly affected individuals (i.e. the father) will survive to adulthood and therefore reproduce.

2 If one or other parent is a known carrier of the deletion, the chance that any individual offspring will inherit that deletion is 50% irrespective of the number of deletion-negative offspring.

Case Study 24

1 A detailed clinical review of that parent would be advisable. There are now a number of well described cases where unbalanced karyotypes are inherited from one generation to another with variable clinical effects.

2 *De novo* structural rearrangements are more likely to have been inherited from the father. Genotyping of chromosome 1 markers close to and within the deleted region should allow assignment of origin of the deleted chromosome.

Case Study 25

1 Current evidence suggests that the incidence of balanced translocation in one partner of a couple who has experienced two or more miscarriages is 2–3%. This figure increases to 5–10% if the couple has previously had an abnormal or stillborn child, or there is a family history of recurrent miscarriage. These figures indicate that a careful clinical history

may help in selecting appropriate couples for cytogenetic analysis.

2 Chromosome analysis of tissue from any fetal loss would help in confirming that an unbalanced karyotype was present and so was likely to be the cause of the miscarriage.

Case Study 26

1 In a case diagnosed prenatally, the prognosis for the liveborn child would not be so severe if the locus was not deleted.

2 It must be remembered that for all the documented chromosomal syndromes the range of features associated need not all be present and that the severity can be variable. The cases published in the scientific literature are often the most badly affected. However, all cases of short arm 5 deletion involving the critical region for Cri-du-chat syndrome will be more severely affected than those deleted outside the region.

Case Study 27

1 The CFTR gene encodes a cAMP-dependent membrane-spanning chloride channel. Patients with cystic fibrosis have a defect in the CFTR gene, resulting in absence or malfunction of the chloride ion channel and hence deregulation of sodium and chloride ion transport. Elevated levels of these ions can therefore be detected in sweat samples.

2 Population screening: it has been suggested that all children are screened for CF carrier status at birth. The problems with this are that the children cannot give informed consent and there are issues around when and how the children would be told. It would also be an impossibly labour intensive and slow process to screen all children for all known mutations. Therefore, only the presence of common mutations could be screened for and this would only reduce the carrier risk. A couple-targeted strategy would involve screening only those couples

planning to have children or those currently pregnant. Once again this approach would be resource-intensive and because of this would only be able to identify the common mutations.

Case Study 28

1 Hypercalcaemia can cause significant symptoms of constipation, lethargy, nausea and abdominal pain. Her blood biochemistry should be kept under review since treatment may be required.

Neurological signs of spinal cord compression may occur if tumour deposits or fractured vertebral bodies impinge on the cord. A history of either sudden or gradually increasing loss of function of limbs bilaterally in association with sensory loss, bladder and bowel disturbance should alert one to this possibility. Investigation and treatment is urgently required to avoid permanent neurological damage and disability.

Further risk of bone pain and pathological fractures require palliation. Oral bisphosphonates inhibit osteoclast activity and may be given to patients at high risk of these complications in an attempt to control bone resorption.

2 Yes, having a mother or sister with breast cancer increases a woman's risk of breast cancer by 1.5–3 fold that of the general population. There are now two recognized types of breast cancer risk associated with a family history. True inherited breast cancer is actually very rare, accounting for around 5% of cases, and is due to inheritance of a specific germ line mutation in either of the tumour suppressor genes, BRCA1 or BRCA2 (Chapter 22). Families with more than three relatives with breast cancer often occurring at an early age and in association with other cancers such as ovarian cancer may have an inherited gene mutation. Most women with a family history, however, do not fit this pattern and their risk is much lower. Prevention strategies in both groups of women at increased risk are being evaluated.

Case Study 29

1 Plasma urate is derived in part from the break-

down of *adenine* and *guanine*, the purine bases present in nucleic acids, and in part from dietary sources. *Hyperuricaemia* (raised concentration of blood urate) occurs in CML due to a very high rate of nucleic acid breakdown resulting from increased cell turnover. When treatment commences, the rate of cell destruction can be so high that treatment of hyperuricaemia is essential to avoid precipitating gout.

2 Proliferation of large numbers of granulocytes and their precursors is a feature of CML. These cells produce transcobalamin-1, a vitamin B_{12}-carrying protein, which is released into the plasma. High levels of transcobalamin-1 in the plasma are associated with raised vitamin B_{12} concentrations.

3 Myeloproliferative disorders are low-grade neoplastic disorders characterized by proliferation of neoplastic clones of cells derived from haemopoietic stem cells. Examples include primary proliferative polycythaemia (formerly called polycythaemia rubra vera) and myelofibrosis, neither of which are regarded as true leukaemias. Cytochemistry helps to differentiate these conditions from CML, since the NAP score is usually high in myeloproliferative disorders and low in CML. However, a myeloproliferative disorder may transform to leukaemia, often initially to CML, but sometimes directly to an acute form.

Case Study 30

1 Several unfavourable biological features suggest the involvement of more primitive myeloid stem cells in elderly AML patients. These include the following:
• Fewer elderly AML patients have a favourable cytogenetic picture (see Table CS30.3, p. 290).
• A drug-resistant phenotype is more common in the older AML patient.
• Cytological and cytochemical features of blast cell differentiation are less common in elderly AML patients.

2 AML blast cells constitutively express several haemopoietic cytokines including interleukin-1, -3, -6, -8, -11, GM-CSF, M-CSF and tumour necrosis factor-alpha (TNFα). Many of these are believed to act as autocrine growth factors.

Case Study 31

1 Anaplastic large cell lymphoma (ALCL)—Hodgkin's like. These lymphomas mainly affect young females and present with bulky mediastinal disease. Biopsy of ALCL shows marked fibrosis similar to NSHD. Immunophenotyping shows that the large ALCL cells are CD30-positive, and usually CD15-negative. ALCL patients do not respond to conventional HD chemotherapy but they may respond to more aggressive chemotherapy similar to that used for high-grade non-Hodgkin's lymphomas.

2 Patients treated for HD have a significant risk of developing a myelodysplastic syndrome (MDS)/acute myeloid leukaemia (AML) which may occur after both radiotherapy and chemotherapy. The cumulative risk is about 3% after 10 years. Cutaneous malignancy, sarcomas, breast and thyroid carcinomas also occur in radiotherapy fields. The overall incidence of second malignancy is approximately 13%.

Case Study 32

1 Yes, the hoarseness was caused by the tumour spreading outwards and pressing on the recurrent laryngeal nerve which lies near the left main bronchus on its way to supply the larynx. This is an example of a local effect of a tumour.

2 There are two possible causes of hypercalcaemia in malignant disease: (a) when malignant cells metastasize they damage the tissues in which they settle. Hypercalcaemia can be caused by metastatic destruction of bone leading to the release of calcium; and (b) some tumours can influence distant sites in the body by producing hormones or their analogues. For example, some types of lung cancer can make antidiuretic hormone (ADH) causing water retention. Similarly, hypercalcaemia can be caused by secretion of pathyroid hormone or an analogue by the tumour cells. Other remote effects of tumours are less easy to understand, for example abnormalities in peripheral nerves (*neuropathy*) or muscle (*myopathy*). The clubbing of the patient's fingers was a remote effect of his lung disease but the mechan-

ism is not understood and certain non-malignant conditions can cause this.

Case Study 33

1 Although no prostate cancer susceptibility genes have been isolated, there is evidence that hereditary forms of the disease exist. These account for approximately 9% of all cases. Cases may be due to an inherited susceptibility.

2 The BCL-2 protein protects cells from apoptosis (see Chapters 4 and 22). This suggests that the expression of BCL-2 and subsequent protection from apoptosis is important for the progression of androgen sensitive tumours to hormone independency.

Case Study 34

1 Pre-operative techniques include: manual examination of the tumour and the pelvis, rectal ultrasound, CT scanning of the pelvis and abdomen and chest X-ray. Measurement of carcino-embryonic antigen (CEA, a protein produced by many epithelial tumours) in the serum may have some use in detecting recurrence after surgery.

The important factors that determine prognosis are; whether the local excision (peripheral) margins of the specimen that is surgically removed are involved by tumour, the histological degree of differentiation of the carcinoma and the Dukes' stage.

2 Unlike most other solid tumours in the body there is no direct relationship between increasing size of the cancer and either spread to other tissues, lymphatic metastases, or survival. The important feature about these tumours is how far they have spread through the bowel wall at the time of surgery. Some very small cancers can spread rapidly to other sites while large tumours can sometimes be present for a long time and grow only slowly.

3 Although an attractive proposition, the answer is no. Screening programmes for colorectal cancer, which rely on testing the stools for occult blood (blood in the stools that is 'hidden' or not clinically obvious), for example, may aid in reducing the incidence of the disease by detecting premalignant polyps, but this would by no means eliminate the disease. There are other pathways by which colorectal cancer can arise, for example as *de novo* lesions (with no prior evidence of polyps) or alternatively from so-called 'flat' adenomas. It has been estimated that at least 20 adenomas would need to be removed in order to prevent one cancer.

Appendix

Reference ranges

Please note that reference ranges depend upon local factors, including techniques utilized and the population under investigation. Data presented in the case studies reflect this, and in each case reference ranges are presented to indicate the analytical conditions at the time the investigations were performed.

Table A1 Typical haematological values (reference ranges) for normal individuals, the majority expressed as mean + 2 SD (95% range).

Red cell count	
Men	$5.5 \pm 1.0 \times 10^{12}$/L
Women	$4.8 \pm 1.0 \times 10^{12}$/L
Infants (full-term, cord blood)	$6.0 \pm 1.0 \times 10^{12}$/L
Children, 3 months	$4.0 \pm 0.8 \times 10^{12}$/L
Children, 1 yr	$4.4 \pm 0.8 \times 10^{12}$/L
Children, 3–6 yr	$4.8 \pm 0.7 \times 10^{12}$/L
Children, 10–12 yr	$4.7 \pm 0.7 \times 10^{12}$/L
Haemoglobin	
Men	155 ± 25 g/L
Women	140 ± 25 g/L
Infants (full-term, cord blood)	165 ± 30 g/L
Children, 3 months	115 ± 20 g/L
Children, 1 yr	120 ± 15 g/L
Children, 3–6 yr	130 ± 10 g/L
Children, 10–12 yr	130 ± 15 g/L
Packed cell volume (PCV; haematocrit value)	
Men	0.47 ± 0.07 (L/L)
Women	0.42 ± 0.05 (L/L)
Infants (full-term, cord blood)	0.54 ± 0.10 (L/L)
Children, 3 months	0.38 ± 0.06 (L/L)
Children, 3–6 yr	0.04 ± 0.04 (L/L)
Children 10–12 yr	0.41 ± 0.04 (L/L)
Mean cell volume (MCV)	
Adults	87 ± 5 fl
Infants (full-term, neonates)	120 fl (mean)
Children, 3 months	95 fl (mean)
Children, 1 yr	78 ± 8 fl
Children, 3–6 yr	84 ± 8 fl
Children, 10–12 yr	84 ± 7 fl
Mean cell haemoglobin (MCH)	
Adults	29.5 ± 2.5 pg
Children, 3 months	29 ± 5 pg
Children, 1 yr	27 ± 4 pg
Children, 3–6 yr	27 ± 3 pg
Children, 10–12 yr	27 ± 3 pg
Mean cell haemoglobin concentration (MCHC)	
Adults and children	325 ± 25 g/L
Infants (full-term, neonates)	300 ± 27 g/L
Red cell diameter (mean values)	
Adults (dry films)	6.7–7.7 µm
Red cell density	1092–1100 g/L
Reticulocyte count	
Adults and children	0.5–2.5% (c.50–100×10^9/L)
Infants (full-term, cord blood)	2–6% (mean 150×10^9/L)
Blood volume	
Red cell volume, men	30 ± 5 mlL/kg
women	25 ± 5 mL/kg
Plasma volume	45 ± 5 mL/kg
Total blood volume	70 ± 10 mL/kg
Red cell life-span	120 ± 30 days
Leucocyte count	
Adults	$7.5 \pm 3.5 \times 10^9$/L
Infants (full-term, 1st day)	$18 \pm 8 \times 10^9$/L
Infants, l yr	$12 \pm 6 \times 10^9$/L
Children, 4–7 yr	$10 \pm 5 \times 10^9$/L
Children, 8–12 yr	$9 \pm 4.5 \times 10^9$/L
Differential leucocyte count	
Adults:	
Neutrophils	2.0–7.5×10^9/L (40–75%)
Lymphocytes	1.5–4.0×10^9/L (20–45%)
Monocytes	0.2–0.8×10^9/L (2–10%)
Eosinophils	0.04–0.4×10^9/L (1–6%)
Basophils	0.02–0.1×10^9/L (1%)
Infants (1st day):	
Neutrophils	5.0–13.0×10^9/L
Lymphocytes	3.5–8.5×10^9/L
Monocytes	0.5–1.5×10^9/L

(continued on p. 313)

Table A1 (*continued*)

Eosinophils	$0.1–2.5 \times 10^9$/L	
Basophils	$0.02–0.1 \times 10^9$/L	
Infants (3 days):		
Neutrophils	$1.5–7.0 \times 10^9$/L	
Lymphocytes	$2.0–5.0 \times 10^9$/L	
Monocytes	$0.3–1.1 \times 10^9$/L	
Eosinophils	$0.2–2.0 \times 10^9$/L	
Basophils	$0.02–0.1 \times 10^9$/L	
Children (6 yr):		
Neutrophils	$2.0–6.0 \times 10^9$/L	
Lymphocytes	$5.5–8.5 \times 10^9$/L	
Monocytes	$0.7–1.5 \times 10^9$/L	
Eosinophils	$0.3–0.8 \times 10^9$/L	
Basophils	$0.02–0.1 \times 10^9$/L	
Platelet count	$150–400 \times 10^9$/L	
Bleeding time (Ivy's method)	2–7 min	
(Template method)	2.5–9.5 min	
Prothrombin time	11–16 s	
Partial thromboplastin time (PTTK)	30–40 s	
Prothrombin-consumption index	0–10%	
Plasma fibrinogen	1.5–4.0 g/L	
Fibrinogen titre	≥128	
Plasminogen	80–120 U/dL	
Euglobulin lysis time	90–240 min	
Antithrombin III	75–125 U/dL	
β-thromboglobulin	<50 ng/mL	
Platelet factor 4	<10 ng/mL	
Protein C	70–140%	
Protein S	70–140%	
Heparin co-factor II	55–145%	

Osmotic fragility (at 20°C and pH 7.4)

NaCl(g/L)	Before incubation (% lysis)	After incubation for 24 h at 37°C (% lysis)
2.0	100	95–100
3.0	97–100	85–100
3.5	90–99	75–100
4.0	50–95	65–100
4.5	5–45	55–95
5.0	0–6	40–85
5.5	0	15–70
6.0	0	0–40
6.5	0	0–10
7.0	0	0–5
7.5	0	0
8.0	0	0
8.5	0	0

Median corpuscular fragility (MCF) (g/L NaCl)

4.0–4.45	4.65–5.9

Autohaemolysis (37°C)	
48 h, without added glucose	0.2–4.0%
48 h, with added glucose	0–0.5%
Cold-agglutinin titre (4°C)	<64
Serum iron	13–32 μmol/L
	(0.7–1.8 mg/L)
Total iron-binding capacity	45–70 μmol/L
	(2.5–4.0 mg/L)
Transferrin	2.0–3.0 g/L
Ferritin	
Adults	15–300 μg/L
Children	15–140 μg/L
Serum vitamin B_{12} (as cyanocobalamin)	160–760 ng/L
Serum folate	3–20 μg/L
Red cell folate	160–640 μg/L
Plasma haemoglobin	10–40 mg/L
Serum haptoglobin (Hb-binding)	0.3–2.0 g/L

Sedimentation rate (Westergren, 1 h at $20 \pm 3°C$)
(upper limits)

Men	17–50 yr	10 mm
	>50 yr	12–14 mm
Women	17–50 yr	12 mm
Women	>50 yr	19–20 mm
Plasma viscosity		
(25°C)		1.50–1.72 mPa/s
(37°C)		1.16–1.33 mPa/s
Heterophile (anti-sheep red cell)		<80
agglutinin titre		
After absorption with guinea-pig kidney		<10

Table A2 Typical clinical biochemistry values (reference ranges) for normal individuals.

Acid phosphatase	1–5 U/L	Potassium	3.5–5.0 mmol/L
Alanine aminotransferase (ALT)	5–40 U/L	Prostate-specific antigen	up to 4.0 μg/L
Albumin	34–48 g/L	Protein (total)	62–80 g/L
Alkaline phosphatase	25–115 U/L	Sodium	135–146 mmol/L
Amylase	<220 U/L	Urate	0.18–0.42 mmol/L
Angiotensin-converting enzyme	10–70 U/L		(3.0–7.0 mg/dL)
α_1-Antitrypsin	2–4 g/L	Urea	2.5–6.7 mmol/L (8–25 mg/dL)
Aspartate aminotransferase (AST)	10–40 U/L	Vitamin A	0.5–2.01 μmol/L
Bicarbonate	22–30 mmol/L	Vitamin D	
Bilirubin	<17 μmol/L (0.3–1.5 mg/dL)	25-hydroxy	37–200 nmol/L (0.15–0.80 ng/L)
Caeruloplasmin	0.20–0.45 g/L	1,25-dihydroxy	60–108 pmol/L (0.24–0.45 pg/L)
Calcium	2.20–2.67 mmol/L	Zinc	7–18 μmol/L
	(8.5–10.5 mg/dL)	*Lipids and lipoproteins*	
Chloride	95–106 mmol/L	Cholesterol	3.5–6.5 mmol/L
Cholinesterase	2.25–7.0 U/L		(ideal <5.2 mmol/L)
Copper	12–25 μmol/L (100–200 mg/dL)	HDL cholesterol	
C-reactive protein	<10 mg/L	Male	0.95–2.15 mmol/L
Creatinine	0.06–0.12 mmol/L	Female	0.70–2.00 mmol/L
	(0.6–1.5 mg/dL)	Lipids (total)	4.0–10.0 g/L
Creatine kinase (CPK)		Lipoproteins	
Female	24–170 U/L	VLDL	0.128–0.645 mmol/L
Male	24–195 U/L	LDL	1.55–4.4 mmol/L
CK-MB fraction	25 U/L (<60% of total activity)	HDL	
C3	0.55–1.20 g/L	Male	0.70–2.1 mmol/L
C4	0.20–0.50 g/L	Female	0.50–1.70 mmol/L
Ferritin	5.8–144 nmol/L (15–300 μg/L)	Non-esterified fatty acids	
α-Fetoprotein	<10 kU/L	Male	0.19–0.78 mmol/L
Glucose (fasting)	4.5–5.6 mmol/L (70–110 mg/L)	Female	0.06–0.9 mmol/L
Fructosamine	up to 285 μmol/L	Phospholipid	2.9–5.2 mmol/L
Gamma glutamyltransferase (γ-GT)		Triglycerides	
Male	11–50 U/L	Male	0.70–2.1 mmol/L
Female	7–32 U/L	Female	0.50–1.70 mmol/L
Glycosylated haemoglobin (HbA$_{Ic}$)	3.8–8.5%	*Blood gases*	
Hydroxybutyric dehydrogenase (HBD)	40–150 U/L	Arterial P_{CO_2}	4.8–6.1 kPa (36–46 mmHg)
Immunoglobulins (11 years and over)		Arterial P_{O_2}	10–13.3 kPa (75–100 mmHg)
IgA	0.8–4 g/L	Arterial [H$^+$]	35–45 nmol/L
IgG	7.0–18.0 g/L	Arterial pH	7.35–7.45
IgM	0.4–2.5 g/L	*Urine values*	
Iron	13–32 μmol/L (50–150 μg/dL)	Calcium	7.5 mmol daily or less
Iron binding capacity (total) (TIBC)	42–80 μmol/L (250–410 μg/dL)		(<300 mg daily)
Lactate dehydrogenase	240–460 U/L	Copper	0.2–1.0 μmol daily
Lead	<0.7 μmol/L	Creatinine	0.13–0.22 mmol/kg body weight, daily
Magnesium	0.7–1.1 mmol/L		
β_2-Microglobulin	1.0–3.0 mg/L	5-Hydroxyindole acetic acid	5–75 μmol daily; amounts lower in females than males
Osmolality	280–296 mosmol/kg		
Phosphate	0.8–1.5 mmol/L	Protein (quantitative)	<0.15 g per 24 h

Index